ONCOLOGY OF THE EYE AND ADNEXA

✳

ONCOLOGIE DE L'ŒIL ET DES ANNEXES

✳

ONKOLOGISCHE DIAGNOSTIK IN DER OPHTHALMOLOGIE

Monographs in Ophthalmology

Oncology of the Eye and Adnexa

Atlas of Clinical Pathology

*

Oncologie de l'Œil et des Annexes

Atlas Anatomo-Clinique

*

Onkologische Diagnostik in der Ophthalmologie

Vergleichender Klinisch-Pathologischer Atlas

A. Brini
Clinique Ophtalmologique
Centre Hospitalier Régional
Strasbourg, France

P. Dhermy
Service d'Ophtalmologie
Hôtel-Dieu, Paris
Paris, France

J. Sahel
Clinique Ophtalmologique
Centre Hospitalier Régional
Strasbourg, France

Kluwer Academic Publishers

Dordrecht / Boston / London

Library of Congress Cataloging-in-Publication Data

Brini, A.
   Oncology of the eye and adnexa : atlas of clinical pathology =
Oncologie de l'oeil et des annexes : atlas anatomo-clinique =
Onkologische Diagnostik in der Ophthalmologie : vergleichender
klinisch-pathologischer atlas / A. Brini, P. Dhermy, J. Sahel.
      p.   cm. -- (Monographs in ophthalmology ; 13)
   Bibliography: p.
   Includes index.

   1. Eye--Tumors--Atlases. 2. Eye--Tumors--Histopathology--Atlases.
3. Adnexa oculi--Tumors--Atlases.   I. Dhermy, Pierre. II. Sahel,
J. III. Title. IV. Title: Oncologie de l'oeil et des annexes.
V. Title: Onkologische Diagnostik in der Ophthalmologie.
VI. Series.
   [DNLM: 1. Eye Neoplasms--atlases.   W1 MO568D v. 13 / WW 17 8858o]
RC280.E9B75 1990
616.99'2840758--dc20
DNLM/DLC
for Library of Congress   89-15496

ISBN-13: 978-94-010-6692-1   e-ISBN-13: 978-94-009-0461-3
DOI: 10.1007/978-94-009-0461-3

Published by Kluwer Academic Publishers,
P.O. Box 17, 3300 AA Dordrecht, The Netherlands.

Kluwer Academic Publishers incorporates the publishing programmes of
D. Reidel, Martinus Nijhoff, Dr W. Junk and MTP Press.

Sold and distributed in the U.S.A. and Canada by
Kluwer Academic Publishers,
101 Philip Drive, Norwell, MA 02061, U.S.A.

In all other countries, sold, and distributed by
Kluwer Academic Publishers Group,
P.O. Box 322, 3300 AH Dordrecht, The Netherlands.

Printed on acid-free paper

Contents

Introduction   vii

Acknowledgements   viii

Detailed table of
contents   ix

Part A: I-IX
Tumours of the eyelids and the
conjunctiva
Plate 1–28   1

Part B: X-XXI
Orbital and orbito-palpebral
tumours
Plate 29–42   59

Part C: XXII-XXIV
Tumours of the uvea
Plate 43–54   91

Part D: XXV-XXXI
Tumours of the retina
and the optic disc
Plate 55–64   117

Technical appendix   139

Literature   143

Alphabetical index of
subjects   145

Table des matières générale

Introduction   vii

Remerciements   viii

Table des matières
détaillée   xiii

Partie A: I-IX
Tumeurs palpébro-
conjonctivales
Planche 1–28   1

Partie B: X-XXI
Tumeurs de l'orbite et
orbito-palpébrales
Planche 29–42   59

Partie C: XXII-XXIV
Tumeurs de l'uvée
Planche 43–54   91

Partie D: XXV-XXXI
Tumeurs de la rétine et
de la papille optique
Planche 55–64   117

Appendice technique   139

Littérature   143

Index alphabétique des
sujets   148

Inhaltsübersicht

Einführung   vii

Danksagungen   viii

Detailliertes
Inhaltsverzeichnis   xvii

Teil A: I-IX
Geschwülste der Augen-
lider und der Bindehaut
Tafel 1–28   1

Teil B: X-XXI
Orbitale und orbito-
palpebrale Geschwülste
Tafel 29–42   59

Teil C: XXII-XXIV
Geschwülste der Uvea
Tafel 43–54   91

Teil D: XXV-XXXI
Geschwülste der Netzhaut
und der Papille
Tafel 55–64   117

Technischer Anhang   139

Literatur   143

Alphabetisches
Sachwörterverzeichnis   151

Introduction

This atlas is the fruit of a many years' experience in the application of anatomico-clinical methods to ophthalmological oncology.

In the field of ophthalmology, as in other medical areas, oncology has progressively increased in importance with the gradual lengthening of life expectation. Apart from rare tumours and certain malformations in children, neoformations in ophthalmology are largely confined to ageing patients. Any of the intraocular tissues may be affected: those of the iris, the ciliary body, the choroid or the retina, as well as of the orbit and the eyelid. In consequence, such neoformations are the reason for a large number of consultations. Thanks to the transparence of the ocular media, the ophthalmologist has the almost unique advantage of being able to examine most intraocular tumours under the biomicroscope. Histopathological examination of the specimen obtained by biopsy or surgical excision continues to be an irreplaceable adjunct to clinical procedure.

Hence the idea of putting together, side by side in an atlas, clinical and histopathological aspects of the various neoformations likely to be encountered in eye pathology, including those most recently discovered as well as those most frequently met with. Some of these notions are already to be found in other works; but they are usually dealt with separately in specialized clinical or pathology studies.

That this atlas is the response to a real need is amply proven by the increasing number of eye oncology consultations. Many ophthalmologists encounter difficulties when faced with tumours. Our aim has thus been to provide them with a reference manual, conceived so as to permit rapid access to essential concepts in current eye oncology.

Our constant concern in preparing this atlas was its usefulness for teaching purposes. Rapid and easy consultation has been made possible through the use of a comprehensive set of colour illustrations, with a concise accompanying text and a detailed alphabetical index. A select bibliography lists the basic studies on oncology and pathology of the eye.

Not only students beginning work in ophthalmology, but also experienced ophthalmologists will find this work most useful. At the same time, it should be of considerable assistance to pathologists and dermatologists, practicians frequently finding themselves faced with ophthalmological problems.

Introduction

Cet atlas est le fruit d'une longue expérience de la méthode anatomo-clinique appliquée à l'oncologie ophtalmologique.

En Ophtalmologie comme dans les autres disciplines médicales, l'allongement progressif de l'espérance de vie donne davantage d'importance à l'oncologie. En effet, mises à part les rares tumeurs de l'enfant et certaines malformations, les néoformations en Ophtalmologie sont l'apanage préférentiel du sujet âgé. Elles peuvent toucher tous les tissus intra-oculaires: iris, corps ciliaire, choroïde, rétine, ainsi que ceux de l'orbite et des paupières, et représentent ainsi une cause fréquente de consultation. La transparence des milieux oculaires donne à l'ophtalmologiste le privilège quasi-unique de pouvoir examiner biomicroscopiquement la plupart des tumeurs intra-oculaires. L'examen histo-pathologique de la biopsie ou de la pièce d'exérèse reste le complément indispensable de l'acte clinique.

Nous avons donc jugé utile de confronter côte à côte, dans un atlas, les aspects cliniques et histo-pathologiques des diverses néoformations susceptibles d'être rencontrées dans le domaine oculaire, aussi bien les plus fréquentes que celles plus récemment connues. Une partie de ces notions se trouve déjà dans d'autres ouvrages; mais elles sont habituellement traitées séparément dans des livres spécialisés de clinique ou d'anatomie pathologique.

Cet atlas répond à un besoin, dont témoigne la fréquentation croissante des consultations d'oncologie oculaire. Nombre d'ophtalmologistes rencontrent des difficultés en présence d'une pathologie tumorale. Nous avons donc souhaité leur fournir un manuel de référence, conçu pour permettre un accès rapide aux notions essentielles de l'oncologie ophtalmologique courante.

Au cours de la rédaction de cet atlas, notre préoccupation constante a été le but didactique. Une excellente iconographie en couleurs, un texte d'accompagnement concis et un index alphabétique détaillé en rendent la consultation aisée et rapide. Une bibliographie sommaire renvoie aux monographies de base en oncologie et en anatomie pathologique oculaires.

Cet ouvrage intéressera non seulement les étudiants qui abordent l'Ophtalmologie, mais aussi les ophtalmologistes confirmés; les anatomo-pathologistes et les dermatologistes, souvent confrontés à des problèmes d'ophtalmologie, y trouveront eux aussi une aide efficace.

Einführung

Dieser Atlas ist das Ergebnis langjähriger Erfahrung mit der auf die ophthalmologische Onkologie angewandten anatomisch-klinischen Methode.

Wie auch in anderen Disziplinen gewinnt die Onkologie in der Ophthalmologie mit der steigenden Lebenserwartung immer mehr an Bedeutung. Von den wenigen Tumoren des Kindes und gewissen Mißbildungen abgesehen sind Neubildungen in der Ophthalmologie in erster Linie dem älteren Menschen vorbehalten. Sie können an sämtlichen intraokularen Geweben, Iris, Ziliarkörper, Aderhaut, Netzhaut, ebenso wie an denen der Augenhöhle und der Lider auftreten und sind somit häufiger Konsultationsgrund. Durch die Transparenz der Augenteile hat der Ophthalmologe das quasi ausschließliche Privileg, die meisten intraokularen Tumoren biomikroskopisch untersuchen zu können. Die pathologische Untersuchung der Biopsie oder des Exhäreseteils bleibt weiterhin unerläßliche Ergänzung der klinischen Diagnose.

Wir hielten es daher für angebracht, in einem Atlas die klinischen und pathologischen Aspekte der verschiedenen im Augenbereich anzutreffenden Neubildungen, und zwar der häufigsten wie auch der erst seit kurzem bekannten gegenüberzustellen. Diese sind teilweise schon in anderen Werken enthalten, werden aber gewöhnlich in der klinischen oder anatomisch-pathologischen Fachliteratur getrennt behandelt.

Für diesen Atlas besteht ein Bedarf, der an der zunehmenden Inanspruchnahme der augenonkologischen Konsultation zu ersehen ist. Für viele Ophthalmologen ist die Tumorpathologie mit Schwierigkeiten verbunden. Wir wollten ihnen deshalb ein Nachschlagewerk zur Verfügung stellen, das einen raschen Einblick in die wesentlichen Begriffe der geläufigen ophthalmologischen Onkologie ermöglicht.

Wir waren bei der Zusammenstellung dieses Atlasses stetig um ein didaktisches Ziel bemüht. Eine ausgezeichnete farbige Ikonographie, ein kurzgefaßter Begleittext und ein detaillierter alphabetischer Index sorgen für einen einfachen und raschen Zugang. Die summarische Bibliographie verweist auf die Basismonographien in Onkologie und Augenpathologie.

Dieses Buch interessiert nicht nur Studenten, die sich als Anfänger mit der Ophthalmologie befassen, sondern auch erfahrene Ophthalmologen, Pathologen und Dermatologen, die oft mit ophthalmologischen Problemen konfrontiert sind.

Acknowledgements

The illustrations to this atlas were, in part, put together over the last thirty years at the Clinique Ophtalmologique de l'Hôtel-Dieu in Paris (Professor P. Dhermy) and at the Clinique Ophtalmologique in Strasbourg (Professor A. Brini), for teaching purposes. They have considerably added to the already existing collections of slides made by Professor Offret (Paris) and Professors Redslob and Nordmann (Strasbourg). We have also had access to the files of clinical photographs made in the departments of Professor Y. Pouliquen (Paris) and Professor A. Bronner (Strasbourg).

Our gratitude also goes to our colleagues and friends who have provided certain rare slides. They are listed below under "Remerciements".

We would also like to thank M. L. Sanner (Strasbourg), S. Teychenné, J. P. Laurens and M. Delacour (Paris), for their accurate technical work in eye pathology, as well as F. Stoeckel (Strasbourg), who was responsible for many of the clinical illustrations.

The atlas could not have been published were it not for the excellent work of our secretary, M. Ott, who managed to decipher our medical scrawl and produced perfectly typed texts in three languages. The help of Mrs. M. Aunis in typing the Index was appreciated.

The German version is the work of G. Gissy and the English version was revised by M. Stuart.

We are particularly grateful to our two colleagues, Professor E. Landolt of Zurich and Dr. R. Barry of Birmingham, members of the European Ophthalmic Pathology Society, who not only reread and corrected the text but also helped us with their experience in clinicopathology.

Finally, we are very grateful for the generous help provided by several pharmaceutical firms: Chauvin-Blanche, M.S.D. Chibret, Dulcis, Faure and Servier.

Remerciements

L'iconographie de cet atlas a été réalisée progressivement au cours des trente dernières années dans un but pédagogique à la Clinique Ophtalmologique de l'Hôtel-Dieu à Paris (Pr P. Dhermy), et à la Clinique Ophtalmologique de Strasbourg (Pr A. Brini). Ces apports relativement récents n'ont fait qu'augmenter les collections déjà existantes de diapositives et de coupes d'anatomie pathologique du Professeur Offret à Paris, des Professeurs Redslob et Nordmann à Strasbourg. Nous avons profité aussi des collections de photos cliniques des deux services (Pr Y. Pouliquen à Paris, Pr A. Bronner à Strasbourg).

En outre de nombreux collègues et amis nous ont aidé à combler certaines lacunes. Ainsi, nous exprimons notre reconnaissance à: Ch. Arnesen (54c); R. Barry (41c); J.A. Bernard (8d); B. Daicker (46e, 46f); Ph. Demailly (24b); J. Ganem (29d); A. Garner (35d); B. Guiberteau (64a,b,c); Ch. Haye (1a, 19e, 32c, 35e, 39a); E. Heid (58b); J. Hungerford (55e); E. Mary-Offenstein (49d-e); G. Merg (59a); S. Morax (19a, 24a, 24d); G.O.H. Naumann (46c, 46d); H. Offret (42c, 43d); J.C. Patillon (53c, 53d); J.P. Rollin (45e, 45f); J.P. Roulland (44a); Schwab (48e); G. Soubrane (62c); A. Tarkkanen (45c); J. Vignaud (36a).

Nous tenons à remercier pour le minutieux travail technique d'anatomie pathologique oculaire: Mme M.L. Sanner (Strasbourg), Mme S. Teychenné (Paris), Mr J.P. Laurens (Paris), Mlle M. Delacour (Paris), ainsi que l'auteur d'une grande partie des illustrations cliniques: Mr F. Stoeckel (Strasbourg).

Ce travail n'aurait pas pu être réalisé sans l'aide fidèle et constante de notre excellente secrétaire Mme M. Ott (Strasbourg). Grâce à elle des manuscrits souvent difficilement lisibles ont abouti à une dactylographie sans faute en trois langues. L'aide apportée par Mme M. Aunis à la mise en forme de l'index a été appréciée.

La traduction en allemand a été assurée grâce à la compétence de Mme G. Gissy, la relecture de l'anglais grâce au travail patient et précis de Mr Malcolm Stuart.

Nous sommes particulièrement reconnaissants à nos deux collègues membres de l'European Ophthalmic Pathology Society, versés à la fois en ophtalmologie et en anatomie pathologique, qui ont relu et corrigé notre texte; ils nous ont apporté non seulement leur compétence linguistique mais aussi le fruit de leur expérience personnelle, anatomo-clinique: le Professeur Ernest Landolt de Zurich et le Docteur René Barry de Birmingham.

Enfin, nous avons apprécié la générosité de plusieurs laboratoires pharmaceutiques qui ont contribué sous diverses formes à la réalisation de cet atlas: Chauvin-Blanche, M.S.D. Chibret, Dulcis, Faure, Servier.

Danksagung

Das Bildmaterial zu diesem Atlas wurde im Lauf der vergangenen dreißig Jahre zu pädagogischen Zwecken in der Klinik für Ophthalmologie des Hôtel-Dieu in Paris (Prof. P. Dhermy) und in der Klinik für Ophthalmologie in Strassburg (Prof. A. Brini) zusammengestellt. Diese relativ neuen Beiträge kamen zu den bereits bestehenden Diapositiv- und Pathologieschnittsammlungen Professor Offrets in Paris, der Professoren Redslob und Nordmann in Strassburg hinzu. Wir haben uns außerdem die klinischen Fotosammlungen von zwei Stationen (Prof. Y. Pouliquen in Paris, Prof. A. Bronner, Strassburg) zunutze gemacht.

Zahlreiche Kollegen und Freunde haben uns geholfen, einige Lücken zu schließen. Ihre Namen sind im französischen Text aufgeführt.

Für die sorgfältige technische Ausführung der augenpathologischen Arbeit danken wir Frau M.L. Sanner (Strassburg), Frau S. Teychenné (Paris), Herrn J.P. Laurens (Paris), Frl. M. Delacour (Paris), sowie Herrn F. Stoeckel (Strassburg), der für einen Großteil der klinischen Illustrationen verantwortlich zeichnet.

Ohne die zuverlässige und andauernde Mithilfe unserer ausgezeichneten Sekretärin, Frau M. Ott (Strassburg), wäre diese Arbeit nicht möglich gewesen. Sie brachte oft schwer leserliche Manuskripte in eine fehlerfreie maschinenschriftliche Fassung in drei Sprachen. Wir haben Frau M. Aunis' freundliche Hilfe bei der Zusammenstellung des Index sehr geschätzt.

Für die deutsche Übersetzung sorgte mit Kompetenz Frau G. Gissy, die Durchsicht des Englischen ist der geduldigen und präzisen Arbeit von Herrn Malcolm Stuart zu verdanken.

Unsere besondere Dankbarkeit gebührt zwei unserer Kollegen der European Ophthalmic Pathology Society, die in der Ophthalmologie wie auch in der Pathologie versiert sind und unseren Text nachgelesen und korrigiert haben; sie unterstützten uns nicht nur mit ihrer sprachlichen Kompetenz, sondern brachten auch ihre persönliche anatomisch-klinische Erfahrung mit ein: Professor Ernest Landolt aus Zürich und Dr. René Barry aus Birmingham.

Schließlich wußten wir die Großzügigkeit mehrerer pharmazeutischer Labors zu schätzen, die in unterschiedlicher Form zur Herstellung dieses Atlasses beigetragen haben: Chauvin-Blanche, M.S.D. Chibret, Dulcis, Faure, Servier.

Detailed table of contents

Plate		PART A: TUMOURS OF THE EYELIDS AND THE CONJUNCTIVA	Page
	I.	Tumours of the epithelium and adnexa	
		1. Benign tumours	2
1		1.1 Benign tumours of the epithelium (without adnexa)	2
		1.1a Papillomas of the eyelid	2
		1.1b Seborrheic keratosis	2
2		1.1c Conjunctival papillomas	4
		1.1d Molluscum contagiosum	4
3		1.1e Kerato-acanthoma	6
4		1.2 Cysts	8
		1.2a Epidermal and pilar cysts	8
		1.2b Conjunctival cysts	8
5		1.3 Benign pilar tumours	10
		1.3a Trichilemmoma	10
		1.3b Tricho-epithelioma	10
6		1.3c Pilomatricoma	12
7		1.4 Benign sebaceous gland tumours	14
		1.4a "Senile" sebaceous naevus of the eyelid	14
		1.4b "Senile" sebaceous naevus of the caruncle	14
		1.4c Meibomian adenoma	14
8		1.5 Sweat gland benign tumours	16
		1.5a Hidrocystoma	16
		1.5b Papillary syringadenoma	16
9		1.5c Syringomas	18
		1.5d Eccrine acrospiroma	18
		1.6 Oncocytoma of the caruncle	18
		2. Precancerous epithelial tumours	20
10		2.1 Palpebral actinic keratosis	20
		2.2 Conjunctival actinic keratosis	20
11		2.3 Conjunctival carcinoma *in situ*	22
		2.4 Xeroderma pigmentosum	22
		3. Malignant epithelial tumours	24
12–13		3.1 Basal cell carcinomas of the lids	24
14		3.2 Squamous cell (epidermoid) carcinoma of the lids	28
15		3.3 Squamous cell (epidermoid) carcinoma of the conjunctiva	30
		3.4 Muco-epidermoid carcinoma of the conjunctiva	30
16		3.5 Sebaceous carcinomas	32
		3.6 Sweat gland carcinomas	32
	II.	Pigmented tumours of the lids and the conjunctiva	
17		1. Benign pigmented tumours	34
		1.1 Junctional naevus	34
		1.2 Compound naevus	34
18		1.3 Intradermal naevus	36
		1.4 Cystic benign naevus	36
		1.5 Balloon cell naevus	36
19		1.6 Giant pigmented naevus	38
		1.7 Juvenile melanoma of S. Spitz	38
		1.8 Blue naevus of Tièche	38
		2. Malignant melanomas of the eyelids and the conjunctiva	40
20		2.1 Precancerous Hutchinson-Dubreuilh melanosis	40
21		2.2 Superficial spreading melanoma	42
		2.3 Nodular melanoma	42

	III.	Xanthomatous tumours	
22		1. Tuberous xanthoma of the lid	44
		2. Xanthelasma	44
		3. Juvenile xanthogranuloma of the eyelid and conjunctiva	44
	IV.	Vascular benign tumours	
23		1. Palpebro-conjunctival lymphangiomas	46
	V.	Vascular malignant tumours	
		1. Kaposi's sarcoma	46
	VI.	Tumours of adipose tissue	
		1. Lipoma of the conjunctiva	46
	VII.	Palpebro-conjunctival tumours of nerve tissue	
24		1. Neurofibroma	48
		2. Schwannoma	48
		3. Merkel cell tumour	48
	VIII.	Dysgenetic tumours of the conjunctiva, lids and orbit	
25		1. Dermoid cyst	50
		2. Dermoid of the limbus and dermis-like choristoma	50
26		3. Dermolipoma	52
		4. Complex choristoma	52
		5. Epibulbar osteoma	52
	IX.	Inflammatory and degenerative pseudo-tumoral lesions	
		1. Chalazion	52
		2. Pyogenic granuloma	54
27		3. Pinguecula	54
		4. Pterygium	54
28		5. Palpebro-conjunctival amyloidosis	56

PART B: ORBITAL AND ORBITO-PALPEBRAL TUMOURS

	X.	Fibrohistiocytic tumours	
29		1. Benign fibrohistiocytoma	60
		2. Malignant fibrohistiocytoma	60
		3. Nodular fasciitis	60
	XI.	Tumours of muscular tissue	
30		1. Embryonal rhabdomyosarcoma	62
	XII.	Benign palpebro-orbital vascular tumours	
31		1. Cavernous haemangioma	64
		2. Benign haemangio-endothelioma	64
32		3. Haemangio-pericytoma	66
		4. Flat haemangioma	66
		5. Intravascular vegetating haemangio-endothelioma	66
	XIII.	Tumours of adipose orbital tissue	
		1. Lipoma	66
		2. Liposarcoma	66

33	XIV.	Bone tumours	
		1. Osteoma	68
		2. Bone haemangioma	68
		3. Giant cell tumour	68
		4. Osteosarcoma	68
		5. Mesenchymatous chondrosarcoma	68
34	XV.	Pseudo-tumorous bone dysplasias	
		1. Fibrous dysplasia and ossifying fibroma	70
		2. Bone cyst aneurysm	70
35	XVI.	Tumours of the neural tissue or neural-like tumours	
		1. Schwannoma	72
35+24		2. Orbital neurofibroma	72
		3. Granular cell tumour	72
		4. Alveolar soft part sarcoma	72
		5. Sympathoblastoma	72
36	XVII.	Tumours of the intra-orbital optic nerve	
		1. Glioma	74
		2. Meningiomas	74
37	XVIII.	Haemato-sarcomas	
		1. Lymphomas	77
38		2. Plasmacytomas	80
		3. Granulocytic sarcoma	80
39	XIX.	Tumours of the lacrimal gland	
		1. Benign mixed tumour	82
		2. Malignant tumours of the lacrimal gland	84
40		2.1 Adenoid cystic carcinoma	84
		2.2 Carcinoma within a pleomorphic adenoma	84
		2.3 Other carcinomas	84
41	XX.	Tumours of the lacrimal sac	86
42	XXI.	Pseudo-tumorous histiocytic lesions (X Histiocytoses)	
		1. Eosinophilic granuloma of bone	88
		2. Hand-Schüller-Christian disease	88
		3. Sinus histiocytosis	88

PART C: TUMOURS OF THE UVEA

43	XXII.	Iris tumours	
		1. Iris cysts	92
		1.1 Primary cysts of the iris pigment epithelium	92
		1.2 Secondary cystic proliferation	92
		2. Iris pigmented tumours	92
		2.1 Adenomas of the iris pigment epithelium	92
43–44		2.2 Melanocytic tumours of the iris stroma	92
45		3. Iris myogenic tumours	96
		4. Juvenile xanthogranuloma	96
		5. Metastases to the iris	96

Plate		PART C: TUMOURS OF THE UVEA (continued)	Page

	XXIII.	Tumours of ciliary body	
46		1. Epithelial tumours	98
		1.1 Tumours of non-pigmented epithelium	98
		1.1a Medullo-epitheliomas	98
		1.1b Adult-type tumours	98
		1.2 Tumours of the ciliary pigment epithelium	98
47		2. Melanocytic tumours of the ciliary body stroma	100
		2.1 Benign tumours	100
		2.2 Ciliary body melanomas	100
	XXIV.	Choroidal tumours	
48		1. Melanocytic tumours and other neural crest-derived-tumours	102
		1.1 Choroidal naevi	102
		1.2 Choroidal tumours in neurofibromatosis	102
49		1.3 Melanosis oculi and naevus of Ota	104
50–52		1.4 Choroidal melanomas	106
53		2. Vascular tumours	112
		2.1 Haemangiomas	112
		3. Choroidal osteomas	112
54		4. Leukaemias and lymphomas	114
		5. Metastatic carcinomas	114

PART D: TUMOURS OF THE RETINA AND THE OPTIC DISC

55–57	XXV.	Malignant tumour: Retinoblastoma	118
	XXVI.	Glial tumours of the retina and the optic disc	
58		1. Astrocytoma	124
	XXVII.	Vascular tumours	
59		1. Coats disease	126
60		2. Von Hippel's disease	128
61	XXVIII.	Retina and disorders of the blood and blood forming organs	130
62	XXIX.	Tumours of the retinal pigment epithelium	132
63	XXX.	Melanocytoma of the optic disc	134
64	XXXI.	Drusen of the optic disc	136
		Technical appendix	139
		Literature	143
		Alphabetical index of subjects	145

Table des matières détaillée

Planche	PARTIE A: TUMEURS PALPÉBRO-CONJONCTIVALES	Page
	I. Tumeurs épithéliales et annexielles	
	1. Tumeurs bénignes	2
1	1.1 Tumeurs bénignes épithéliales (non annexielles)	2
	1.1a Papillome palpébral	2
	1.1b Verrue séborrhéïque	2
2	1.1c Papillome conjonctival	4
	1.1d Molluscum contagiosum	4
3	1.1e Kérato-acanthome	6
4	1.2 Kystes	8
	1.2a Kystes épidermiques et pilaires	8
	1.2b Kystes conjonctivaux	8
5	1.3 Tumeurs bénignes pilaires	10
	1.3a Trichilemmome	10
	1.3b Tricho-épithéliome	10
6	1.3c Pilomatrixome	12
7	1.4 Tumeurs bénignes d'origine sébacée	14
	1.4a Adénome sébacé "senile" de la paupière	14
	1.4b Adénome sébacé "senile" de la caroncule	14
	1.4c Adénome meibomien	14
8	1.5 Tumeurs bénignes sudorales	16
	1.5a Hidrocystome	16
	1.5b Syringadénome papillaire	16
9	1.5c Syringomes	18
	1.5d Acrospirome eccrine	18
	1.6 Tumeur caronculaire d'origine lacrymale	18
	2. Tumeurs précancéreuses épithéliales	20
10	2.1 Kératose actinique palpébrale	20
	2.2 Kératose actinique conjonctivale	20
11	2.3 Carcinome *in situ* de la conjonctive	22
	2.4 Xeroderma pigmentosum	22
	3. Tumeurs malignes épithéliales	24
12–13	3.1 Carcinomes baso-cellulaires des paupières	24
14	3.2 Carcinome spino-cellulaire (épidermoïde) des paupières	28
15	3.3 Carcinome spino-cellulaire (épidermoïde) de la conjonctive	30
	3.4 Carcinome muco-épidermoïde de la conjonctive	30
16	3.5 Carcinomes sébacés	32
	3.6 Carcinomes sudoraux	32
	II. Tumeurs mélaniques palpébro-conjonctivales	
	1. Tumeurs mélaniques bénignes	34
17	1.1 Naevus jonctionnel	34
	1.2 Naevus composé	34
18	1.3 Naevus intradermique ou profond	36
	1.4 Naevus kystique bénin	36
	1.5 Naevus à cellules ballonisantes	36
19	1.6 Naevus pigmentaire géant	38
	1.7 Mélanome juvénile de Spitz	38
	1.8 Naevus bleu de Tièche	38
	2. Tumeurs mélaniques malignes palpébro-conjonctivales	40
20	2.1 Mélanome sur mélanose précancéreuse de Hutchinson-Dubreuilh	40
21	2.2 Mélanome superficiel extensif	42
	2.3 Mélanome nodulaire	42

	III.	Tumeurs xanthomateuses	
22		1. Xanthome tubéreux palpébral	44
		2. Xanthélasma	44
		3. Xanthogranulome juvénile de la paupière et de la conjonctive	44
	IV.	Tumeurs vasculaires bénignes	
23		1. Lymphangiomes palpébro-conjonctivaux	46
	V.	Tumeurs vasculaires malignes	
		1. Sarcome de Kaposi	46
	VI.	Tumeurs du tissu adipeux	
		1. Lipome de la conjonctive	46
	VII.	Tumeurs du tissu nerveux palpébro-conjonctival	
24		1. Neurofibrome	48
		2. Schwannome	48
		3. Tumeur à cellules de Merkel	48
	VIII.	Tumeurs dysgénétiques de la conjonctive, des paupières et de l'orbite	
25		1. Kyste dermoïde	50
		2. Dermoïde du limbe et "dermis-like choristoma"	50
26		3. Dermolipome	52
		4. Choristome complexe	52
		5. Ostéome épibulbaire	52
	IX.	Lésions inflammatoires et dégénératives pseudo-tumorales	
		1. Chalazion	52
27		2. Granulome pyogénique	54
		3. Pinguécula	54
		4. Ptérygion	54
28		5. Amylose palpébro-conjonctivale	56

PARTIE B: TUMEURS DE L'ORBITE ET ORBITO-PALPÉBRALES

	X.	Tumeurs fibrohistiocytaires	
29		1. Fibrohistiocytome bénin	60
		2. Fibrohistiocytome malin	60
		3. Fasciite nodulaire	60
	XI.	Tumeurs musculaires	
30		1. Rhabdomyosarcome embryonnaire	62
	XII.	Tumeurs vasculaires bénignes palpébro-orbitaires	
31		1. Angiome caverneux	64
		2. Hémangio-endothéliome bénin	64
32		3. Hémangio-péricytome	66
		4. Angiome plan	66
		5. Hémangio-endothéliome végétant intravasculaire	66
	XIII.	Tumeurs du tissu adipeux orbitaire	
		1. Lipome	66
		2. Liposarcome	66

	XIV.	Tumeurs osseuses	
33		1. Ostéome	68
		2. Hémangiome de l'os	68
		3. Tumeur à cellules géantes	68
		4. Ostéosarcome	68
		5. Chondrosarcome mésenchymateux	68
	XV.	Dysplasies osseuses pseudo-tumorales	
34		1. Dysplasie fibreuse et fibrome ossifiant	70
		2. Kyste anévrysmal de l'os	70
	XVI.	Tumeurs du tissu nerveux ou assimilées	
35		1. Schwannome	72
35+24		2. Neurofibrome de l'orbite	72
		3. Tumeurs à cellules granuleuses	72
		4. Sarcome alvéolaire des parties molles	72
		5. Sympathoblastome	72
	XVII.	Tumeurs du nerf optique intra-orbitaire	
36		1. Gliome	74
		2. Méningiomes	74
	XVIII.	Hématosarcomes	
37		1. Lymphomes	77
38		2. Plasmocytomes	80
		3. Sarcome granulocytaire	80
	XIX.	Tumeurs de la glande lacrymale	
39		1. Tumeur mixte bénigne	82
40		2. Tumeurs malignes de la glande lacrymale	84
		2.1 Carcinome adénoïde kystique	84
		2.2 Carcinome dans un adénome pléomorphe	84
		2.3 Autres carcinomes	84
41	XX.	Tumeurs du sac lacrymal	86
	XXI.	Lésions histiocytaires pseudo-tumorales (Histiocytoses X)	
42		1. Granulome éosinophile de l'os	88
		2. Maladie de Hand-Schüller-Christian	88
		3. Histiocytose sinusale	88

PARTIE C: TUMEURS DE L'UVÉE

	XXII.	Tumeurs iriennes	
43		1. Kystes iriens	92
		1.1 Kystes spontanés de l'épithélium pigmentaire irien	92
		1.2 Proliférations secondaires kystiques	92
		2. Tumeurs pigmentées de l'iris	92
		2.1 Adénomes de l'épithélium pigmentaire irien	92
43–44		2.2 Tumeurs mélaniques du stroma irien	92
45		3. Tumeurs d'origine musculaire	96
		4. Xanthogranulome juvénile	96
		5. Métastases iriennes	96

Planche	PARTIE C: TUMEURS DE L'UVÉE (suite)	Page

	XXIII.	Tumeurs du corps ciliaire	
46		1. Tumeurs épithéliales	98
		1.1 Tumeurs de l'épithélium non pigmenté	98
		1.1a Médullo-épithéliomes	98
		1.1b Tumeurs de type adulte	98
		1.2 Tumeurs de l'épithélium pigmenté ciliaire	98
47		2. Tumeurs mélaniques du stroma ciliaire	100
		2.1 Tumeurs bénignes	100
		2.2 Mélanomes	100

	XXIV.	Tumeurs choroïdiennes	
48		1. Tumeurs mélaniques et autres tumeurs dérivées de la crête neurale	102
		1.1 Naevi choroïdiens	102
		1.2 Tumeurs choroïdiennes dans la neurofibromatose	102
49		1.3 Melanosis oculi et naevus de Ota	104
50–52		1.4 Mélanomes choroïdiens	106
53		2. Tumeurs vasculaires	112
		2.1 Hémangiomes	112
		3. Ostéomes choroïdiens	112
54		4. Leucémies et lymphomes	114
		5. Carcinomes métastatiques	114

PARTIE D: TUMEURS DE LA RÉTINE ET DE LA PAPILLE OPTIQUE

| 55–57 | XXV. | Tumeur maligne: Rétinoblastome | 118 |

| | XXVI. | Tumeurs gliales de la rétine et de la papille | |
| 58 | | 1. Astrocytome | 124 |

	XXVII.	Tumeurs vasculaires	
59		1. Maladie de Coats	126
60		2. Maladie de Von Hippel	128

| 61 | XXVIII. | Rétine et maladies du sang et des organes hématopoïétiques | 130 |

| 62 | XXIX. | Tumeurs de l'épithélium pigmentaire de la rétine | 132 |

| 63 | XXX. | Mélanocytome de la papille | 134 |

| 64 | XXXI. | Verrucosités hyalines (druses) de la papille | 136 |

| | | **Appendice technique** | 139 |

| | | **Littérature** | 143 |

| | | **Index alphabétique des sujets** | 148 |

Detailliertes Inhaltsverzeichnis

Tafel	TEIL A: GESCHWÜLSTE DER AUGENLIDER UND DER BINDEHAUT	Seite
	I. Geschwülste des Epithels und der Anlagen	
	1. Gutartige Epithelgeschwülste	2
1	1.1 Gutartige Geschwülste des Epithels (ohne die Anlagen)	2
	1.1a Lidpapillom	2
	1.1b Seborrhoische Warze	2
2	1.1c Papillom der Bindehaut	4
	1.1d Molluscum contagiosum	4
3	1.1e Keratoakanthom	6
4	1.2 Zysten	8
	1.2a Zysten der Epidermis und der Haare	8
	1.2b Zysten der Bindehaut	8
5	1.3 Gutartige Haargeschwülste	10
	1.3a Trichilemmom	10
	1.3b Tricho-epitheliom	10
6	1.3c Pilomatrixom	12
7	1.4 Gutartige Talgdrüsengeschwülste	14
	1.4a "Seniles Steatoadenom"	14
	1.4b "Steatoadenom" der Karunkel	14
	1.4c Meibomsches Adenom	14
8	1.5 Gutartige Geschwülste der Schweißdrüsen	16
	1.5a Hidrozystom	16
	1.5b Papillares Syringozystadenom	16
9	1.5c Syringome	18
	1.5d Ekkrines Akrospirom	18
	1.6 Onkozytom der Karunkel	18
	2. Präkanzeröse Epithelgeschwülste	20
10	2.1 Aktinische Lidkeratose	20
	2.2 Aktinische Keratose der Konjunktiva	20
11	2.3 Carcinoma *in situ* der Konjunktiva	22
	2.4 Xeroderma pigmentosum	22
	3. Maligne epitheliale Tumoren	24
12–13	3.1 Basalzellkarzinome des Lides	24
14	3.2 Stachelzellkarzinom (Plattenepithelkarzinom) des Lides	28
15	3.3 Plattenepithelkarzinom der Bindehaut	30
	3.4 Muko-epidermoides Karzinom der Bindehaut	30
16	3.5 Karzinom der Talgdrüsen	32
	3.6 Schweißdrüsenkarzinom	32
	II. Pigmentierte Tumoren der Lider und Bindehaut	
	1. Gutartige pigmentierte Tumoren	34
17	1.1 Junctionaler Naevus	34
	1.2 Compound naevus	34
18	1.3 Intradermaler Naevus	36
	1.4 Gutartiger zystischer Naevus	36
	1.5 Ballonzellnaevus	36
19	1.6 Riesenpigmental	38
	1.7 Juveniles Spitz Melanom	38
	1.8 Naevus bleu nach Tièche	38
	2. Maligne pigmentierte Tumoren (Melanome) der Lider und Bindehaut	40
20	2.1 Melanom auf prekanzeröser erworbener Melanose nach Hutchinson-Dubreuilh	40
	2.2 Sich oberflächlich ausbreitendes Melanom	42
21	2.3 Noduläres Melanom	42

Tafel	TEIL A: GESCHWÜLSTE DER AUGENLIDER UND DER BINDEHAUT (Fortsetzung)	Seite

III. Xanthomatöse Tumoren

22
1. Tuberöses Xanthom des Lides   44
2. Xanthelasma des Lides   44
3. Juveniles Xanthogranulom des Lides und der Konjunktiva   44

IV. Gutartige Gefäßtumoren

23
1. Palpebral-konjunktivale Lymphangiome   46

V. Maligne Gefäßtumoren
1. Kaposi Sarkom   46

VI. Tumore des Fettgewebes
1. Lipom der Bindehaut   46

VII. Palpebro-konjunktivale Nerventumoren

24
1. Neurofibrom   48
2. Schwannom   48
3. Merkel-Zell-Tumor   48

VIII. Dysgenetische Tumoren der Lider und Orbita

25
1. Dermoidzyste   50
2. Dermoid des Limbus und "dermis-like choristoma"   50

26
3. Dermolipom   52
4. Komplexes Choristom   52
5. Epibulbäres Osteom   52

IX. Entzündliche und degenerative Pseudotumoren
1. Chalazion   52

27
2. Granuloma pyogenicum   54
3. Pinguecula   54
4. Pterygium   54

28
5. Amyloidose der Lider und Bindehaut   56

TEIL B: ORBITALE UND ORBITO-PALPEBRALE GESCHWÜLSTE

X. Fibrohistiozytäre Tumoren

29
1. Gutartiges Fibrohistiozytom   60
2. Bösartiges Fibrohistiozytom   60
3. Fasciitis nodularis   60

XI. Muskeltumoren

30
1. Embryonales Rhabdomyosarkom   62

XII. Gutartige Gefäßtumoren der Lider und Orbita

31
1. Kavernöses Hämangiom   64
2. Gutartiges Hämangio-Endotheliom   64

32
3. Hämangio-Perizytom   66
4. Flaches Angiom   66
5. Wucherndes intravasales Hämangio-Endotheliom   66

XIII. Tumoren des orbitalen Fettgewebes
1. Lipom   66
2. Liposarkom   66

	XIV.	Knochentumoren	
33		1. Osteom	68
		2. Knochenhämangiom	68
		3. Riesenzellentumor	68
		4. Osteosarkom	68
		5. Mesenchymatöses Chondrosarkom	68

	XV.	Pseudo-tumorale Knochendysplasien	
34		1. Fibröse Dysplasie und verknöcherndes Fibrom	70
		2. Aneurysmatische Knochenzyste	70

	XVI.	Geschwülste des Nervengewebes und verwandter Gewebsarten	
35		1. Schwannom	72
35+24		2. Neurofibrom der Orbita	72
		3. Granulosazell-Tumor	72
		4. Alveoläres Weichteilsarkom	72
		5. Sympathoblastom	72

	XVII.	Geschwülste des Intraorbitalen Sehnervs	
36		1. Gliom	74
		2. Meningiome	74

	XVIII.	Hämatosarkome	
37		1. Lymphome	77
38		2. Plasmozytome	80
		3. Granulozytäres Sarkom	80

	XIX.	Tumoren der Tränendrüse	
39		1. Gutartiger Tumor	82
40		2. Bösartige Tumoren der Tränendrüse	84
		2.1 Adenoidzystisches Karzinom	84
		2.2 Karzinom in einem pleomorphen Adenom	84
		2.3 Andere Karzinome	84

| 41 | XX. | Tumoren des Tränensacks | 86 |

	XXI.	Pseudotumorale histiozytäre Läsionen (X-Histiozytosen)	
42		1. Eosinophilisches Granulom des Knochens	88
		2. Hand-Schüller-Christian Krankheit	88
		3. Sinus Histiozytose	88

TEIL C: GESCHWÜLSTE DER UVEA

	XXII.	Tumoren der Regenbogenhaut	
43		1. Iriszysten	92
		1.1 Spontane Zysten des Pigmentepithels der Iris	92
		1.2 Sekundäre Zysten	92
		2. Pigmentierte Tumoren der Iris	92
		2.1 Adenom des Pigmentepithels der Iris	92
43–44		2.2 Melanotische Tumoren des Irisstromas	92
45		3. Myogene Tumoren	96
		4. Juveniles Xanthogranulom	96
		5. Iris Metastasen	96

	XXIII.	Tumoren des Ziliarkörpers	
46		1. Epitheliale Geschwülste	98
		1.1 Tumoren des nichtpigmentierten Ziliarepithels	98
		1.1a Medullo-Epitheliome	98
		1.1b Adulte Tumoren	98
		1.2 Tumoren des pigmentierten Ziliarepithels	98
47		2. Melanotische Tumoren des Ziliarstromas	100
		2.1 Gutartige Tumoren	100
		2.2 Maligne Melanome	100
	XXIV.	Aderhauttumoren	
48		1. Melanotische Geschwülste und andere von der Neuralleiste ausgehende Geschwülste	102
		1.1 Aderhautnaevi	102
		1.2 Aderhauttumoren bei Neurofibromatose	102
49		1.3 Melanosis oculi und Naevus von Ota	104
50–52		1.4 Maligne Melanome der Aderhaut	106
53		2. Gefäßtumoren	112
		2.1 Hämangiome	112
		3. Osteom der Aderhaut	112
54		4. Leukämien und Lymphome	114
		5. Metastasen	114

TEIL D: GESCHWÜLSTE DER NETZHAUT UND DER PAPILLE

55–57	XXV.	Bösartige Geschwülste der Netzhaut: Retinoblastom	118
	XXVI.	Gliageschwülste der Netzhaut und der Papille	
58		1. Astrozytom	124
	XXVII.	Gefäßtumoren der Netzhaut	
59		1. Morbus Coats	126
60		2. Von Hippelsche Erkrankung	128
61	XXVIII.	Retina und Erkrankungen des Blutes und der blutbildenden Organe	130
62	XXIX.	Geschwülste des Pigmentepithels der Netzhaut	132
63	XXX.	Melanozytom der Papille	134
64	XXXI.	Drusen der Papille	136
		Technischer Anhang	139
		Literatur	143
		Alphabetisches Sachwörterverzeichnis	151

A

Tumours of the eyelids and the conjunctiva

*

Tumeurs palpébro-conjonctivales

*

Geschwülste der Augenlider und der Bindehaut

PLATE 1   PLANCHE 1   TAFEL 1

I. TUMOURS OF THE EPITHELIUM AND ADNEXA

I.1 Benign tumours

I.1.1 Benign tumours of the epithelium (without adnexa)

I.1.1a Papillomas of the eyelid
Clinical features. They usually involve the lid skin or margin. In children, grayish, dry, warty lesions may occur in a linear pattern (linear naevus verrucosus).

Histopathology. Epidermal papillae are numerous and elongated, hence the term "papilloma". The proliferation is characterized by a thickening of the squamous layer (acanthosis) and of the keratin layer (hyperkeratosis); however the different epidermal layers keep their orderly arrangement without any disturbance of their polarity or cell atypia.

I.1.1b Seborrheic keratosis
Clinical features. Among papillomatous lesions, seborrheic keratosis, occurring frequently on the eyelids after the age of fifty, is often misdiagnosed. Indeed, this small brownish elevated lesion may be confused with a melanoma.

Histopathology. This acanthotic and hyperkeratotic proliferation is composed of small basophilic cells akin to the cells seen in basal cell carcinomas (basal cell papilloma). These are squamous cells with fewer intercellular junctions. The two main types are:
– the keratotic type;
– the adenoid type.
Invariably melanocytes from the basal layer are activated and tattoo neighbouring cells with melanin granules. This accounts for the occasional clinical aspect. Any suspicious lesion should be removed surgically to allow histopathologic examination.

I. TUMEURS ÉPITHÉLIALES ET ANNEXIELLES

I.1 Tumeurs bénignes

I.1.1 Tumeurs bénignes épithéliales (non annexielles)

I.1.1a Papillome palpébral
Clinique. Il siège sur la face cutanée ou sur la marge palpébrale. Chez l'enfant des formations verruqueuses grises, sèches se déposent parfois de façon linéaire ("naevus verruqueux linéaire").

Histopathologie. Les papilles épidermiques sont plus nombreuses et plus allongées que normalement d'où le nom de papillome. La prolifération se caractérise par un épaississement de la couche de Malpighi (hyperacanthose) et de la couche cornée (hyperkératose); mais les diverses couches conservent leur ordonnance habituelle sans bouleversement de leur polarisation ni anomalies cytologiques.

I.1.1b Verrue séborrhéique
Clinique. Dans le cadre des papillomes la verrue séborrhéique, fréquente aux paupières surtout après la cinquantaine, est souvent source d'erreurs de diagnostic.
En effet cette petite excroissance brunâtre peut être confondue avec un mélanome.

Histopathologie. C'est une prolifération hyperacanthosique et hyperkératosique constituée de petites cellules basophiles ressemblant un peu à celles d'un épithélioma baso-cellulaire ("papillome basocellulaire" des anglosaxons). Ce sont bien des cellules malpighiennes avec des ponts d'union mais moins nombreux que normalement. On distingue deux formes principales:
– la forme kératosique;
– la forme adénoïde.
Quoiqu'il en soit les mélanocytes de la basale participent souvent activement à la prolifération, tatouant les cellules voisines de grains de mélanine ce qui explique l'aspect clinique occasionnel. Au moindre doute il faut préférer l'exérèse chirurgicale qui permet le contrôle histologique.

I. GESCHWÜLSTE DES EPITHELS UND DER ANLAGEN

I.1 Gutartige Epithelgeschwülste

I.1.1 Gutartige Geschwülste des Epithels (ohne die Anlagen)

I.1.1a Lidpapillom
Klinik. Es tritt auf der Hautseite oder am Lidrand auf. Beim Kind setzen sich trockene, graue Warzengebilde manchmal linienförmig ab ("linearer Warzennaevus").

Histopathologie. Die Epidermisleisten sind zahlreicher und länger als gewöhnlich, daher der Name *"Papillom"*. Die Wucherung ist erkenntlich an einer Verdickung der Malpighischicht (Hyperakanthose) und der Hornschicht (Hyperkeratose); aber die verschiedenen Schichten behalten ihre gewöhnliche Anordnung ohne Veränderung ihrer Polarisierung und ohne zytologische Anomalien bei.

I.1.1b Seborrhoische Warze
Klinik. Unter den Papillomen ist die Alterswarze, die hauptsächlich im Alter von über fünfzig an den Augenlidern auftritt, eine häufige Ursache für Fehldiagnosen. Der kleine, bräunliche Auswuchs kann in der Tat mit einem Melanom verwechselt werden.

Histopathologie. Es handelt sich um eine Hyperakanthose und Hyperkeratose kleiner basophiler Zellen, die ein wenig denen eines Basalzellkarzinoms (angelsächsisch "Basalzellpapillom") gleichen. Es sind Zellen der Malpighi-Schicht mit Verbindungspunkten, aber in geringerer Zahl als normalerweise. Man unterscheidet zwei Hauptformen:
– die keratöse Form;
– die adenoide Form.
Oft sind die basalen Pigmentzellen aktiv mitbeteiligt, wobei sie die Nachbarzellen mit Melaningranula tätowieren, woraus sich der gelegentliche klinische Aspekt erklärt. Beim geringsten Zweifel ist die operative Entfernung, die eine histologische Kontrolle ermöglicht, vorzuziehen.

PLATE 1   PLANCHE 1   TAFEL 1

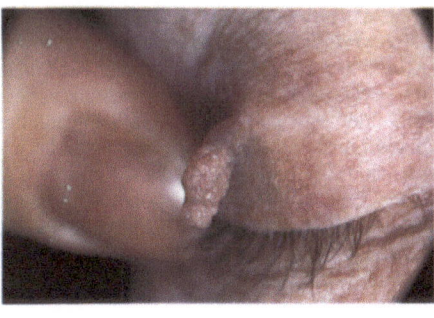

a

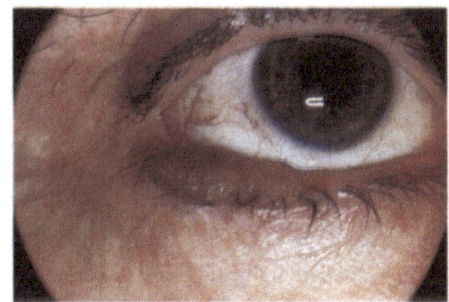

b

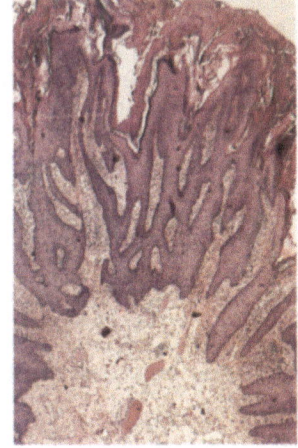

c

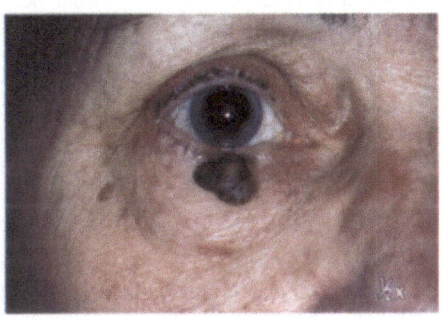

d

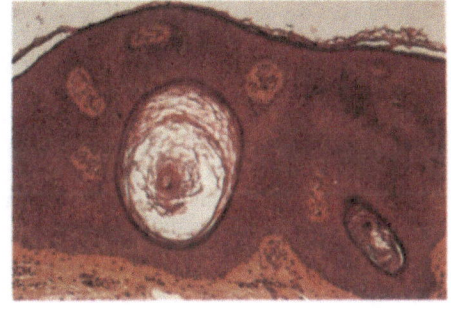

e

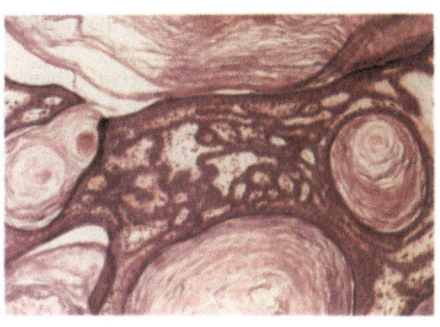

f

Fig. a. Pedunculated papilloma of the lid.
Pedunculated outgrowth with a keratin cap on the apex.

Fig. b. Sessile, warty papilloma at the margin with a greasy irregular surface. No induration. No loss of eyelashes.

Fig. c. Lid papilloma: histology.
Hyperplastic papillae centered on a fibrovascular core. Hyperkeratosis.

Fig. d. Seborrheic wart.
Black excrescence with elevated, sharp margins; the surface is covered with a crust of keratin giving a greasy aspect.

Fig. e. Seborrheic keratosis, keratotic type.
Within the hyperplastic epidermis, uniformly basophilic, scattered pseudo-horncysts are punched out. These concentric keratin lamellae represent invaginations of the surface keratin.

Fig. f. Seborrheic keratosis, adenoid type.
The arrangement of the basophilic cells in interweaving rows accounts for the lace-like pattern of the proliferation; pseudo-horncysts are irregularly scattered.

Fig. a. Papillome pendulaire de la paupière.
Excroissance pédiculée recouverte à son extrêmité d'une coiffe de kératine.

Fig. b. Verrue séborrhéïque.
Papillome verruqueux de la marge palpébrale, sessile, à surface irrégulière d'aspect onctueux. Pas d'induration. Pas de chute des cils.

Fig. c. Papillome palpébral: histologie.
Exagération des papilles centrées par un axe conjonctivo-vasculaire. Hyperkératose.

Fig. d. Verrue séborrhéïque.
Excroissance à bords nets surélevés, noirâtre; la surface est recouverte d'une squame kératosique lui donnant un aspect onctueux.

Fig. e. Verrue séborrhéïque, forme kératosique.
L'hyperplasie épidermique, d'une teinte basophile uniforme, est parsemée de pseudo-kystes cornés, à "l'emporte-pièce", lamelles concentriques de kératine, (sections des invaginations de l'hyperkératose de surface).

Fig. f. Verrue séborrhéïque, forme adénoïde.
Les cellules basophiles en travées entrecroisées, donnent à la prolifération un aspect "en dentelle", avec de place en place quelques pseudo-kystes cornés.

Abb. a. Pendelpapillom des Augenlids.
Gestielter Auswuchs, dessen Ende mit einer Keratinhaube bedeckt ist.

Abb. b. Warzenartiges Papillom.
Am Lidrand, festhaftend, mit unregelmäßiger, ölig aussehender Oberfläche. Keine Verhärtung. Kein Wimpernausfall.

Abb. c. Lidpapillom: Histologie.
Vermehrung der um eine Konjunktivagefäßachse angeordneten Papillen. Hyperkeratose.

Abb. d. Seborrhoische Warze.
Auswuchs mit deutlichen, angehobenen Rändern, schwärzlich; die Oberfläche ist mit einer keratösen Squama bedeckt, die ihr ein öliges Aussehen verleiht.

Abb. e. Seborrhoische Warze, Keratöse Form.
Die Epidermisverdickung mit gleichmäßiger basophiler Färbung ist übersät mit falschen Hornzysten, "wie ausgestanzt", konzentrischen Keratinlamellen, Einstülpungsabschnitten der Oberflächen-Hyperkeratose.

Abb. f. Seborrhoische Warze, adenoide Form.
Die sich überkreuzenden basophilen Zellen geben der Wucherung ein "spitzenartiges" Aussehen mit einzelnen falschen Hornzysten.

PLATE 2   PLANCHE 2   TAFEL 2

I.1.1c Conjunctival papillomas
Clinical features. When located on the palpebral conjunctiva, in the fornix or the semilunar fold, these lesions are prominent, sessile or pedunculated, sometimes with a cauliflower-like surface. They may be covered by a purulent mucus layer, if an infection is associated. At the limbus, they tend to remain flat and are less vascularized.

Histopathology. Elevated papillomas have a variable goblet cell component. Mitotic figures are not exceptional in the basal layers. At the limbus, papillomas have a flat base and few goblet cells.

I.1.1d Molluscum contagiosum
Clinical features. Secondary to a viral infection by Pox virus, it may occur either in childhood, as multiple lesions, or in adults as a solitary, often large tumour. The latter may be misdiagnosed as kerato-acanthoma. Follicular conjunctivitis is often associated; it will resolve only after excision of the tumour.

Histopathology. The characteristic pattern stems from the lobular structure with a heavy content of rounded figures: the molluscum bodies. These result from the degeneration of virus infected squamous cells.

I.1.1c Papillome conjonctival
Clinique. Lorsqu'il siège sur la conjonctive palpébrale, au fornix ou sur le pli semi-lunaire il est saillant, pendulaire, ou sessile parfois framboisé et peut être recouvert d'une lame de mucus purulent en cas d'infection surajoutée. Au limbe il peut être plus étalé et moins vascularisé.

Histopathologie. Les papillomes saillants sont plus ou moins riches en cellules muqueuses. Ils peuvent être le siège d'une exocytose à polynucléaires; les mitoses ne sont pas rares dans les couches basales.
Au limbe les papillomes ont une basale plus rectiligne et sont pauvres en cellules muqueuses.

I.1.1d Molluscum contagiosum
Clinique. Dû à un virus du groupe Pox virus il peut se rencontrer aussi bien chez l'enfant, où il est rarement unique, que chez l'adulte où il est plutôt solitaire, parfois de grande taille. Il peut dans ces cas se confondre avec le kérato-acanthome. Il s'accompagne souvent d'une conjonctivite folliculaire que seule l'exérèse de la tumeur peut faire disparaître.

Histopathologie. L'aspect en lobules remplis de formations arrondies est caractéristique, (les "corps du molluscum"). Ils traduisent la dégénérescence complète des cellules malpighiennes infectées par le virus.

I.1.1c Papillom der Bindehaut
Klinik. Wenn es in der palpebralen Bindehaut, im Fornix oder in der Plica semilunaris liegt, so bildet es einen Vorsprung, ist pendelnd-papillomatös oder breit aufsitzend und manchmal himbeerartig und kann im Fall einer zusätzlichen Infektion mit einem schleimig-eitrigen Belag überzogen sein. Am Limbus kann es ausgebreitet und weniger vaskularisiert sein.

Histopathologie. Die vorstehenden Papillome sind mehr oder weniger reich an Schleimzellen. Sie können von gelappt kernigen Leukozyten durchsetzt sein. Mitosen sind in den Basalschichten keine Seltenheit. Am Limbus haben Papillome eine eher geradlinige Basalschicht und sind arm an Schleimzellen.

I.1.1d Molluscum contagiosum
Klinik. Durch ein Virus aus der Gruppe der Pockenviren verursacht, ist es sowohl beim Kind, wo es selten in der Einzahl vorkommt, als auch beim Erwachsenen, wo es eher einzeln ist, aber manchmal groß sein kann, anzutreffen. Es kann in diesen Fällen mit dem Keratoacanthom verwechselt werden. Es geht häufig mit einer Follikularkonjunktivitis einher, die nur mit der Beseitigung des Tumors zu heilen ist.

Histopathologie. Charakteristisch ist das Auftreten von mit rundlichen Gebilden gefüllten Knötchen, den "Molluscum-Körperchen". Sie weisen auf die völlige Degeneration der vom Virus infizierten Malpighi-Zellen hin.

PLATE 2 PLANCHE 2 TAFEL 2

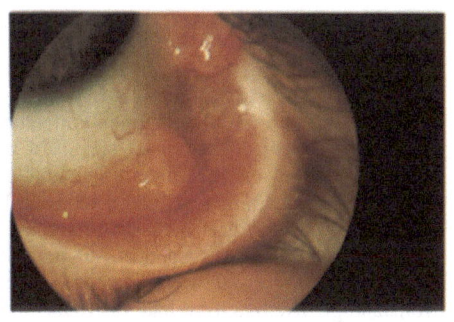

a

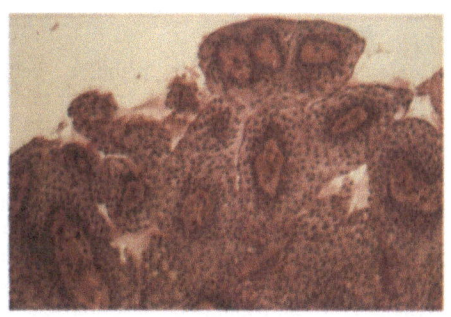

b

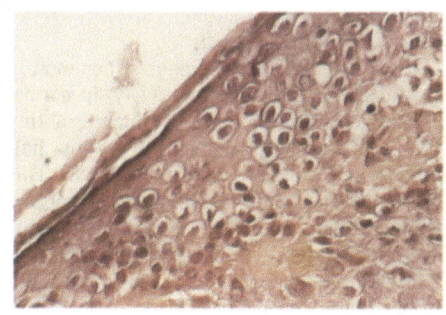

c

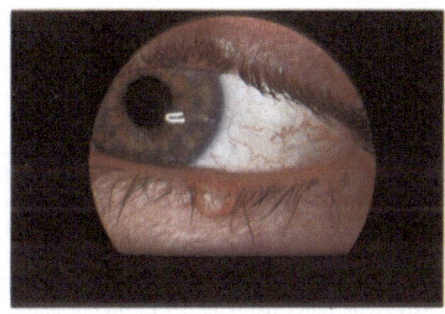

d

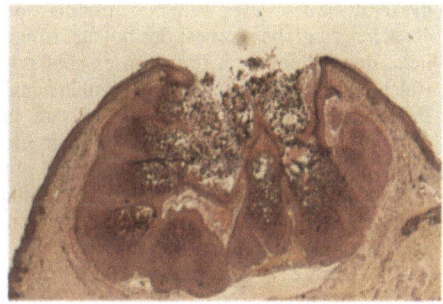

e

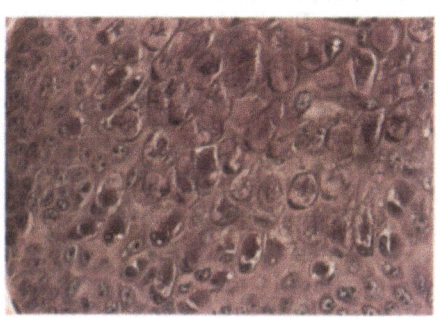

f

Fig. a. These fornix papillomas are indurated, vascular and may appear vivid red.

Fig. b. Histology of a cauliflower-like conjunctival papilloma with an overlying thickened, regular epithelium, raised by vascular cores.

Fig. c. Koïlocytes: clear cytoplasm, small, hyperchromatic central nucleus.
They are suggestive when located in the squamous cell layer. They may be evidence of a papilloma virus infection.

Fig. d. Molluscum nodules.
These small, painless, pinkish nodules of a variable size, from a pinpoint to the size of a pea, are often umbilicated.

Fig. e. Concentric, pear shaped lobules filled with molluscum bodies, breaking out to the surface into a true pore (Fig. f).

Fig. f. Molluscum bodies.

Fig. a. Papillomes conjonctivaux des culs-de-sac, sessiles, non indurés, vascularisés, pouvant parfois prendre une teinte rouge vif.

Fig. b. Histologie d'un papillome conjonctival framboisé recouvert d'un épithélium épaissi, régulier, soulevé par des axes conjonctifs vascularisés.

Fig. c. Koïlocytes: cytoplasme clair, petit noyau central hyperchromatique.
Ils sont surtout évocateurs lorsqu'ils siègent dans la couche de Malpighi. Ils témoigneraient d'une infection virale à papilloma virus.

Fig. d. Nodule de molluscum.
Petit nodule indolore dont la taille peut aller de celle d'une tête d'épingle à un petit pois, de couleur nacrée ou rosée, souvent ombiliqué.

Fig. e. Lobules piriformes, concentriques s'ouvrant à la surface par un véritable pore, remplis de "corps du molluscum" (Fig. f).

Fig. f. Corps du molluscum.

Abb. a. Bindehaut-Papillome im Fornix, breitbasig, nicht verhärtet, vaskularisiert, die manchmal eine leuchtend rote Färbung annehmen können.

Abb. b. Histologie eines himbeerartigen Bindehaut-Papilloms, das mit einem verdickten, regelmäßigen, durch vaskularisiertes Bindegewebe angehobenen Epithel bedeckt ist.

Abb. c. Koilozyten: helles Zytoplasma, kleiner zentraler hyperchromer Kern.
Bezeichnend sind sie vor allem, wenn sie in der Malpighi-Schicht auftreten. Sie lassen angeblich einen viralen Infekt mit Papilloma virus erkennen.

Abb. d. Molluscum-Knötchen.
Kleine schmerzlose Knötchen, stecknadelkopf- bis erbsengroß, perlmutter- oder rosafarben, häufig eingedellt.

Abb. e. Birnförmige, konzentrische Knötchen, die sich an der Oberfläche durch eine richtige Pore öffnen und mit "Molluscum-Körperchen" (Abb. f) gefüllt sind.

Abb. f. Molluscum-Körperchen.

PLATE 3   PLANCHE 3   TAFEL 3

I.1.1e Kerato-acanthoma
Clinical features. This tumour is common in the lid and appears spontaneously, in normal skin, after fifty. In the early stages, a tiny papule forms and invaginates at the top, hollowing into a crater filled with keratin. This crater enlarges progressively and disappears spontaneously, sometimes leaving no visible scar. The total cycle of the lesion extends over a 6 week period. Despite the benign character of this lesion, recurrences can occur.

Histopathology. During the maturation period, the diagnosis is easy, provided that the excision is complete and that the sections examined comprise the centre of the lesion. The latter is prominent, crater-like, limited by two spurs overhanging a cavity filled with keratin lamellae.
The epithelial walls are thickened and acanthotic. The cells show dyskeratotic features, even sometimes with squamous eddies; irregular nuclei, with atypia and mitoses may be present. The basal membrane is regular, although often eroded by inflammatory infiltrates, including sometimes eosinophils. The deeper tumour lobules always stay above the level of the sweat glands, accounting for the exophytic nature of the lesion.

I.1.1e Kérato-acanthome
Clinique. Fréquente à la paupière, cette tumeur apparaît spontanément, en peau saine, chez des sujets ayant, en général, dépassé la cinquantaine. C'est au départ, une petite papule qui va bientôt former un nodule qui s'ombiliquera à son sommet pour se creuser d'un cratère rempli de kératine. Ce cratère va s'élargir progressivement pour s'éliminer spontanément sans parfois laisser de trace visible. Le cycle complet de la lésion se sera étendu sur 6 semaines environ. En dépit de sa bénignité, cette lésion peut récidiver.

Histopathologie. A la période de maturation le diagnostic est facile à condition que le prélèvement ait été complet et que les coupes examinées passent par le centre de la lésion. Celle-ci est surélevée, cratériforme, limitée latéralement par deux éperons surplombant une cavité remplie de lamelles de kératine.
Les parois épithéliales sont épaissies, hyperacanthosiques. Les cellules sont souvent dyskératosiques avec même parfois des ébauches de globes cornés; des noyaux irréguliers, dystrophiques et des mitoses sont possibles. La basale est cependant régulière mais souvent effacée, comme rongée par un infiltrat inflammatoire pouvant contenir des éosinophiles. Les lobules tumoraux les plus profonds restent toujours au dessus du plan des glandes sudorales ce qui atteste du caractère exophytique de la lésion.

I.1.1e Keratoakanthom
Klinik. Diese häufig am Augenlid auftretende Geschwulst entsteht spontan auf gesunder Haut bei meist über fünfzigjährigen Patienten. Die anfangs kleine Papel bildet sich bald zu einem Knötchen aus, das oben eingedellt ist und einen mit Keratin angefüllten Krater bildet. Dieser Krater erweitert sich nach und nach und verschwindet spontan, ohne eine sichtbare Spur zu hinterlassen. Der vollständige Krankheitsverlauf erstreckt sich auf ungefähr 6 Wochen, kann aber auch mehrere Monate dauern. Trotz ihrer Gutartigkeit, kann diese Läsion jedoch rezidivieren.

Histopathologie. Während der "Reifung" (im typischen Stadium) fällt die Diagnose leicht, vorausgesetzt die Exzision war vollständig und die untersuchten Schnitte verlaufen durch die Mitte der Läsion. Diese ist erhöht, kraterförmig, seitlich abgegrenzt durch zwei Sporne, die in eine mit Keratinlamellen gefüllte Aushöhlung hineinragen.
Diese Epithelwände verdicken sich durch eine übermäßige Stachelzellenbildung. Die Zellen weisen oft eine abnorme Verhornung auf, manchmal mit Ansätzen zu kleinen Hornkugeln; unregelmäßige, dystrophische Kerne und Mitosen können vorkommen. Die Basalschicht ist indessen regelmäßig, aber oft verwischt, wie angefressen von einem entzündlichen Infiltrat, das Eosinophile enthalten kann. Die tiefsten Tumorzellen bleiben stets über der Schweißdrüsenebene, was den exophytischen Charakter der Läsion bestätigt.

PLATE 3   PLANCHE 3   TAFEL 3

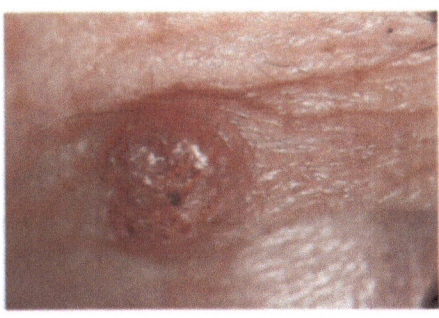

a

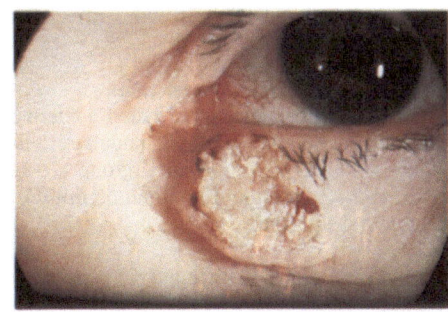

b

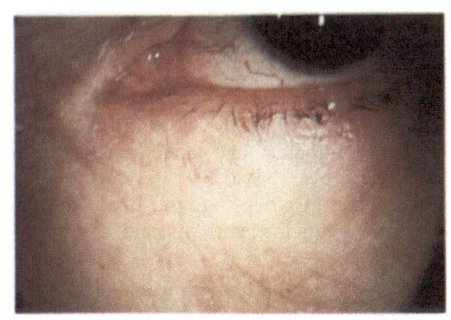

c

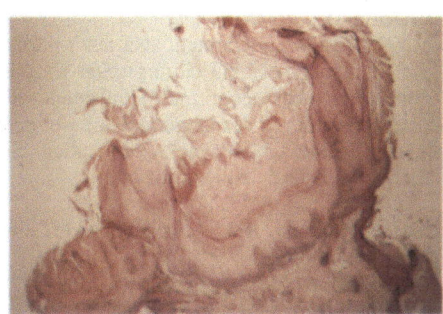

d

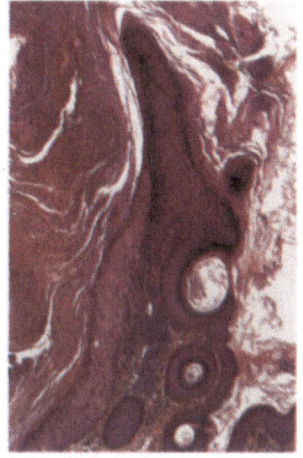

e

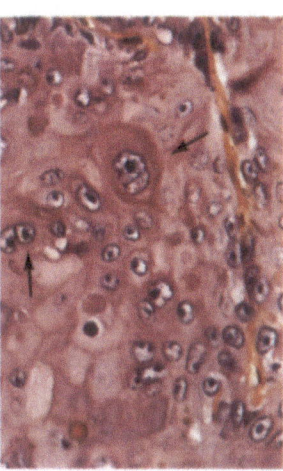

f

Fig. a. "Mature" kerato-acanthoma.
Firm, hemispherical, rounded, insensitive, pinkish nodule with overlying dilated blood vessels. The top is hollowed with a keratin-filled crater.

Fig. b-c. Spontaneous evolution of a kerato-acanthoma.
The lesion evolves toward its regression (fig. b); a few weeks later (fig. c) no scar is visible.

Fig. d. Kerato-acanthoma, overall view.
Central crater filled with keratin, yet elevated, exophytic.

Fig. e. Epithelial "spur" overhanging the central cavity, well demarcated from the peripheral normal epidermis.

Fig. f. Cytologic features of the crater walls.
Dyskeratosis, nuclear abnormalities are noted (→).
Such features could suggest the diagnosis of squamous cell carcinoma, if the excision is not performed in toto.

Fig. a. Kérato-acanthome "mature".
Nodule hémisphérique, ferme, d'aspect "rebondi", indolore, de teinte rosée, sillonné de télangiectasies. Son sommet est creusé d'un cratère rempli de kératine.

Fig. b-c. Evolution spontanée d'un kérato-acanthome.
Sur la fig. b la lésion entame sa régression; quelques semaines après, tout a disparu sans cicatrice visible.

Fig. d. Kérato-acanthome, vue d'ensemble.
Cratère central rempli de kératine et néanmoins surélevé, exophytique.

Fig. e. "Eperon" épithélial surplombant latéralement la cavité, se continuant de façon abrupte avec l'épiderme normal.

Fig. f. Cellules de la paroi du cratère.
On distingue une cellule dyskératosique et des noyaux nettement dystrophiques (→). De telles images peuvent évoquer un carcinome spino-cellulaire surtout si l'examen n'intéresse qu'une partie de la lésion. Aussi faut-il exiger une exérèse totale.

Abb. a. "Reifes" Keratoakanthom.
Halbkugelförmiges, festes Knötchen, "prall" aussehend, schmerzlos, rosafarben, von Telangiektasien durchzogen. Es hat oben eine kraterförmige, mit Keratin gefüllte Vertiefung.

Abb. b-c. Spontaner Verlauf eines Keratoakanthoms.
In Abb. b ist die Läsion im Rückgang begriffen; ein paar Wochen danach ist alles ohne sichtbare Narbe verschwunden.

Abb. d. Keratoakanthom, Gesamtansicht.
Zentraler, mit Keratin gefüllter, aber dennoch erhabener Krater, exophytisch.

Abb. e. Epithelial-"Sporn", seitlich über die Vertiefung ragend, setzt sich abrupt in die normale Epidermis fort.

Abb. f. Zellen der Kraterwand.
Man erkennt eine abnorm verhornende Zelle und deutlich dystrophische Kerne (→). Solche Bilder lassen an ein Stachelzellarzinom denken, besonders wenn für die Untersuchung nur ein Teil der Läsion vorliegt. Es muß deshalb eine vollständige operative Entfernung verlangt werden.

7

I.1.2 Cysts

I.1.2a Epidermal and pilar cysts
Clinical features. They are embedded in the epidermis, nodular and painless, and can be mobilized over the deeper layers. Some of them, often in groups, are the size of a millet granule, giving the name "milium".

Histopathology. Pinkus distinguishes two varieties:
– epidermal, or infundibular cysts, arising from the distal end (or infundibulum) of pilar follicules. Milia are the smallest among epidermal cysts;
– pilar cysts (or tricholemmal) arising from the pilar sheat.
Rupture of their wall may induce an inflammatory foreign body reaction.

I.1.2b Conjunctival cysts
Clinical features. They may appear spontaneously or as a consequence of trauma, surgical or non surgical. They may arise on the bulbar conjunctiva or in a fornix, most often the inferior one. They are easy to identify clinically.

Histopathology. Two types exist histopathologically:
– conjunctival inclusion cysts;
– cysts of lacrymal origin.
Inclusion cysts are lined by a mucous epithelium, which, in cases of severe distension, may be reduced to a monolayer of flattened cells. Lacrymal cysts arise frequently in the fornix, from the excretory duct of an accessory lacrymal gland and are surrounded by two layers of cells: cubical internally, flat externally.
The perfectly transparent elevated lesions of the bulbar conjunctiva usually known as lymphatic cysts, are actually telangiectases.

I.1.2 Kystes

I.1.2a Kystes épidermiques et pilaires
Clinique. Ils sont enchassés dans l'épiderme, mobiles sur le plan profond, nodulaires, indolores. Certains, souvent groupés, ne dépassent pas la taille d'un grain de mil d'où leur nom de milium.

Histopathologie. On distingue à la suite de Pinkus:
– les kystes épidermiques ou infundibulaires car ils se développent aux dépens de la partie distale (ou infundibulum) du follicule pilaire. Les grains de milium sont les plus petits des kystes épidermiques;
– les kystes pilaires dits aussi tricholemmiques car ils tirent leur origine de la gaine du poil.
La rupture de leur paroi peut donner lieu à une réaction inflammatoire à corps étranger.

I.1.2b Kystes conjonctivaux
Clinique. Ils peuvent être d'apparition spontanée ou succéder à un traumatisme, chirurgical ou non. Ils siègent soit sur la conjonctive bulbaire soit dans un cul-de-sac surtout l'inférieur. Ils sont facilement identifiés cliniquement.

Histopathologie. Il existe deux types histologiques:
– les kystes conjonctivaux par inclusion;
– les kystes d'origine lacrymale.
Les kystes par inclusion sont bordés d'un épithélium de type muqueux qui, en cas de distension importante, peut être réduit à une seule couche de cellules aplaties.
Les kystes d'origine lacrymale, fréquents dans le cul-de-sac, se développent aux dépens du canal excréteur d'une glande lacrymale accessoire et sont donc bordés de deux couches de cellules: les internes cubiques, les externes aplaties.
Les lésions surélevées parfaitement transparentes de la conjonctive bulbaire connues sous le nom de kystes lymphatiques sont en réalité des lymphangiectasies.

I.1.2 Zysten

I.1.2a Zysten der Epidermis und der Haare
Klinik. Sie sind in die Epidermis eingelassen, über den tieferen Schichten beweglich, knötchenförmig, schmerzlos. Manche treten in Gruppen in Erscheinung und sind meist nicht mehr als hirsegroß, daher der Name Hirsekorn.

Histopathologie. Man unterscheidet nach Pinkus:
– Epidermoid- oder Infundibulumzysten, da sie sich auf dem trichterförmigen Teil (oder Infundibulum) des Haarfollikels entwickeln. Hirsekörner sind die kleinsten Epidermoidzysten;
– Haar- oder auch Tricholem-Zysten, die aus der Haarhülle entstehen.
Ein Riß ihrer Wandung kann eine entzündliche Fremdkörperreaktion verursachen.

I.1.2b Zysten der Bindehaut
Klinik. Sie können spontan, aber auch infolge eines Traumas, das ein chirurgischer Eingriff sein kann (aber nicht muß), auftreten. Sie sitzen entweder in der Conjunktiva bulbi oder in der Umschlagsfalte, vor allem unten. Sie sind klinisch leicht zu identifizieren.

Histopathologie. Es bestehen zwei histologische Typen:
– Konjunktiva-Einschlußzysten;
– von den Tränenorganen herrührende Zysten.
Einschlußzysten sind von einem Epithel mit Schleimzellen überzogen, das bei starker Dehnung auf eine einzige Schicht abgeflachter Zellen beschränkt sein kann. Von den Tränendrüsen herrührende Zysten treten häufig in den Umschlagsfalten auf und entwickeln sich aus dem Ausführungsgang einer akzessorischen Tränendrüse; sie sind also von zwei Zellschichten eingesäumt, von denen die innere kubisch, die äußere abgeflacht ist.
Anmerkung: Die erhabenen, völlig transparenten Läsionen der Conjunctiva bulbi, die unter dem Namen lymphatische Zysten bekannt sind, sind in Wirklichkeit Lymphangiektasien.

PLATE 4 PLANCHE 4 TAFEL 4

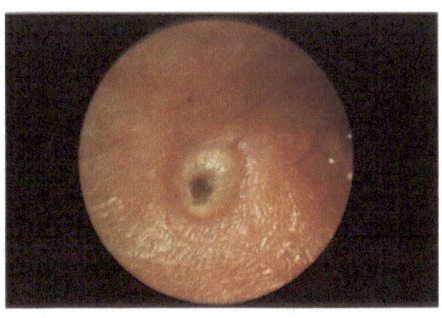

a

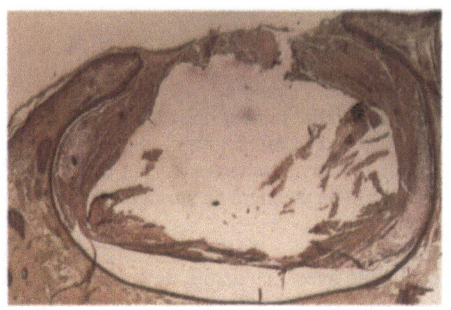

b

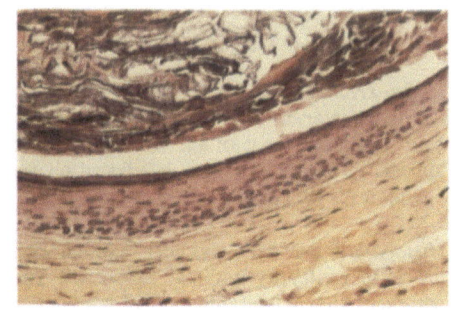

c

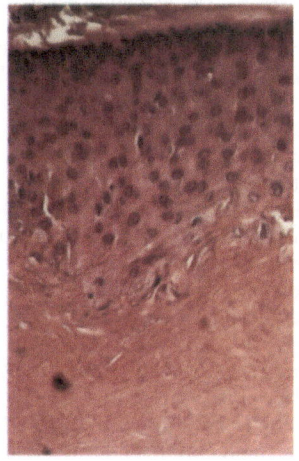

d

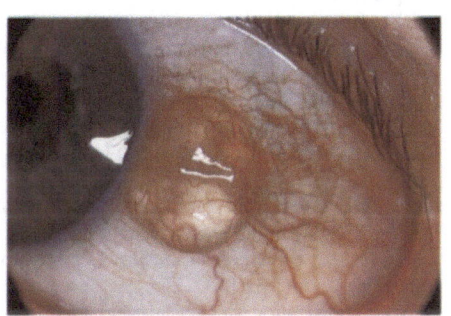

e

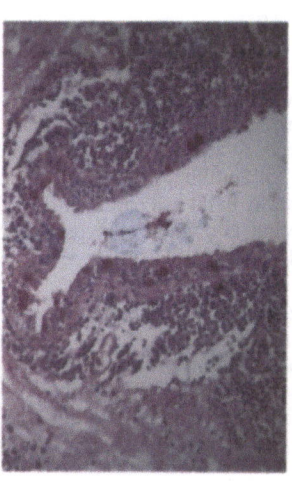

f

Fig. a. Epidermal cyst opening through an orifice with a blackened plug (oxydated keratin).

Fig. b. Epidermal cyst with its orifice and keratin issuing through it.

Fig. c. Wall of an epidermal cyst.
Normal epidermis with a granular layer, a keratin layer and keratin lamellae.

Fig. d. Wall of pilar cyst.
Absence of granular layer, vacuolar swollen squamous cells, transforming progressively into an amorphous, eosinophilic material, a soft keratin, or sebum.

Fig. e. Conjunctival inclusion cyst (post-surgical) of juxta-limbal conjunctiva.
A cystic, rounded, translucent, insensitive mass, with a liquid content, can be mobilized on deep layers.

Fig. f. Conjunctival inclusion cyst: histopathology.
Stratified epithelium with mucous cells (PAS).

Fig. a. Kyste épidermique s'ouvrant par un orifice noirâtre (kératine oxydée).

Fig. b. Kyste épidermique avec son orifice d'où s'échappe la kératine.

Fig. c. Paroi de kyste épidermique.
Épiderme normal avec une couche granuleuse, une couche cornée et les lamelles de kératine.

Fig. d. Paroi de kyste pilaire.
Absence de couche granuleuse; les cellules malpighiennes gonflées, vacuolaires, se transforment progressivement en un matériel amorphe éosinophile (kératine grasse ou sébum).

Fig. e. Kyste conjonctival par inclusion (post-opératoire) de la conjonctive juxta-limbique.
Masse kystique, arrondie, translucide, à contenu liquidien, rénitente et indolore, mobile sur les plans profonds.

Fig. f. Kyste conjonctival par inclusion: histopathologie.
Épithélium pavimenteux stratifié, présence de quelques cellules muqueuses (PAS).

Abb. a. Epidermoidzyste mit einer schwärzlichen Öffnung (oxydiertes Keratin).

Abb. b. Epidermoidzyste mit Öffnung, aus der das Keratin fließt.

Abb. c. Wand einer Epidermoidzyste.
Normale Epidermis mit einer Körnerschicht, Hornschicht und Keratinlamellen.

Abb. d. Wand einer Haarzyste.
Die Körnerschicht fehlt, die angeschwollenen Malpighi-Zellen mit Vakuolen verwandeln sich nach und nach in einen amorphen, eosinophilen Stoff (fettes Keratin oder Sebum).

Abb. e. Postoperative Konjunktiva-Einschlußzyste der an den Limbus grenzenden Konjunktiva.
Zystische Masse, abgerundet, durchscheinend, mit flüssigem Inhalt, renitent und schmerzlos, beweglich auf den tieferen Schichten.

Abb. f. Konjunktiva-Einschlußzyste: Histopathologie.
Mehrschichtiges Pflasterepithel, mit einigen Schleimzellen (PAS).

I.1.3 Benign pilar tumours

I.1.3a Trichilemmoma

Clinical features. This small tumour derives from the outer sheat of the hair follicle and appears as a papule or nodule located on the eyelid or the lid margin.

Histopathology. This nodular proliferation grows in continuity with the epidermis. The periphery shows palisading of columnar cells with a thick basal membrane, well stained with PAS. It contains abortive hair follicles and glycogen-rich clear cells.

I.1.3b Tricho-epithelioma

Clinical features. This tumour may occur in two varieties:
- a hereditary type with multiple localizations (face, scalp): this is Brooke's cystic adenoid epithelioma. The first tumours occur during the first two decades;
- a solitary tumour, occurring later in life and resembling the picture observed in keratotic basal cell carcinoma.

This lesion is nodular or papular and not ulcerated.

Histopathology. The tumour is well demarcated and contains keratinized formations resembling abortive hair follicles. Tumour strands may be bristling with intricating epithelial excrescences forming a network within a dense fibrous stroma.

I.1.3 Tumeurs bénignes pilaires

I.1.3a Trichilemmome

Clinique. Petite tumeur dérivée de la gaine externe du poil (d'où son nom), c'est une lésion papuleuse ou nodulaire siégeant sur la face cutanée de la paupière ou sur la marge.

Histopathologie. Prolifération nodulaire en continuité avec l'épiderme de surface, bordée par une rangée de cellules hautes palissadiques reposant sur une basale épaisse bien colorée par le PAS. Elle contient des ébauches pilaires et des cellules claires surchargées de glycogène.

I.1.3b Tricho-épithéliome

Clinique. Cette tumeur peut se présenter sous deux formes:
- l'une héréditaire à localisations multiples (face, cuir chevelu): c'est l'épithélioma adénoïde kystique de Brooke dont les premiers éléments se manifestent dès l'enfance ou l'adolescence;
- l'autre isolée apparaissant plus tardivement et que certains assimilent à un épithélioma baso-cellulaire kératinisant.

Macroscopiquement la lésion est nodulaire ou papuleuse, non ulcérée.

Histopathologie. Il s'agit d'une tumeur bien délimitée contenant des formations kératinisées à type d'ébauches pilaires. Les boyaux tumoraux sont parfois hérissés d'excroissances épithéliales s'anastomosant en réseau au sein d'un stroma dense et fibreux.

I.1.3 Gutartige Haargeschwülste

I.1.3a Trichilemmom

Klinik. Die von der äußeren Haarhülle ausgehende kleine Geschwulst ist bläschen- oder knötchenförmig und tritt auf der Lidaußenseite oder am Lidrand auf.

Histopathologie. Knötchenförmige Proliferation in Verbindung mit der Epidermis, gesäumt von einer Schicht aus hohen palissadenartigen Zellen, die auf einer dicken, stark PAS-positiven Basalmembran liegen. Sie enthält Haaransätze und klare, stark glycogenhaltige Zellen.

I.1.3b Tricho-epitheliom

Klinik. Dieser Tumor kann sich in zwei Formen zeigen:
- einerseits hereditär mit vielfältiger Lokalisation (Gesicht, Kopfhaut). Es handelt sich um die Brookesche zystische Epithelioma adenoides, dessen erste Zeichen von der Kindheit oder Adoleszenz an auftreten;
- andererseits isoliert, später auftretend und von gewissen Autoren dem verhornenden Basalzellkarzinom gleichgestellt.

Makroskopisch ist die Läsion knötchen- oder bläschenförmig, nicht ulzerös.

Histopathologie. Gut abgegrenzte Geschwulst, die verhornte haaransatzartige Abschnitte enthält. Von den Tumorschläuchen gehen bisweilen zahlreiche Epithelstränge ab, die im dichten und fibrösen Stroma anastomisieren und ein Netz bilden.

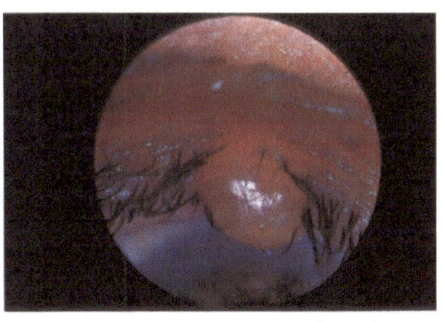

a

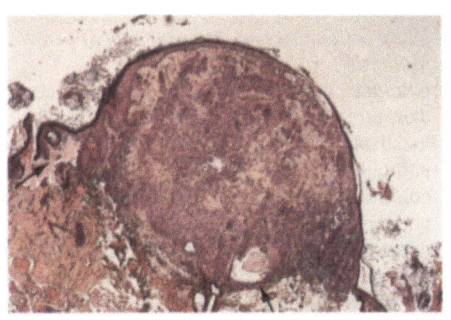

b

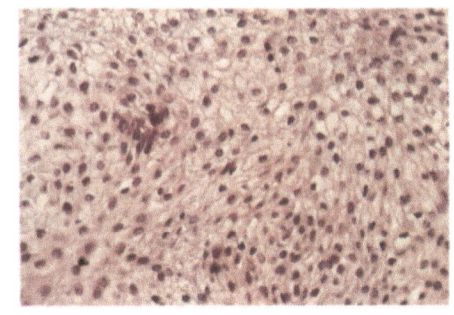

c

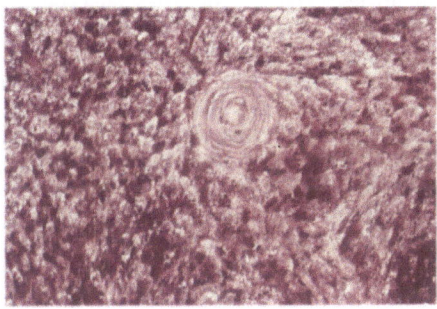

d

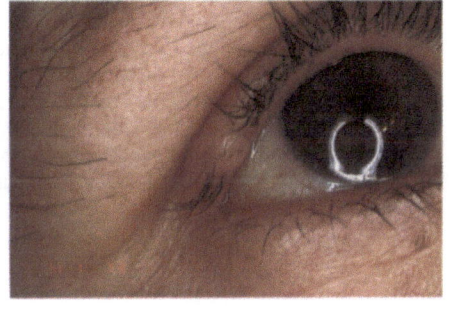

e

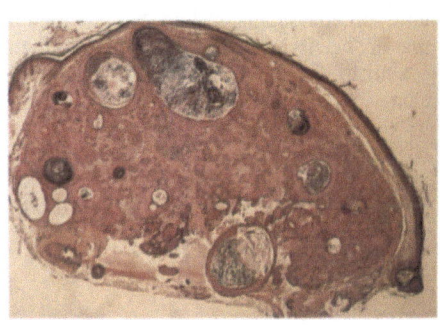

f

Fig. a. Clinical features of a trichilemmoma.
These prominent nodules, with a smooth, pinkish surface, separating the lashes, may mimic a basal cell carcinoma or a tricho-epithelioma.

Fig. b. Trichilemmoma.
Nodular lesion located in the superficial dermis; collagen septa budding from the basal membrane. Pilar formation at the periphery of the lesion. (→).

Fig. c. Trichilemmoma.
Clear, well defined cells, resembling cells of the outer sheath of the hair follicle.

Fig. d. Trichilemmoma.
Strong positivity of the PAS stain confirming the presence of glycogen.

Fig. e. Trichoepithelioma of the lid margin.
Small, smooth, soft, insensitive nodule with colour identical to that of surrounding skin.

Fig. f. Trichoepithelioma: histology.
Intricate sheaths containing horn cysts with abrupt and complete keratinization forming abortive hair follicles.

Fig. a. Aspect clinique du trichilemmome.
Nodule saillant, à surface lisse, de teinte rosée, écartant les cils, pouvant simuler un épithélioma baso-cellulaire ou un trichoépithéliome.

Fig. b. Trichilemmome.
Lésion nodulaire siégant dans le derme superficiel; des cloisons collagènes la segmentent. Formation pilaire à la périphérie de la lésion (→).

Fig. c. Trichilemmome.
Cellules claires à limites nettes rappelant les cellules de la gaine externe du poil.

Fig. d. Trichilemmome.
Forte positivité de la coloration au PAS confirmant la présence de glycogène.

Fig. e. Trichoépithéliome de la marge palpébrale.
Petit nodule lisse indolore non induré dont la teinte ne tranche pas sur celle de la peau voisine.

Fig. f. Trichoépithéliome: histologie.
Boyaux plus ou moins anastomosés contenant des kystes cornés à kératinisation abrupte et complète ébauchant des follicules pilaires.

Abb. a. Klinischer Aspekt des Trichilemmoms.
Vorstehendes Knötchen mit glatter Oberfläche, rosafarben, das die Wimpern auseinanderdrückt, kann ein Basalzellenkarzinom oder Trichoepitheliom vortäuschen.

Abb. b. Trichilemmom, Gesamtansicht.
Knötchenförmige, in der oberen Dermis liegende Läsion; von der Basalschicht ausgehende Kollagenwände unterteilen sie. Haarbildung an der Peripherie der Läsion (→).

Abb. c. Trichilemmom.
Klare Zellen mit deutlichen Abgrenzungen, die an die Zellen der äußeren Haarhülle erinnern.

Abb. d. Trichilemmom.
Stark positive PAS-Färbung bestätigt das Vorhandensein von Glycogen.

Abb. e. Trichoepitheliom am Lidrand.
Glattes, schmerzloses, nicht verhärtetes Knötchen, dessen Farbe sich nicht von der umliegenden Haut abhebt.

Abb. f. Trichoepitheliom: Histologie.
Mehr oder weniger anastomosierende Schläuche, Hornzysten mit abrupter und vollständiger Keratinisierung, Haarfollikel andeutend.

PLATE 6   PLANCHE 6   TAFEL 6

I.1.3c Pilomatricoma (Malherbe's calcifying epithelioma)

Clinical features. This childhood tumour may sometimes occur in adults. The common site of involvement is the face, particularly the eyebrow where it can be mistaken for a dermoid cyst. The nodule is of variable size but never exceeds that of a hazelnut. This freely moveable subcutaneous nodule may be of characteristic stony hardness. It is covered by normal skin.

Histopathology. In the early stages the lesion is well limited and contains two distinct areas: a peripheral hyperbasophilic zone, composed of small epithelial cells of the basal type; a central eosinophilic area composed of clearer cells called shadow cells. The latter may contain calcium or may even ossify, eliciting a giant cell granulomatous reaction. Some histochemical data provide evidence of a dysembryoplastic origin of the tumour from the primitive hair matrix cells. Therefore the term pilomatricoma should be preferred to that of "calcifying epithelioma" used formerly – a misleading term since this is a benign lesion.

I.1.3c Pilomatrixome (tumeur momifiée de Malherbe)

Clinique. Tumeur de l'enfant, elle peut cependant être parfois rencontrée chez l'adulte. Sa localisation préférentielle est la face et particulièrement le sourcil où elle est souvent confondue avec un kyste dermoïde. De forme nodulaire elle est de taille variable ne dépassant cependant guère celle d'une noisette. Ensachée dans le derme mais mobile sur les plans profonds, elle est d'une dureté parfois véritablement "pierreuse" caractéristique. Elle est recouverte d'une peau normale parfois érythémateuse.

Histopathologie. Au début de son évolution la lésion a des limites encore nettes et présente deux zones différentes: l'une périphérique très basophile formée de petites cellules de type épithélial basal, l'autre centrale éosinophile constituée de cellules plus claires dites "momifiées". Ces dernières peuvent se surcharger de calcaire voire s'ossifier et être le point de départ de réactions de résorption macrophagique. Divers arguments histochimiques orientent vers une origine dysembryoplasique à partir des cellules de la matrice pilaire et c'est pourquoi le terme de pilomatrixome a été préféré à l'ancienne dénomination d'"épithélioma calcifié" qui peut prêter à confusion, d'autant qu'il s'agit d'une tumeur toujours bénigne.

I.1.3c Pilomatrixom (verkalkendes Epithelioma Malherbe)

Klinik. Die beim Kind anzutreffende Geschwulst kann manchmal auch beim Erwachsenen auftreten. Sie ist vorzugsweise im Gesicht und insbesondere an der Braue lokalisiert und wird häufig mit einer Dermoidzyste verwechselt. Sie ist knotenförmig, von unterschiedlicher Größe, aber selten größer als eine Haselnuß. In der Derma liegend, aber beweglich gegenüber der Unterlage kann sie bis zu "steinharter" Konsistenz sein. Die darüberliegende Haut ist normal, manchmal gerötet.

Histopathologie. Zu Beginn des Verlaufs ist die Läsion noch deutlich abgegrenzt und weist zwei verschiedene Zonen auf: eine periphere, sehr basophile, aus kleinen Zellen vom Epithelial-Basal-Typ bestehende und eine zentrale eosinophile, aus helleren, sogenannten "mumifizierten" Zellen bestehende. Diese letzteren können sich mit Kalk aufladen, sogar ossifizieren und zum Ausgangspunkt von makrophagen Resorptionsreaktionen werden. Verschiedene histochemische Argumente sprechen für ein aus den Zellen der Haarmatrix ausgehendes Hamartom, weshalb die Bezeichnung Pilomatrixom den Vorrang erhielt vor der früheren Benennung "verkalkendes Epitheliom", die irreführend sein kann, zumal es sich immer um einen gutartigen Tumor handelt.

PLATE 6 PLANCHE 6 TAFEL 6

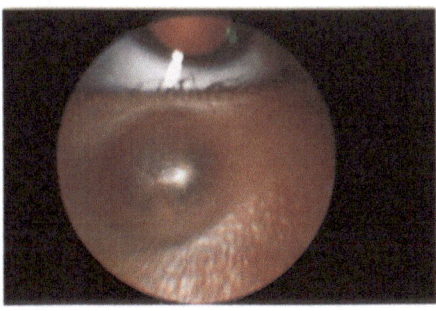

a

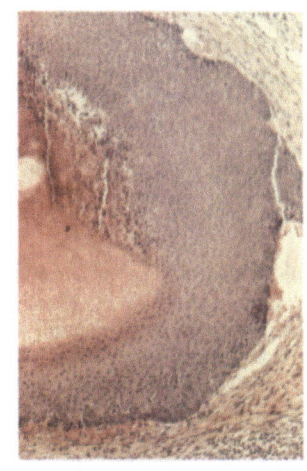

b

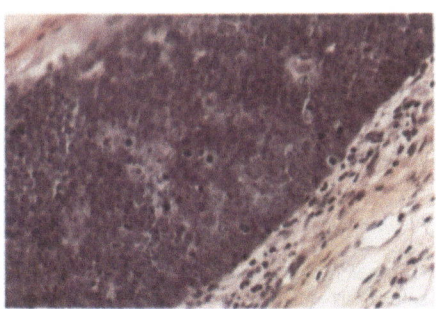

c

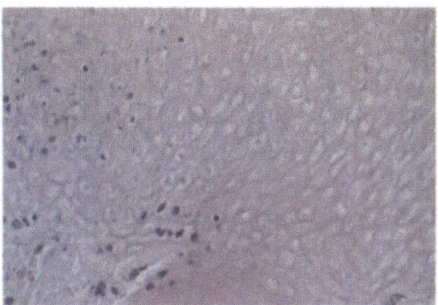

d

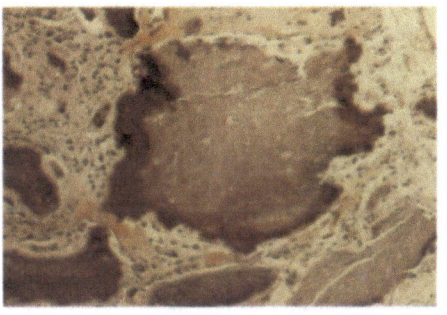

e

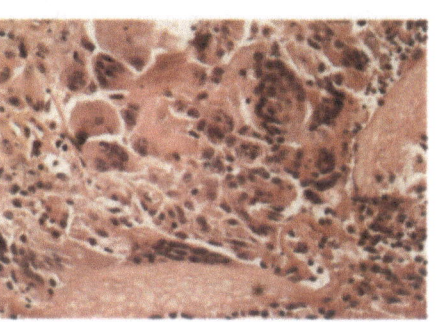

f

Fig. a. Pilomatricoma of the lower eyelid.
Its purplish colour results from the secondary inflammatory process; the lesion may then become painful.

Fig. b. Irregular but sharp borders of the lesion.
At the periphery, the germinative area mingles progressively with the central, eosinophilic area.

Fig. c. Germinative area.
Small, hyperbasophilic cells with indistinct borders, no intercellular bridges, and abundant mitoses.

Fig. d. "Shadow" cells composing the central part of the lesion.
Cells with distinct borders, clear cytoplasm, small pycnotic nuclei, sometimes absence of nuclei, lending them their "ghost cell" appearance.

Fig. e. Area of calcifying "ghost cells".

Fig. f. Foreign body granulomatous inflammatory reaction with large multinucleated cells around areas of "ghost cells".

Fig. a. Pilomatrixome de la paupière inférieure.
Sa teinte violacée est liée à une réaction inflammatoire surajoutée; la lésion peut alors devenir douloureuse.

Fig. b. Limites irrégulières mais nettes.
La partie périphérique de la lésion ou zone germinative se continue insensiblement avec la partie centrale légèrement éosinophile.

Fig. c. Zone germinative.
Petites cellules très basophiles à limites peu distinctes, sans ponts d'union, riches en mitoses.

Fig. d. Cellules "momifiées" formant la partie centrale de la lésion.
Limites bien marquées mais cytoplasme clair, petit noyau picnotique; parfois absence de noyau leur donnant une allure de "cellules fantômes".

Fig. e. Plage de cellules momifiées en voie de calcification.

Fig. f. Réaction de résorption macrophagique avec de grandes plasmodes plurinucléées autour de plages de cellules momifiées.

Abb. a. Pilomatrixom des Unterlids.
Seine ins Violette spielende Färbung rührt von einer zusätzlichen entzündlichen Reaktion her; die Läsion kann dann schmerzhaft werden.

Abb. b. Unregelmäßige, aber deutliche Abgrenzungen: Gesamtansicht.
Der periphere Teil der Läsion oder Keimzone geht unmerklich auf den zentralen, leicht eosinophilen Teil über.

Abb. c. Keimzone.
Kleine, sehr basophile Zellen mit kaum erkennbaren Zellgrenzen, ohne Interzellularbrücken, reich an Mitosen.

Abb. d. "Mumifizierte" Zellen, die den mittleren Teil der Läsion bilden.
Deutliche Abgrenzungen, aber helles Zytoplasma, kleiner, manchmal verschwindender piknotischer Kern, der ihnen etwas "Phantomhaftes" verleiht.

Abb. e. Ansammlung in Kalzifizierung begriffener, mumifizierter Zellen.

Abb. f. Makrophage Resorptionsreaktion mit mehrkernigen Riesenzellen um die mumifizierten Zellen herum.

13

PLATE 7   PLANCHE 7   TAFEL 7

I.1.4 Benign sebaceous gland tumours

I.1.4a "Senile" sebaceous naevus of the eyelid (adenomatoid sebaceous hyperplasia)

I.1.4b "Senile" sebaceous naevus of the caruncle (adenomatoid sebaceous hyperplasia)

Clinical features. This lesion may affect the sebaceous glands of the eyelid or of the caruncle in patients over fifty years of age. In the *lids*, it appears as a small, slightly raised yellowish, round or oval, nodule or papule, sometimes umbilicated. At the *caruncle* (I.1.4b) it may appear merely as a yellowish thickening.

Histopathology. This lesion is a hyperplasia rather than an adenoma. Sebaceous glands are more numerous and larger but display a normal structure. Mainly 1) they are located in the superficial dermis instead of their normal situation in the medium dermis; 2) they are grouped around a unique, centrally located dilated duct, unrelated to a hair follicle.

I.1.4c Meibomian adenoma
(This lesion is rare)
Clinical features. It appears as a localized lid thickening, at first recalling a chalazion.

Histopathology. Meibomian glands are hypertrophic but remain located at the tarsal level, the acini being separated by vascularized connective septa. Pseudo-cystic dilatation of excretory ducts may occur, particularly when the corresponding acini have been destroyed either by a chronic inflammatory process e.g. trachomatous tarsal inflammation, or by a tumour e.g. basal cell carcinoma extending deeply.

I.1.4 Tumeurs bénignes d'origine sébacée

I.1.4a Adénome sébacé "senile" de la paupière

I.1.4b Adénome sébacé "senile" de la caroncule

Clinique. Il se rencontre en général chez les sujets ayant dépassé la cinquantaine. A la *paupière* ils se présente comme une petite tumeur nodulaire ou papuleuse, arrondie ou ovalaire, de 1 à 2 cm de diamètre, légèrement surélevée de teinte jaunâtre, parfois ombiliquée. A la *caroncule* (I.1.4b) il se manifeste parfois simplement par une augmentation de volume de la caroncule, de teinte jaunâtre.

Histopathologie. C'est plus une hyperplasie qu'un véritable adénome. Des glandes sébacées de structure normale sont augmentées de volume et plus nombreuses, mais surtout 1) elles sont groupées dans le derme superficiel d'où normalement elles sont absentes car elles siègent en règle dans le derme moyen; 2) elles se groupent en grappe autour d'un unique canal collecteur central dilaté et non relié à un follicule pilaire.

I.1.4c Adénome meibomien
(Cette tumeur est relativement rare)
Clinique. Elle pose le problème d'un épaississement palpébral localisé et évoque au premier abord un chalazion.

Histopathologie. Les glandes de Meibomius sont hypertrophiques mais demeurent dans le plan tarsal, les acini étant séparés par des septa conjonctifs vascularisés. On peut parfois rencontrer des dilatations pseudo-kystiques de canaux excréteurs lorsque notamment les acini dont ils dépendent ont été détruits soit par un processus inflammatoire chronique tel qu'une tarsite trachomateuse soit par une tumeur telle qu'un carcinome baso-cellulaire s'étendant en profondeur.

I.1.4 Gutartige Talgdrüsengeschwülste

I.1.4a "Seniles Steatoadenom" (Talgdrüsenhyperplasie)

I.1.4b "Steatoadenom" der Karunkel

Klinik. Es ist im allgemeinen bei über Fünfzigjährigen anzutreffen. Am Augenlid erscheint es als kleiner knötchen- oder papelförmiger Tumor, abgerundet oder leicht oval, von 1 bis 2 cm Durchmesser, leicht erhaben, mit gelblicher Färbung, manchmal eingedellt. Auf der *Karunkel* (I.1.4b) vergrößert es manchmal einfach das Volumen der gelblich gefärbten Caruncula.

Histopathologie. Es handelt sich eher um eine Hyperplasie als um ein tatsächliches Adenom. Talgdrüsen mit normaler Struktur nehmen zu an Umfang und Zahl, vor allem aber 1) gruppieren sie sich in der oberflächlichen Dermis, wo sie normalerweise fehlen (sie sind in der Regel in der mittleren Derma angesiedelt); 2) gruppieren sie sich traubenartig um einen einzigen zentralen, ausgeweiteten und nicht mit einem Haarbalg verbundenen Sammelkanal.

I.1.4c Meibomsches Adenom
(Dieses Adenom ist verhältnismäßig selten)
Klinik. Klinisch stellt es das Problem einer lokalisierten palpebralen Verdickung und lässt zunächst an ein Chalazion denken.

Histopathologie. Die Meibomschen Drüsen sind hypertrophisch, bleiben jedoch im tarsalen Bereich, da die Acini durch vaskularisierte Bindegewebesepten getrennt sind. Mitunter trifft man auf pseudozystische Erweiterungen der Ausscheidungskanäle, hauptsächlich wenn die Acini, zu denen sie gehören, entweder durch einen chronischen Entzündungsprozeß (trachomatöse Tarsitis) oder durch einen Tumor (zum Beispiel ein tief ausgedehntes Basalzellkarzinom) zerstört wurden.

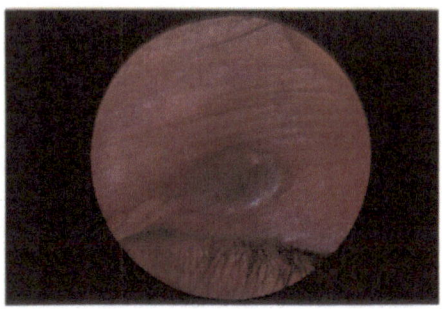

a

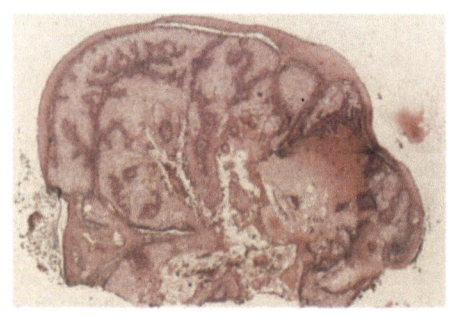

b

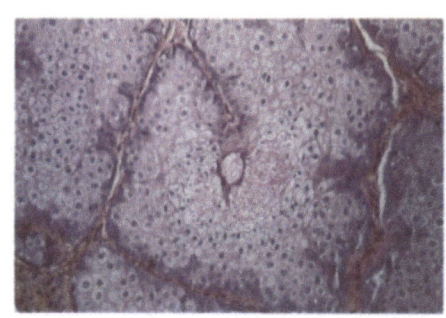

c

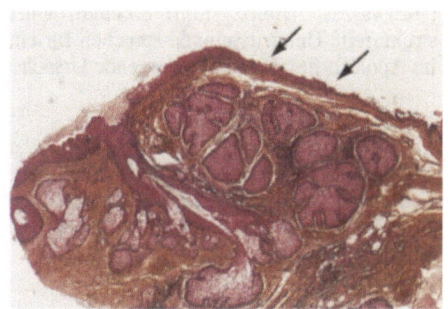

d

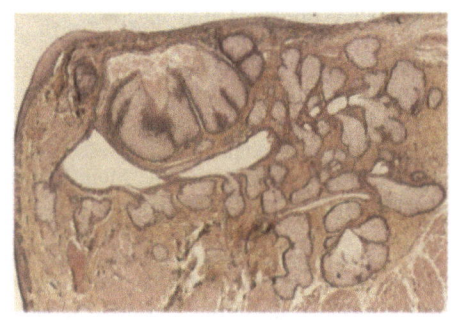

e

Fig. a. Lid sebaceous adenoma.
Small grayish, oval, slightly raised and well demarcated papule.

Fig. b. Lid sebaceous adenoma (low power).
Hyperplastic acini grouped in the superficial dermis.

Fig. c. Sebaceous adenoma.
The acini display a strictly normal structure and are composed of typical sebaceous cells with no cytologic atypia.

Fig. d. Sebaceous adenoma of the caruncle (low power).
The acini can be seen abnormally grouped in the superficial dermis (⇉).

Fig. e. Meibomian adenoma.
The overall structure of a meibomian gland can be recognized; yet, the acini are larger and apparently more numerous. They collect into a dilated excretory duct.

Fig. a. Adénome sébacé palpébral.
Petite papule ovalaire grisâtre légèrement surélevée, bien limitée.

Fig. b. Adénome sébacé palpébral (faible grossissement).
Acini hyperplasiques groupés dans le derme superficiel.

Fig. c. Adénome sébacé.
Acinus de structure strictement normale, constitué de cellules sébacées typiques sans anomalies cytologiques.

Fig. d. Adénome sébacé de la caroncule (faible grossissement).
On trouve les acini groupés anormalement dans le derme superficiel (⇉).

Fig. e. Adénome meibomien.
On reconnaît la structure générale d'une glande de Meibomius; les acini sont cependant de plus grande taille et apparemment plus nombreux, se drainant dans un canal excréteur dilaté.

Abb. a. Talgdrüsenhyperplasie des Lides.
Kleine, ovale, graue, leicht erhabene, gut abgegrenzte Papel.

Abb. b. Talgdrüsenhyperplasie des Lides (schwache Vergrößerung).
Hyperplastische Acini, in der oberflächlichen Dermis gruppiert.

Abb. c. Talgdrüsenhyperplasie.
Acinus mit völlig normaler Struktur, aus typischen Talgdrüsenzellen bestehend, ohne zytologische Anomalien.

Abb. d. Talgdrüsenhyperplasie der Karunkel (schwache Vergrößerung).
Die Acini sind abnorm in der oberen Derma gruppiert (⇉).

Abb. e. Meibomsches Adenom.
Die allgemeine Struktur einer Meibomschen Drüse ist zu erkennen; die Acini sind jedoch größer und offenbar zahlreicher und münden in einen erweiterten Ausscheidungskanal.

15

PLATE 8   PLANCHE 8   TAFEL 8

I.1.5 Sweat gland benign tumours

I.1.5a Hidrocystoma
Clinical features. This cystic, well limited tumour, grows in the deep layers of the lid, at the margin or close to it. Its cystic nature can be confirmed by transillumination.

Histopathology. This cystic, uni- or multifocal structure is surrounded by two layers of cells: cuboid internally, flattened, darker, externally (myoepithelial cells). The wall may present some papillary projections forming villosities. The lumen contains a protein-like eosinophilic substance or a PAS-positive secretory product.
Intracystic haemorrhage or pigmentation of the sweat (chromhidrosis) accounts for the blackish colour sometimes observed ("black" hidrocystoma). Ultrastructural studies suggest a secretory-apocrine origin.

I.1.5b Papillary syringadenoma
(Syringocystadenoma papilliferum)
Clinical features. This congenital, naevoid lesion, may be papular or verrucous. It arises from the excretory duct of a Moll's gland and develops most often after puberty.

Histopathology. Pseudocystic projections with papillary vegetations extend into the dermis. The lesion opens to the surface through a channel. Beneath the tumour, lobules of Moll's glands suggest the apocrine origin of the lesion.

I.1.5 Tumeurs bénignes sudorales

I.1.5a Hidrocystome
Clinique. Tumeur kystique bien limitée développée dans l'épaisseur de la paupière, dans la marge ou à son voisinage. La transillumination peut confirmer son caractère kystique.

Histopathologie. Structure kystique uni ou multiloculaire bordée de deux couches de cellules: internes cubiques, externes aplaties plus sombres (cellules myoépithéliales). La paroi présente parfois des replis papillaires formant des villosités.
La cavité contient une substance protéinacée éosinophile ou une sécrétion prenant le PAS. Une hémorragie intrakystique ou la pigmentation de la sécrétion sudorale (chromhidrose) rend compte de la teinte noirâtre observée parfois (hidrocystome "noir"). Les études ultrastructurales sont en faveur d'une origine sécréto-apocrine.

I.1.5b Syringadénome papillaire
(Syringocystadénome papillifère)
Clinique. Lésion congénitale papuleuse ou verruqueuse dont le point de départ est le segment excréteur d'une glande de Moll. Elle se développe surtout après la puberté.

Histopathologie. La lésion s'ouvre en surface par un pertuis et envoie dans le derme sous-jacent des expansions pseudokystiques occupées par des végétations papillaires. Sous-jacents à la lésion, des lobules de glandes de Moll viennent souvent attester de son origine apocrine.

I.1.5 Gutartige Geschwülste der Schweißdrüsen

I.1.5a Hidrozystom
Klinik. Gut abgegrenzte zystische Geschwulst, die sich im Lidinnern, am Lidrand oder in seiner Umgebung entwickelt. Mit Transillumation läßt sich der zystische Charakter bestätigen.

Histopathologie. Zystische Struktur, multipel oder einzeln auftretend, von zwei Zellschichten eingesäumt; innen kubische, außen abgeflachte, dunklere Zellen (Muskelepithelzellen). Die Wand weist manchmal papillomatöse Windungen auf, die ein zottenartiges Aussehen haben.
Die Vertiefung enthält eine eosinophile, proteinhaltige Substanz oder ein PAS-positives Sekret. Aus einer Blutung im Zysteninnern oder einer gefärbten Schweißabsonderung (Chromhidrose) läßt sich die manchmal beobachtete schwärzliche Färbung ("schwarzes" Hidrozystom) erklären. Ultrastrukturelle Untersuchungen sprechen für eine im Apokrin-Sekret-Bereich liegende Ursache.

I.1.5b Papillares Syringozystadenom
Klinik. Kongenitale, nävoide, papel- oder warzenförmige Läsion, die vom sezernierenden Teil einer Mollschen Drüse ausgeht. Sie entwickelt sich hauptsächlich nach der Pubertät.

Histopathologie. Die Läsion öffnet sich an der Oberfläche und wächst in die Dermis mit pseudozystischen, mit papillären Strängen gefüllten Strukturen ein. Läppchen der Mollschen Drüsen bestätigen oft den apokrinen Charakter der Läsion.

PLATE 8   PLANCHE 8   TAFEL 8

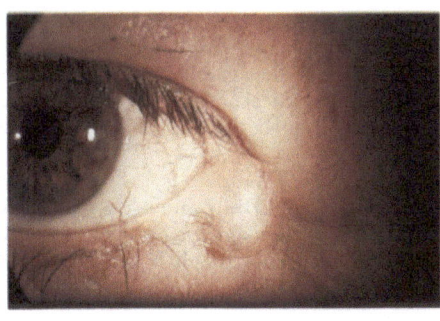

a

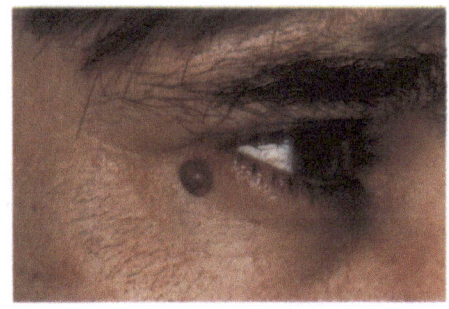

b

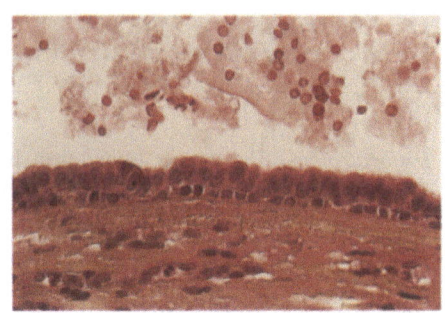

c

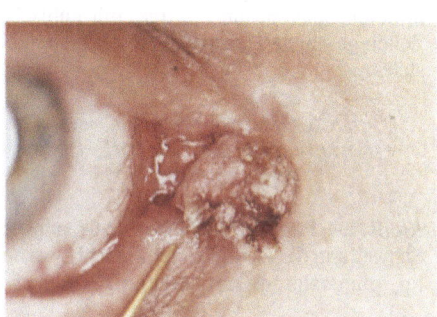

d

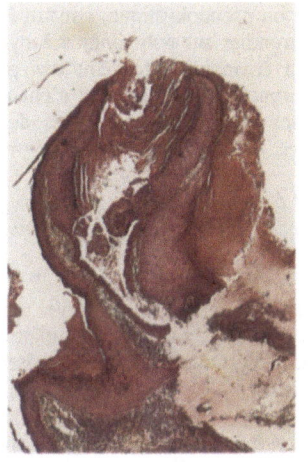

e

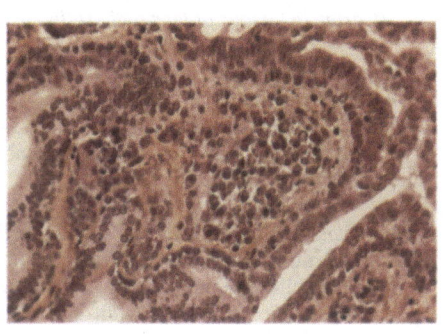

f

Fig. a. Hidrocystoma of the inferior lid at the canthus.
This small, clear, translucent tumour, represents the common transparent cyst of the lids.

Fig. b. Black hidrocystoma.
Small, round lesion, showing a blackish discoloration (see text).

Fig. c. Wall of a hidrocystoma with its two cellular layers.

Fig. d. Syringocystadenoma papilliferum of the inner canthus.
(The stylet points toward the location of the inferior lacrymal canaliculus.) The lesion is slightly raised and verrucous. In other instances it may appear as a papule with a central umbilication and fistulization.

Fig. e. Syringocystadenoma papilliferum.
Surface opening, communicating more deeply with a large lumen lined by a glandular epithelium.

Fig. f. Syringocystadenoma papilliferum.
Villuslike projections covered with a double cell layer: columnar internally, cuboid externally.
An inflammatory infiltrate, principally plasmacytic, occupies the connective core of these villosities.

Fig. a. Hidrocystome de l'angle externe, paupière inférieure.
Petite tumeur claire, translucide. C'est le classique kyste transparent des paupières.

Fig. b. Hidrocystome noir.
Petite lésion arrondie ayant pris une teinte noirâtre (voir texte).

Fig. c. Paroi d'un hidrocystome avec ses deux couches de cellules.

Fig. d. Syringocystadénome papillifère de l'angle interne des paupières.
(Le stylet marque la situation du canalicule lacrymal inférieur.) Lésion légèrement surélevée et verruqueuse. Dans d'autres cas c'est une papule ombiliquée et fistuleuse en son centre.

Fig. e. Syringocystadénome papillifère.
Pertuis ouvert en surface, se continuant en profondeur par une large cavité tapissée d'un épithélium glandulaire.

Fig. f. Syringocystadénome papillifère.
Villosités tapissées d'une double couche de cellules: internes cylindriques et externes cubiques.
Un infiltrat inflammatoire à prédominance plasmocytaire occupe l'axe conjonctif de ces villosités.

Abb. a. Hidrozystom am äußeren, unteren Lidwinkel.
Kleiner, heller, durchsichtiger Tumor. Es ist dies die klassische, durchsichtige Lidzyste.

Abb. b. Schwarzes Hidrozystom.
Kleine rundliche Läsion, die eine schwarze Färbung angenommen hat (siehe Text).

Abb. c. Wand eines Hidrozystoms mit seinen beiden Zellschichten.

Abb. d. Papilläres Syringozystadenom des inneren Lidwinkels.
(Die Kanüle zeigt die Lage des unteren Tränenkanälchens.) Leicht erhabene, warzenförmige Läsion. In anderen Fällen kann es eine scheibenförmige Papel mit nabelartiger Einziehung und Fistel in der Mitte sein.

Abb. e. Papilläres Syringozystadenom.
Enge Öffnung an der Oberfläche, die sich in der Tiefe in einen weiten, von Drüsenepithel ausgekleideten Hohlraum fortsetzt.

Abb. f. Papilläres Syringozystadenom.
Mit einer doppelten Zellschicht ausgepolsterte Zotten: innen zylindrische, außen kubische Zellen.
Ein entzündliches, vorwiegend plasmozytisches Infiltrat weist auf die Bindegewebsachse dieser Zotten hin.

PLATE 9 PLANCHE 9 TAFEL 9

I.1.5c Syringomas
Clinical features. These multiple yellowish papules, no bigger than a pinhead, occur principally on the eyelids.

Histopathology. The dermis is occupied by ductal formations of sudoral type, i.e. lined by two rows of cubical cells.

I.1.5d Eccrine acrospiroma (clear cell hydradenoma)
Clinical features. This small tumour, with no specific feature, appears as a small, solid nodule, mobile under a normal skin.

Histopathology. This tumour, well circumscribed, lobulated or pseudocystic, is composed of round or polyhedral cells with an eosinophilic or clear cytoplasm forming areas in which ductal lumina lined by cuboidal cells are developing.

I.1.6 Oncocytoma of the caruncle
(Caruncle tumour of lacrimal origin;
oxyphil cell adenoma;
oxyphilic granular cell adenoma)

Clinical features. The lesion appears as a yellowish painless, slightly vascularized, sometimes cystoid swelling of the caruncle.

Histopathology. The tumour is round, well limited, surrounded by a connective capsule. It is often hollowed out by a pseudocystic lumen, more or less filled with papillary growth. In other instances, it is more dense, of solid aspect. It is composed of large cells with well defined borders and granular cytoplasm. These cells are often grouped into acini and the lumen may be filled with a material rich in acid mucopolysaccharides. These tumours are widely seen as arising from accessory lacrimal glands.

I.1.5c Syringomes
Clinique. Les paupières semblent être une des localisations préférentielles de ces papules jaunâtres de la grosseur d'une tête d'épingle disséminées sur toute la surface cutanée.

Histopathologie. Le derme est occupé par des formations à caractère sudoral c'est-à-dire bordées de deux rangées de cellules cubiques.

I.1.5d Acrospirome eccrine (hidradénome à cellules claires)
Clinique. Petite tumeur sans caractère bien spécifique se présentant comme un petit nodule de consistance ferme, mobile, sous une peau normale.

Histopathologie. Tumeur bien circonscrite lobulée ou pseudokystique, constituée de cellules arrondies ou polygonales à cytoplasme clair ou éosinophile formant des plages au sein desquelles on peut voir s'ébaucher des structures canaliculaires bordées de cellules cuboïdes.

I.1.6 Tumeur caronculaire d'origine lacrymale (Oncocytome; Adénome oxyphile)

Clinique. La lésion se présente comme un gonflement de la caroncule, jaunâtre, parfois d'aspect kystique, indolore, discrètement vascularisée.

Histopathologie. Tumeur arrondie bien limitée entourée d'une capsule conjonctive, elle est souvent creusée d'une cavité pseudokystique plus ou moins comblée de végétations papillaires. Dans d'autres cas elle est plus dense, d'aspect "solide". Les cellules qui la composent sont de grande taille, à limites nettes et présentent un cytoplasme granuleux. Elles se groupent volontiers en formations acineuses dont la lumière peut contenir une substance riche en mucopolysaccharides acides. L'origine de l'oncocytome à partir des glandes lacrymales accessoires est la plus communément admise.

I.1.5c Syringome
Klinik. Die Lider scheinen eine der bevorzugten Stellen für diese gelblichen Papeln von der Größe eines Stecknadelkopfs, die auf der gesamten Hautoberfläche verstreut sind, zu sein.

Histopathologie. Die Dermis ist von Strukturen mit Schweißdrüsencharakter, die also mit zweireihigen kubischen Zellen bedeckt sind, durchsetzt.

I.1.5d Ekkrines Akrospirom (klarzelliges Hidradenom)
Klinik. Kleiner Tumor ohne besonders ausgeprägte Merkmale, erscheint wie ein Knötchen mit fester Konsistenz, beweglich, unter normaler Haut.

Histopathologie. Gut umrissener, gelappter oder pseudozystischer Tumor, aus rundlichen oder polygonalen Zellen mit hellem oder eosinophilem Zytoplasma, die Flächen bilden, in deren Innerem lumenartige, mit kubischen Zellen gesäumte Strukturen zu sehen sind, bestehen.

I.1.6 Onkozytom der Karunkel
(Karunkeltumor lakrimaler Herkunft;
oxyphiles Adenom)

Klinik. Die Läsion zeigt sich als eine gelbliche Schwellung der Karunkel, manchmal zystenartig, schmerzlos, diskret vaskularisiert.

Histopathologie. Abgerundeter, gut abgegrenzter, von einer Bindegewebskapsel umschlossener Tumor, oft mit einer mehr oder weniger mit proliferierten Zellsträngen aufgefüllten Pseudozyste. In anderen Fällen ist er dichter, erscheint "fester". Die Zellen, aus denen er besteht, sind groß, mit deutlichen Grenzen und haben ein granuläres Zytoplasma. Sie schließen sich leicht zu Schläuchen zusammen, deren Lumen eine an sauren Mukopolysacchariden reiche Substanz enthalten kann. Allgemein wird die Entstehung des Onkozytoms auf die akzessorischen Tränendrüsen zurückgeführt.

PLATE 9 PLANCHE 9 TAFEL 9

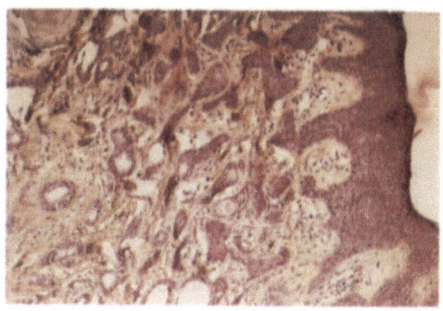

a

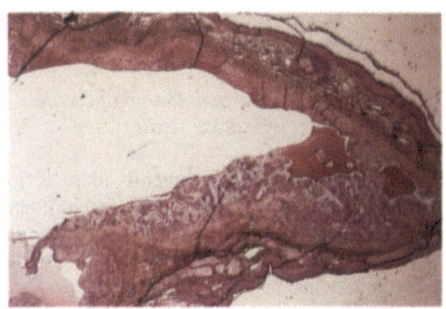

b

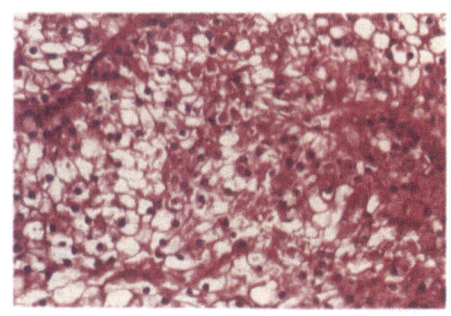

c

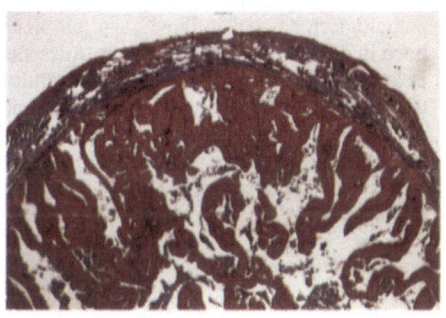

d

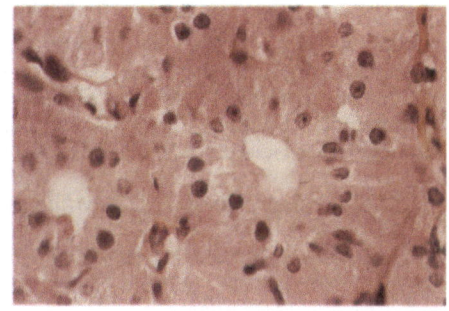

e

Fig. a. Syringoma.
Dermal cellular sheats, most often lining a channel-like tumour. Some of these channels possess a comma-shaped tail and resemble tadpoles.
Notice that, when no glandular lumen is present, this tumour can be confused with a morphealike basal cell carcinoma.

Fig. b. Eccrine acrospiroma (low power).

Fig. c. Eccrine acrospiroma.
PAS stain. Clear, glycogen-rich, well limited cells (clear cell hidradenoma).

Fig. d. Oncocytoma with a pseudocystic structure, partly filled with papillary growth.

Fig. e. Oncocytic cells.
Large, well limited with a small, dark nucleus, an eosinophilic granular cytoplasm, corresponding ultrastructurally to the accumulation of giant mitochondria.

Fig. a. Syringome.
Travées cellulaires dermiques le plus souvent occupées par une lumière de type canaliculaire. Certaines de ces travées possèdent un prolongement caudiforme qui leur donne un aspect "en têtard". La confusion peut être parfois possible avec un épithélioma baso-cellulaire sclérodermiforme.

Fig. b. Acrospirome eccrine (faible grossissement).

Fig. c. Acrospirome eccrine.
Coloration au PAS. Cellules claires à limites nettes, riches en glycogène (hidradénome à cellules claires).

Fig. d. Oncocytome pseudokystique dont la cavité est en partie comblée par des végétations papillaires.

Fig. e. Cellules oncocytaires.
Cellules de grande taille à petit noyau foncé, à cytoplasme éosinophile granuleux, du fait de l'accumulation de mitochondries géantes ainsi que l'a montré l'ultrastructure.

Abb. a. Syringom.
Zellstränge in der Dermis, in denen sich meist ein röhrenförmiges Lumen befindet. Einige dieser Röhrenanlagen besitzen eine kanalförmige Verlängerung, die ihnen ein "kaulquappenartiges" Aussehen geben. Es sei darauf hingewiesen, daß bei Fehlen der Hohlräume eine Verwechslung mit dem sklerodermiformen Basalzellkarzinom möglich ist.

Abb. b. Ekkrines Akrospirom (schwacher Vergrößerung).

Abb. c. Ekkrines Akrospirom.
PAS-Fährbung. Klare, deutlich abgegrenzte, glycogenreiche Zellen (klarzelliges Hidradenom).

Abb. d. Onkozytom mit Pseudozyste, die zum Teil mit papillenartigen Wucherungen gefüllt ist.

Abb. e. Große Onkozytenzellen.
Deutlich abgegrenzt, mit kleinem dunklem Kern, granulösem, eosinophilem Zytoplasma infolge der Ansammlung von Riesenmitochondrien, wie die Ultrastruktur gezeigt hat.

19

PLATE 10 PLANCHE 10 TAFEL 10

I.2 Precancerous epithelial tumours

I.2.1 Palpebral actinic keratosis (Senile keratosis)

Clinical features. This is the most common precancerous lesion of the eyelids. It occurs after fifty, sometimes earlier (actinic pathogenesis). A squamous lesion appears above an erythematous basis, later forming a yellowish or brownish scab.

Histopathology. The epidermis, hyperkeratotic, is irregularly thickened. Yet the basement membrane is never disrupted. The cells are less chromophilic than the normal surrounding epithelial cells, due to a disorder of RNA metabolism. The structure of the epidermis is disrupted: squamous cells are no longer regularly oriented, there is a loss of polarity, and there may be intra-epithelial clefts. The mitotic figures are atypical, e.g. located in upper layers, also morphologically. Nuclear aberrations, dyskeratotic figures can be seen. These lesions evolve slowly or rapidly toward carcinomas. A wide excision with histopathologic assessment is therefore essential.

I.2.2 Conjunctival actinic keratosis

Clinical features. This lesion, prominent, pearly, painless, poorly vascularized, is usually located at the limbus.

Histopathology. The thickened mucous membrane is covered with an orthokeratotic keratin layer. Cytologic abnormalities are the same as those of the lid lesions. The basement membrane is spared, lined with an inflammatory infiltrate. Here again, the lesion evolves, through a disruption of basement membrane, toward carcinoma. Thus every keratotic lesion of the limbus should be excised.

I.2 Tumeurs précancéreuses épithéliales

I.2.1 Kératose actinique palpébrale (Kératose sénile)

Clinique. La plus fréquente des lésions précancéreuses palpébrales, elle apparaît après la cinquantaine, parfois plus précocément (pathogénie actinique). Sur une base érythémateuse apparaît une squame qui forme ensuite une croûte jaunâtre ou brunâtre.

Histopathologie. L'épiderme, hyperkératosique, est d'épaisseur irrégulière, mais sa basale n'est jamais rompue. Les cellules sont moins chromophiles que celles de l'épiderme voisin ce qui traduit un trouble du métabolisme de l'ARN. La structure de l'épiderme est bouleversée: les cellules malpighiennes ne sont plus orientées régulièrement, il y a perte de la polarité cellulaire, présence parfois de fentes intra-épidermiques, les mitoses sont anormales dans leur siège (elles sont haut situées) et leur aspect, il existe des dystrophies nucléaires, des images de dyskératose. L'évolution de la kératose sénile se fait plus ou moins rapidement vers le carcinome épidermoïde. L'exérèse large suivie de contrôle histologique est donc indispensable.

I.2.2 Kératose actinique conjonctivale

Clinique. Habituellement à localisation limbique elle est saillante, indolore et peu vascularisée, d'un blanc nacré.

Histopathologie. La muqueuse, épaissie, est recouverte d'une couche de kératine orthokératosique. Les modifications cytologiques sont celles de la localisation palpébrale. La basale reste intacte, bordée d'un infiltrat inflammatoire. Ici aussi l'évolution se fait, par rupture de la basale, vers le carcinome épidermoïde. C'est dire qu'il faut pratiquer l'excision de toute lésion kératosique du limbe.

I.2 Präkanzeröse Epithelgeschwülste

I.2.1 Aktinische Lidkeratose (Alterskeratose)

Klinik. Die häufigste unter den präkanzerösen Lidläsionen tritt nach fünfzig, manchmal auch früher auf (aktinische Pathogenese). Auf einer Erythembasis bildet sich eine Schuppe, die sich sodann in eine gelbliche oder bräunliche Kruste verwandelt.

Histopathologie. Die übermäßig stark verhornende Epidermis ist von unregelmäßiger Dicke, die Basalschicht ist jedoch nie durchbrochen. Die Zellen sind weniger chromophil als die der benachbarten Epidermis, was eine Störung des RNA-Stoffwechsels andeutet. Die Struktur der Epidermis erfährt eine Umwälzung: die Basalzellen sind nicht mehr regelmäßig orientiert, die Zellpolarität geht verloren, manchmal bilden sich Risse innerhalb der Epidermis, die Mitosen sind pathologisch sowohl in ihrer Lage (sie liegen hoch in der Epidermis), als auch im Aussehen, es kommen Kerndystrophien vor, Dyskeratose tritt auf. Die Alterskeratose entwickelt sich mehr oder weniger schnell auf das Plattenepithelkarzinom hin. Eine breite Exzision gefolgt von einer histologischen Kontrolle ist deshalb unerläßlich.

I.2.2 Aktinische Keratose der Konjunktiva

Klinik. Sie ist gewöhnlich am Limbus lokalisiert, vorragend, schmerzfrei und wenig vaskularisiert, perlmutterartig.

Histopathologie. Das verdickte Epithel ist mit einer orthokeratotischen Keratinschicht überzogen. Die zytologischen Veränderungen sind dieselben wie bei der palpebralen Lokalisation. Die Basalschicht bleibt intakt, von einem entzündlichen Infiltrat eingesäumt. Auch hier ist im weiteren Verlauf durch den Bruch der Basalschicht mit einem Plattenepithelkarzinom zu rechnen. Das heißt, daß jegliche keratotische Läsion am Limbus exzidiert werden muß.

PLATE 10 PLANCHE 10 TAFEL 10

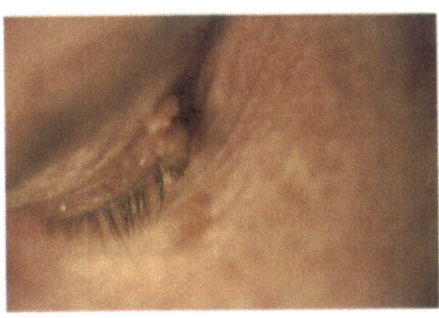

a

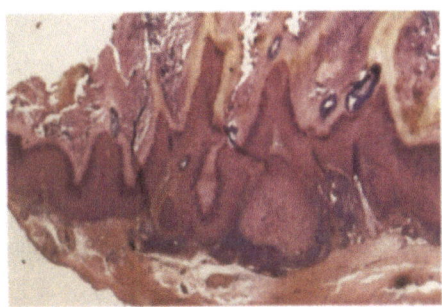

b

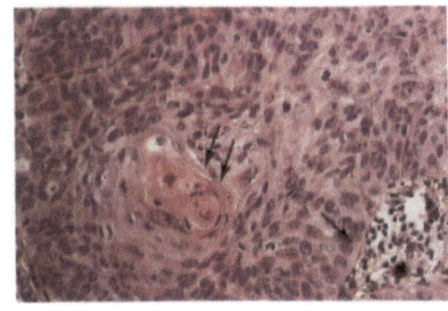

c

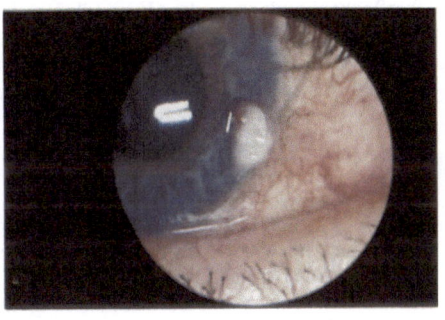

d

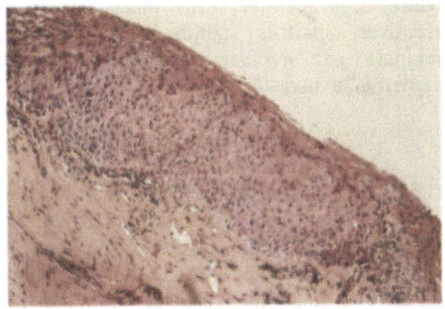

e

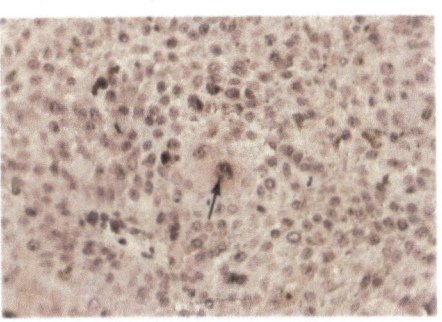

f

Fig. a. Actinic keratosis.
Upper eyelid. Papillomatous lesion, surmounted by a keratin cone. The aspect is that of a "cutaneous horn".

Fig. b. Palpebral actinic keratosis.
The epidermis is thickened and comparatively non-basophilic. Abrupt keratinization due to the lack of granular layer. The basement membrane is lined by an inflammatory infiltrate partly concealing a degeneration of the underlying collagen.

Fig. c. Palpebral actinic keratosis.
The basement membrane is distinctly seen (→). Disruption of the epithelial structure, numerous mitotic figures. Notice a dyskeratotic globe (⇉).

Fig. d. Actinic keratosis at the limbus.
Highly suggestive pearly white colour.

Fig. e. Conjunctival actinic keratosis.
The epithelium is thickened, staining poorly with the usual stains, abnormally keratinized. The basement membrane is regular, uninvolved.

Fig. f. Conjunctival actinic keratosis.
Dyskeratotic cells with a large, deformed nucleus (→). Some melanin-laden cells: pigmented actinic keratosis often encountered in pigmented individuals.

Fig. a. Kératose actinique.
Paupière supérieure. Lésion papillomateuse, surmontée d'un cône de kératine. C'est l'aspect de la "corne cutanée".

Fig. b. Kératose actinique.
Epiderme épaissi, relativement peu basophile. Kératinisation abrupte du fait de l'absence de couche granuleuse. Basale bordée d'un infiltrat inflammatoire qui masque plus ou moins une involution du collagène sous-jacent.

Fig. c. Kératose actinique.
Basale toujours nettement visible (→), mais structure de l'épithélium bouleversée, mitoses nombreuses; notez un globe dyskératosique (⇉).

Fig. d. Kératose actinique du limbe.
Teinte blanc nacré très évocatrice.

Fig. e. Kératose actinique conjonctivale.
Epithélium épaissi prenant mal les colorants habituels, anormalement kératinisé en surface. Basale régulière, intacte.

Fig. f. Kératose actinique conjonctivale.
Cellule dyskératosique à gros noyau dystrophique (→). Quelques cellules chargées de mélanine: kératose actinique pigmentée qui se rencontre surtout chez les mélanodermes.

Abb. a. Papillomatöse Läsion.
Oberlid. Bedeckt von einem Keratinspitz. So sieht das "Hauthorn" aus.

Abb. b. Aktinische Keratose.
Verdickte, verhältnismäßig schwach basophile Epidermis. Abrupte Verhornung auf Grund des Fehlens des Stratum granulosum. Basalschicht von einem entzündlichen Infiltrat eingesäumt, das eine Rückbildung des daruntergelegenen Kollagens mehr oder weniger verdeckt.

Abb. c. Aktinische Keratose.
Basalschicht deutlich sichtbar (→), aber starke Veränderung der Epithelstruktur, zahlreiche Mitosen; auffällig ist das abnorm verhornte, kugelförmige Gebilde (⇉).

Abb. d. Aktinische Keratose am Limbus.
Bezeichnend die perlmutterartige weiße Färbung.

Abb. e. Aktinische Keratose der Konjunktiva.
Verdicktes, die gewohnten Färbemittel schlecht annehmendes, anormal verhorntes Epithel. Regelmäßige, intakte Basalschicht.

Abb. f. Aktinische Keratose der Konjunktiva.
Abnorm verhornende Zellen mit einem großen, dystrophischen Kern (→). Einige melaninhaltige Zellen: pigmentierte aktinische Keratose, die vor allem bei den Dunkelhäutigen auftritt.

21

PLATE 11 PLANCHE 11 TAFEL 11

I.2.3 Conjunctival carcinoma in situ

Clinical features. As with actinic keratosis carcinoma in situ appears in patients over fifty years, mainly at the limbus, i.e. a transition between two types of epithelium, and also an area submitted to mechanical irritations and actinic radiations.

Histopathology. There is a definite thickening of the epithelium, the basement membrane of which remains undamaged, but which shows in its depth the usual precancerous alterations that we have previously described. The term of Bowen's disease of the conjunctiva is based on certain aspects of agglomerated and swollen nuclei ("clumped cells"). However it seems more advisable to keep the denomination of carcinoma in situ, adding "of bowenoid type", if necessary. In any case, the essential feature of carcinoma in situ of the conjunctiva is its tendency to recur without metastasis. These recurrences are sometimes repetitive; but their final stage is always an invasive epidermoid carcinoma.

I.2.4 Xeroderma pigmentosum

Clinical features. This genodermatosis with recessive autosomal transmission is mostly found in people living around the Mediterranean. It is related to a photo-sensitivity due to a faulty repair of DNA after UV exposure. Ocular damage is observed in 50% of cases. Photophobia is often the first sign, associated with a blepharo-conjunctivitis. Later, skin atrophy develops, provoking entropion or ectropion of the lids. Telangiectases, pigmented spots, areas of hyperkeratosis, appear on this atrophic skin. Progressively they will change into a skin carcinoma, mostly of the epidermoid type, but sometimes a malignant melanoma, which may affect the lid or the conjunctiva. In addition a dry eye syndrome may provoke corneal lesions, with the risk of perforation. The treatment is restricted to repetitive surgical excisions of the recurrences as and when necessary, and the vital prognosis is very poor.

I.2.3 Carcinome in situ de la conjonctive

Clinique. Comme la kératose actinique le carcinome in situ apparaît chez des sujets ayant dépassé la cinquantaine et marque une certaine prédilection pour le limbe, zone de transition entre deux épithéliums, mais aussi exposée aux irritations mécaniques et aux radiations actiniques.

Histopathologie. Il existe un épaississement marqué de l'épithélium dont la basale reste intacte mais qui présente dans son épaisseur les désordres habituels des lésions précancéreuses, décrites plus haut. Certains aspects de noyaux conglomérés ou boursouflés ("clumped cells") ont fait parler de "Bowen" conjonctival. Mais il vaudrait mieux conserver la dénomination de carcinome in situ en ajoutant au besoin: "de type bowenoïde". Quoiqu'il en soit le trait primordial du carcinome in situ de la conjonctive est sa tendance à la récidive, sans métastases. Ces récidives, parfois nombreuses, finissent toujours par évoluer vers le carcinome épidermoïde invasif.

I.2.4 Xeroderma pigmentosum

Clinique. Génodermatose à hérédité autosomale récessive qui frappe surtout les ethnies du pourtour du bassin méditerranéen, elle est liée à une photosensibilisation qu'on sait maintenant être due à un défaut de réparation de l'ADN après exposition aux ultra-violets. Les atteintes oculaires se rencontrent dans 50% des cas. La photophobie est souvent le premier signe, accompagnée de blépharoconjonctivite. Puis apparaît une atrophie cutanée entraînant des déformations palpébrales, entropion ou ectropion. Sur cette peau atrophique surviennent des télangiectasies, des taches pigmentaires, des plages d'hyperkératose qui évolueront plus ou moins rapidement vers le carcinome cutané, épidermoïde le plus souvent, mélanome malin parfois, touchant aussi bien la paupière que la conjonctive. A ces lésions s'ajoute une sécheresse conjonctivale source de kératopathies qui peuvent être perforantes. Le traitement se limite le plus souvent à l'exérèse chirurgicale à la demande, et le pronostic vital est très sombre.

I.2.3 Carcinoma in situ der Konjunktiva

Klinik. Wie die aktinische Keratosis tritt auch das Carcinoma in situ bei über Fünfzigjährigen auf und zwar bevorzugt am Limbus, der Übergangszone zwischen zwei Epithelien, die auch mechanischen Beanspruchungen und aktinischen Strahleneinwirkungen ausgesetzt ist.

Histopathologie. Es besteht eine deutliche Verdickung des Epithels, dessen Basalschicht intakt bleibt, das aber in seiner ganzen Dicke die üblichen, früher beschriebenen Strukturveränderungen der Präkanzerose aufweist. Gewisse Aspekte zusammengeballter oder angeschwollener Kerne ("clumped cells") ließen von einem "Bowen" der Konjunktiva sprechen. Die Beibehaltung der Bezeichnung Carcinoma in situ ist jedoch besser, wobei bei Bedarf "vom Bowenschen Typ" hinzugefügt werden kann. Das Hauptmerkmal des Oberflächenkarzinoms der Konjunktiva ist jedenfalls seine Neigung zum Rezidiv, ohne Metastasen. Diese manchmal zahlreichen Rezidiven entwickeln sich letztlich immer zum invasiven Plattenepithelkarzinom hin.

I.2.4 Xeroderma pigmentosum

Klinik. Genodermatose mit rezessiver autosomaler Heredität, von der vor allem die Völker des Mittelmeerraums betroffen sind. Sie steht mit einer Photosensibilisierung in Zusammenhang, von der man jetzt weiß, daß sie auf einen DNS-Reparationsmangel nach Ultravioletteinwirkung zurückgeht. Augenbeteiligung kommt in 50% der Fälle vor. Lichtscheu ist oft das erste Anzeichen, einhergehend mit einer Lid- und Bindehautentzündung. Sodann tritt eine kutane Atrophie in Erscheinung, die Liddeformationen, Entropium oder Ektropium nach sich zieht. Auf dieser atrophischen Haut entstehen sodann Telangiektasien, Pigmentflecken, hyperkeratotische Bezirke, die sich mehr oder weniger rasch auf ein kutanes, meist ein Plattenepithelkarzinom, manchmal ein malignes Melanom hin entwickeln, wovon sowohl das Lid als auch die Bindehaut betroffen ist. Hinzu kommt häufig Trockenheit der Bindehaut, die zu Keratopathien führt, die perforierend sein können. Die Behandlung beschränkt sich meist auf eine operative Entfernung, wenn verlangt, und die Prognose ist sehr schlecht.

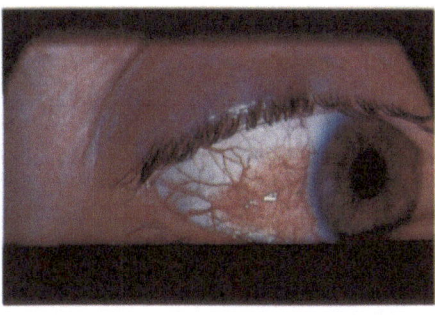

a

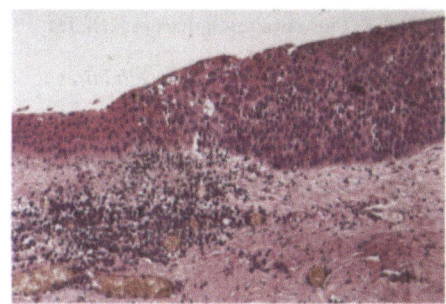

b

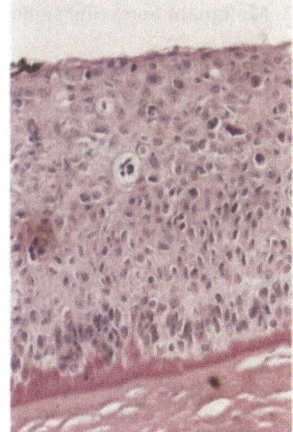

c

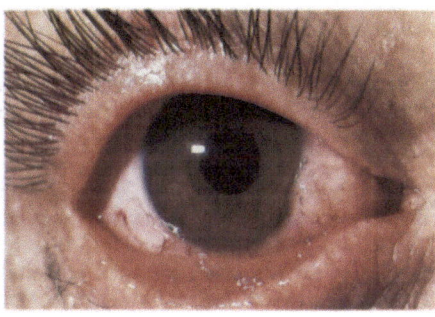

d

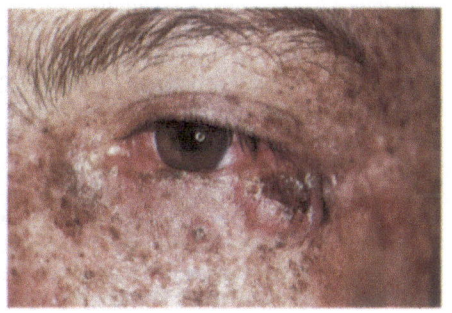

e

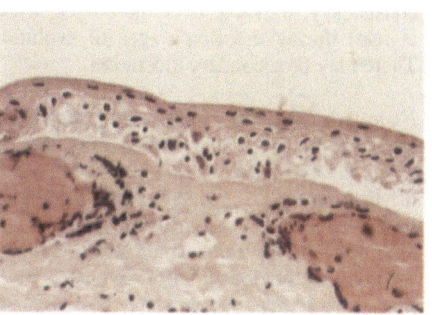

f

Fig. a. Carcinoma in situ of the limbus.
Thickening of the mucous membrane, sometimes mamillate, painless, opalescent, with fine vascularization, of pinkish or salmon colour (as opposed to the mother-of-pearl whiteness of actinic keratosis).

Fig. b. Carcinoma in situ of the conjunctiva (low power).
Sudden thickening of the mucous membrane, with definite borders. The basal membrane is undamaged, lined by an infiltrate of inflammatory cells. Some dystrophic cells may be found at a distance from the lesions, accounting for the frequent recurrences.

Fig. c. Carcinoma in situ of the conjunctiva.
Loss of polarity of the cells and presence of abnormal mitotic figures. The integrity of the basement membrane is emphasized by the PAS stain.

Fig. d. Xeroderma pigmentosum (early stage).
Pronounced conjunctival hyperhemia and incipient ectropion of the eyelid. A thickening of the nasal conjunctiva already recalls the aspect of a carcinoma in situ.

Fig. e. Xeroderma pigmentosum.
More advanced stage with pigmented spots and keratotic lesions disseminated on the lids. At the outer canthus: ulcerated epidermoid carcinoma.

Fig. f. Xeroderma pigmentosum.
Histopathology of the conjunctiva at an early stage: atrophy of the epithelium, telangiectases.

Fig. a. Carcinome in situ du limbe.
Epaississement de la muqueuse, parfois un peu mamelonné, indolore, opalescent, finement vascularisé, de couleur rosée ou saumon (contrastant avec la teinte blanc nacré de la kératose actinique).

Fig. b. Carcinome in situ de la conjonctive (faible grossissement).
Epaississement brutal de la muqueuse, à limites latérales nettes. La basale, intacte, est bordée d'un infiltrat inflammatoire. On peut trouver à distance de la lésion quelques cellules dystrophiques expliquant la fréquence des récidives.

Fig. c. Carcinome in situ de la conjonctive.
Perte de polarité cellulaire et mitoses anormales. L'intégrité de la basale est soulignée par la coloration au PAS.

Fig. d. Xeroderma pigmentosum (au début).
Hyperhémie conjonctivale prononcée et début d'ectropion. Un épaississement de la conjonctive nasale a déjà l'allure d'un carcinome in situ.

Fig. e. Xeroderma pigmentosum.
Stade plus évolué avec des taches pigmentaires et des lésions kératosiques disséminées sur les paupières. A l'angle externe: carcinome épidermoïde ulcéreux.

Fig. f. Xeroderma pigmentosum.
Histopathologie de la conjonctive à un stade précoce: atrophie de l'épithélium, télangiectasies.

Abb. a. Carcinoma in situ am Limbus.
Verdickung der Schleimhaut, manchmal mit ein paar warzenähnlichen Erhebungen, schmerzfrei, opaleszent, fein vaskularisiert, rosa- oder lachsfarben (im Gegensatz zu der perlmuttweißen Färbung der aktinischen Keratose).

Abb. b. Carcinoma in situ der Bindehaut (schwache Vergrößerung).
Abrupte Verdickung des Epithels mit deutlicher seitlicher Abgrenzung, die durch die verschiedene Orientierung der Zellen und ihre oft etwas verstärkte Basophilie hervorgehoben wird. Die Basalschicht ist intakt, von einem entzündlichen Infiltrat gesäumt. In einiger Entfernung von der Läsion sind dystrophische Zellen anzutreffen, aus denen sich die häufigen Rezidiven erklären lassen.

Abb. c. Carcinoma in situ der Bindehaut.
Polaritätsverlust der Zellen und pathologische Mitosen. Die Intaktheit der Basalschicht wird durch die PAS-Färbung hervorgehoben.

Abb. d. Xeroderma pigmentosum (Frühstadium).
Starke Hyperämie der Bindehaut und beginnendes Ektropium. Eine Verdickung der nasalen Bindehaut hat bereits das Aussehen eines Carcinoma in situ.

Abb. e. Xeroderma pigmentosum.
Weiter fortgeschrittenes Stadium mit über die Lider verstreuten Pigmentflecken und Verhornungsläsionen. Am äußeren Winkel: ulzeröses Plattenepithel-karzinom.

Abb. f. Xeroderma pigmentosum.
Histopathologie der Konjunktiva in einem frühen Stadium: Atrophie des Epithels, Telangiektasien.

PLATE 12 PLANCHE 12 TAFEL 12

I.3 Malignant epithelial tumours

I.3.1 Basal cell carcinomas of the lids

85% of the malignant epithelial tumours of the lid are basal cell carcinomas. Their aspect is essentially variable and they may be schematically classified into 4 main anatomo-clinical types:
- nodular;
- ulcerated;
- morphealike;
- pigmented.

These varieties have one typical feature in common: the loss of eyelashes in the area of the lesion. The ulcerous type often presents a thick, uneven rim, made of small epidermal pearls. The latter can be observed also, though rarely, in the nodular and pigmented types.

Nodular basal cell carcinoma
Clinical features. It is prominent and of firm consistency, movable over the deeper layers, at least during the first stages of evolution. There may be secondary ulceration.

Histopathology. The dense tumour masses are related to the epidermal surface and consist of small basophilic cells [recalling the basal cells of the epidermis, whence the designation basal cell carcinoma (Krompecher)], without any optically revealed intercellular bridges; the latter are obvious in ultrastructure.
Some histological varieties may be observed:
- a cystic type;
- an adenoid type: sometimes wrongly called "skin cylindroma" owing to its similarity with the salivary gland cylindroma; in Lever's opinion this type could be of sudoral origin;
- a keratinizing or pilar type.

I.3 Tumeurs malignes épithéliales

I.3.1 Carcinomes baso-cellulaires des paupières

Ils représentent 85% des tumeurs épithéliales malignes des paupières.
Leur aspect est des plus variables et on peut schématiquement distinguer 4 types anatomo-cliniques principaux:
- nodulaire;
- ulcéreux;
- sclérodermiforme;
- tatoué.

Un élément clinique caractéristique est commun à toutes ces formes: la chute des cils dans l'aire de la lésion. La variété ulcéreuse présente souvent une bordure saillante, bosselée, constituée de véritables petites "perles" épidermiques. Ces dernières peuvent se trouver aussi, plus rarement, dans les formes nodulaire ou pigmentée.

Carcinome baso-cellulaire nodulaire
Clinique. Saillant, ferme, il fait corps avec l'épiderme mais est mobile sur les plans profonds, du moins en début d'évolution. Il est susceptible de s'ulcérer secondairement.

Histopathologie. Ce sont des masses denses en relation avec l'épiderme de surface, constituées de petites cellules basophiles [rappelant les cellules basales de l'épiderme d'où le nom de carcinome baso-cellulaire (Krompecher)], sans ponts d'union optiquement visibles; ces derniers sont décelables en ultrastructure.
Quelques variantes histologiques peuvent se rencontrer:
- forme kystique;
- forme adénoïde décrite parfois à tort sous le nom de cylindrome cutané à cause de sa ressemblance avec le cylindrome des glandes salivaires. Il pourrait s'agir pour Lever d'une évolution de type sudoral;
- forme kératinisante ou pilaire.

I.3 Maligne epitheliale Tumoren

I.3.1 Basalzellkarzinome des Lides

Sie machen 85% der malignen Epithelial-tumoren der Lider aus. Sie sind in ihrem Aussehen äußerst verschiedenartig und können schematisch in 4 anatomisch-klinische Haupttypen eingeteilt werden:
- knötchenförmig;
- ulzerös;
- sklerodermieartig;
- pigmentiert.

Alle diese Formen haben ein klinisches Element gemeinsam das typisch ist: den Verlust der Wimpern im Bereich der Läsion. Bei der ulzerösen Form ist öfters an der Peripherie ein erhabener, höckriger, aus richtigen kleinen "Hautperlen" bestehender Rand vorhanden. Letztere kann man auch, jedoch seltener, bei den knötchenförmigen und pigmentierten Typen beobachten.

Knötchenförmiges Basalzellkarzinom
Klinik. Es ist erhaben, fest, auf den tieferen Lagen beweglich, zumindest im anfänglichen Stadium. Es bildet möglicherweise im weiteren Verlauf ein Geschwür.

Histopathologie. Es sind dies kompakte, mit der Epidermis in Verbindung stehende Massen, aus kleinen basophilen Zellen bestehend [die an die Basalzellen der Epidermis erinnern, daher der Name Basalzellkarzinom (Krompecher)], ohne optisch sichtbare Stachel-zellen; letztere sind aber in der Ultrastruktur nachweisbar.
Einige histologische Varianten sind anzutreffen:
- zystisch;
- adenoid, manchmal wegen der Ähnlichkeit mit dem Zylindrom der Speicheldrüsen zu Unrecht als kutanes Zylindrom bezeichnet. Lever zufolge könnte es sich um eine Entwicklung vom sudoralen Typ handeln;
- zur Verhornung neigende Form.

PLATE 12   PLANCHE 12   TAFEL 12

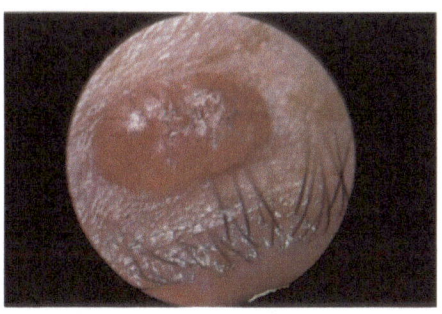

a

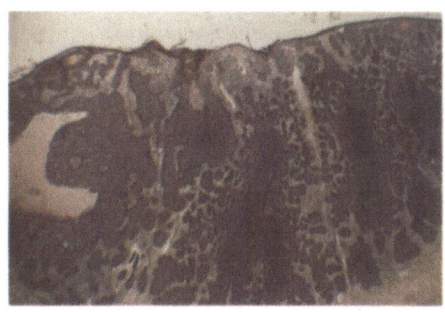

b

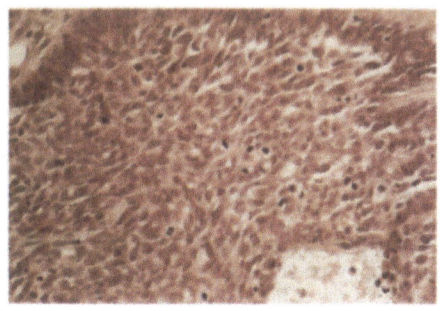

c

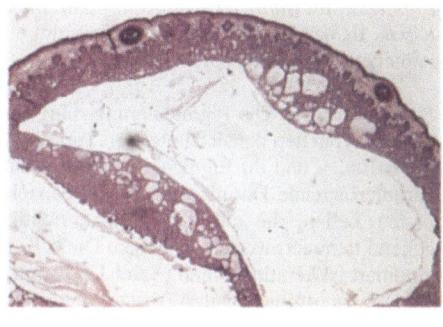

d

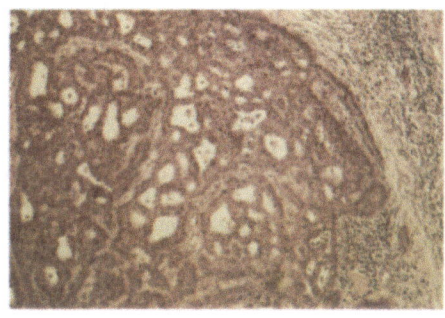

e

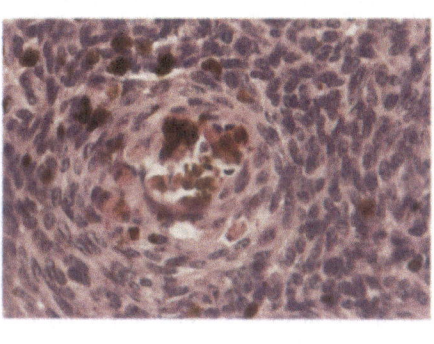

f

Fig. a. Nodular basal cell carcinoma of the lid. Prominent nodule, slightly depressed and squamous at its center, of firm consistency, with small telangiectases on its surface. Presence of epidermic pearls.

Fig. b. Nodular basal cell carcinoma. The tumour consists of massive nodules derived from the epidermis and rimmed with multiple peripheral ramifications. The lesion is endophytic, extensively invading the underlying dermis.

Fig. c. Nodular basal cell carcinoma. Cytology shows small, elongated basophilic cells with small chromatin-rich nuclei, some of them being mitotic. At the periphery they present a palisading pattern.

Fig. d. Nodular basal cell carcinoma, cystic type. The nodule shows a central cavity, surrounded by tumour cells, a consequence of central necrosis, or of degeneration of areas of stroma which are encircled by the tumour.

Fig. e. Nodular basal cell carcinoma, adenoid type. Strands of 2 or 3 layers of cells which intersect and form a network recalling a salivary cylindroma (the prognosis of which is quite different).

Fig. f. Nodular basal cell carcinoma, keratinizing type. Round structures of flat eosinophilic cells, in concentric layers, more or less keratinized centrally, suggesting a developing hair shaft.

Fig. a. Carcinome baso-cellulaire nodulaire de la paupière. Nodule saillant un peu déprimé et squameux au centre, ferme, et dont la surface est parcourue de fines télangiectasies. Présence de perles épidermiques.

Fig. b. Carcinome baso-cellulaire nodulaire. La tumeur est constituée de nodules massifs prenant leur origine dans l'épiderme et hérissés de ramifications périphériques. La lésion est endophytique, envahissant largement le derme sous-jacent.

Fig. c. Carcinome baso-cellulaire nodulaire. Cytologiquement ce sont de petites cellules allongées, basophiles, à petits noyaux riches en chromatine, dont certains sont en mitose. A la périphérie elles prennent une disposition palissadique.

Fig. d. Carcinome baso-cellulaire nodulaire, forme kystique. Le nodule se creuse d'une cavité bordée par les cellules tumorales, conséquence d'une nécrose centrale, ou de la dégénérescence du stroma englobé par la tumeur.

Fig. e. Carcinome baso-cellulaire nodulaire, forme adénoïde. Travées de 2 à 3 couches cellulaires qui s'entrecroisent, formant un réseau rappelant l'aspect d'un cylindrome salivaire, dont le pronostic est tout différent.

Fig. f. Carcinome baso-cellulaire nodulaire, forme kératinisante. Structures arrondies formées de cellules aplaties éosinophiles, en couches concentriques plus ou moins kératinisées en leur centre et évoquant des ébauches pilaires.

Abb. a. Knötchenförmiges Basalzellkarzinom des Lids. Erhabenes, in der Mitte leicht vertieftes und schuppiges, in die Epidermis eingeschlossenes derbes Knötchen, das an der Oberfläche von feinen Telangiektasien durchzogen ist.

Abb. b. Knötchenförmiges Basalzellkarzinom des Lids. Der Tumor besteht aus kompakten Knötchen, die von der Epidermis herrühren und mit peripheren Verzweigungen gespickt sind. Die Läsion ist endophytisch und dringt weitgehend in die darunterliegende Dermis ein.

Abb. c. Knötchenförmiges Basalzellkarzinom des Lids. Zytologisch sind es kleine, längliche basophile Zellen mit kleinen chromatinreichen Kernen, von denen sich einige in Mitose befinden. An der Peripherie nehmen sie eine Palissadenanordnung ein.

Abb. d. Knötchenförmiges Basalzellkarzinom des Lids, zystisch. In dem Knötchen entsteht ein von Tumorzellen eingerahmter Hohlraum als Folge einer zentralen Nekrose oder der Degeneration des vom Tumor umschlossenen Stromas.

Abb. e. Knötchenförmiges Basalzellkarzinom des Lids, adenoide Form. Stränge aus 2 bis 3 Zellschichten, die sich kreuzen und ein Netz bilden, das an ein Zylindrom der Speicheldrüse erinnert. Dessen Prognose ist eine völlig andere.

Abb. f. Zur Verhornung neigende Form eines knötchenförmigen Basalzellkarzinoms. Abgerundete, aus abgeflachten, eosinophilen Zellen gebildete Strukturen mit konzentrischen, in ihrer Mitte mehr oder weniger verhornenden Schichten, die an Haaranlagen denken lassen.

25

PLATE 13 PLANCHE 13 TAFEL 13

Ulcerative basal cell carcinoma

Clinical features. This lesion can be a variant of a nodular carcinoma, or be directly ulcerative. It is chiefly localized at the medial canthus. When it results in the destruction of the underlying dermis it deserves the term of "ulcus rodens".

Histopathology. Proliferating nodular masses or strands of cells grow towards the deeper layers of the skin, beneath an ulceration filled with a fibrino-polymorphonuclear exudate.

Morphealike basal cell carcinoma

Clinical features. Ivory white hard plaque, fixed in the dermis; this is the type which most often recurs.

Histopathology. Fine strands of tumour cells invade the connective tissue beneath the atrophic epidermis.

Pigmented ("tattooed") basal cell carcinoma

Clinical features. This is usually a nodular carcinoma.

Histopathology. The pigmentation is due to the presence, among the tumour cells, of melanocytes which yield their pigment either into the underlying dermis, or into the adjacent cells, which are thus literally "tattooed". This variety of carcinoma is often of a keratinizing type (Plate 12, Fig. f), a point in favour of its pilar origin; according to Lever, hair matrices are indeed specially rich in melanocytes.

Prognosis. The prognosis of basal cell carcinoma is essentially local. But recurrences may develop and both the "ulcus rodens" and the morphealike type may invade the orbit or even the cranial cavity. Their total surgical eradication and/or radiotherapy are necessary.

Carcinome baso-cellulaire ulcéreux

Clinique. Evolution d'un carcinome nodulaire ou ulcéreux d'emblée, il siège de préférence à l'angle interne; lorsqu'il détruit le derme sous jacent il mérite le nom d'"ulcus rodens".

Histopathologie. Sous une ulcération comblée par un exsudat fibrino-leucocytaire prolifèrent des masses nodulaires ou des travées gagnant les plans profonds.

Carcinome baso-cellulaire sclérodermiforme

Clinique. Plaque de teinte blanc ivoire, dure, fixée dans le derme, il représente la forme la plus récidivante.

Histopathologie. Sous un épiderme atrophique de minces travées cellulaires tumorales envahissent le tissu conjonctif.

Carcinome baso-cellulaire pigmenté (tatoué)

Clinique. C'est en général un carcinome nodulaire.

Histopathologie. La pigmentation est liée à la présence parmi les cellules tumorales de mélanocytes qui rejettent leur pigment soit vers le derme sous-jacent soit dans les cellules avoisinantes qui sont véritablement tatouées. Cette variété de carcinome est souvent de type kératinisant (Planche 12, Fig. f) ce qui serait pour Lever en faveur de son origine pilaire, les matrices pilaires étant particulièrement riches en mélanocytes.

Pronostic. Le pronostic des carcinomes baso-cellulaires est purement local. Mais ils peuvent récidiver et les types "ulcus rodens" et sclérodermiforme peuvent envahir l'orbite et même la cavité crânienne. Leur éradication totale par chirurgie et/ou radiothérapie est donc nécessaire.

Ulzeröses Basalzellkarzinom

Klinik. Diese Weiterentwicklung eines knotenförmigen oder gleich von Anfang an geschwürigen Karzinoms tritt vorwiegend im inneren Augenwinkel auf. Wenn es die darunterliegende Dermis zerstört, verdient es den Namen "Ulcus rodens".

Histopathologie. Unter einer von einem fibrinoleukozytären Exsudat aufgefüllten Geschwürbildung wuchern Knotenmassen oder Zellstränge, die sich in tiefere Schichten ausbreiten.

Sklerodermieartiges Basalzellkarzinom

Klinik. Verhärtung von elfenbeinweißer Färbung, in der Dermis festsitzend: die am stärksten rezidivierende Form.

Histopathologie. Unter einer atrophischen Epidermis breiten sich dünne Tumorzellsprossen in das Bindegewebe aus.

Pigmentiertes (tätowiertes) Basalzellkarzinom

Klinik. Es handelt sich im allgemeinen um ein knötchenförmiges Karzinom.

Histopathologie. Die Pigmentierung rührt von Melanozyten her, die sich unter den Tumorzellen befinden und ihr Pigment entweder in die darunterliegende Dermis oder an die benachbarten Zellen, die auf diese Weise richtiggehend tätowiert werden, abgeben. Diese Karzinomart ist keratinisierend (Tafel 12, Abb. f), was Lever zufolge für ihre Abstammung vom Haarsystem spricht, da die Haarmatrices besonders reich an Melanozyten sind.

Prognose. Die Prognose für den Verlauf der Basalzellkarzinome betrifft rein das lokale Verhalten. Sie können jedoch rezidivieren, und die sklerodermieartige Form sowie das "Ulcus rodens" können in die Orbita und sogar in die Schädelhöhle übergreifen. Eine vollständige Entfernung durch Chirurgie und/oder Radiotherapie sind daher notwendig.

PLATE 13 PLANCHE 13 TAFEL 13

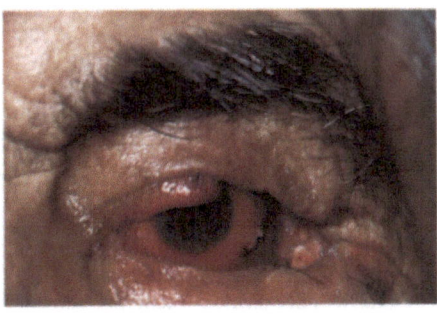

a

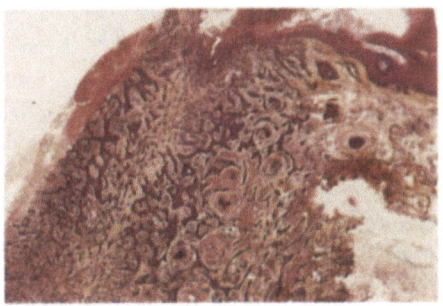

b

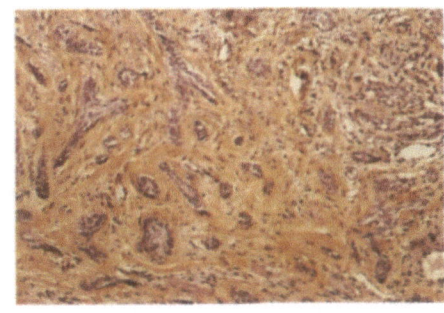

c

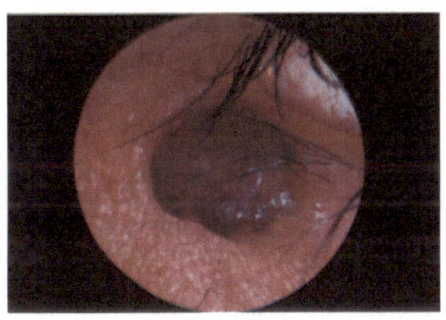

d

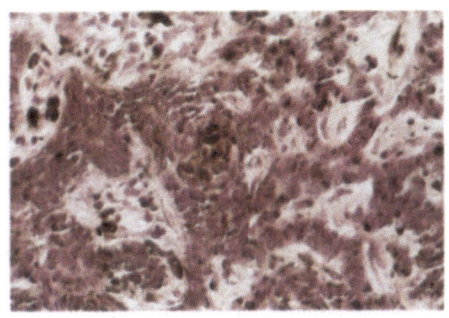

e

Fig. a. Basal cell carcinoma, ulcerative type (ulcus rodens), localized at the left external canthus: deep ulcerous carcinoma, with steep edges, and irregular growth from the floor, which bleeds at the slightest contact. This type of carcinoma is more often found at the inner canthus (the sutures are remnants from a recent biopsy).

Fig. b. Ulcus rodens: histology.
The superficially ulcerated tumour extends deeply into the underlying dermis and forms ramifying and divergent strands.

Fig. c. Morphealike basal cell carcinoma.
Thin cellular strands surrounded by a dense, collagen-rich stroma. This proliferation often grows beyond the limits of the clinical lesion.

Fig. d. Basal cell carcinoma, pigmented type.
Entirely pigmented nodular carcinoma. The colour may vary from a more or less spotted brown to an almost black shade. The diagnosis of malignant melanoma may be considered in this case.

Fig. e. Pigmented basal cell carcinoma.
Melanin is present in the strands of cancerous cells, which are "tattooed", and also in the stroma where it has been taken up by macrophages.

Fig. a. Carcinome baso-cellulaire, type térébrant (ulcus rodens), localisé à l'angle externe de l'oeil gauche: carcinome ulcéreux creusant en profondeur, à bords taillés à pic, à fond végétant et saignant au moindre contact. Ce type de carcinome siège plus souvent à l'angle interne (les fils sont ceux d'une biopsie récente).

Fig. b. Ulcus rodens: histologie.
La tumeur ulcérée en surface envahit profondément le derme sous-jacent sous la forme de travées ramifiées et divergentes.

Fig. c. Carcinome baso-cellulaire, type sclérodermiforme.
Minces travées tumorales dispersées au sein d'un stroma dense, riche en collagène. La prolifération déborde souvent les limites de la lésion clinique.

Fig. d. Carcinome baso-cellulaire, type pigmenté.
Carcinome nodulaire entièrement pigmenté. La teinte peut aller d'un brun plus ou moins moucheté à des tons franchement noirâtres qui peuvent faire discuter alors un mélanome malin.

Fig. e. Carcinome baso-cellulaire pigmenté.
Le pigment mélanique est présent aussi bien dans les travées épithéliomateuses qui en sont "tatouées" que dans le stroma où il est repris par les macrophages.

Abb. a. Basalzellkarzinom, invasiver Typ (Ulcus rodens), im linken äußeren Augenwinkel lokalisiert: ulzeröses, in die Tiefe dringendes Karzinom mit steil abfallenden Rändern, wucherndem Grund, das bei der geringsten Berührung blutet. Dieser Karzinomtyp ist meist am inneren Winkel anzutreffen (die Fäden stammen von einer kurz zuvor durchgeführten Biopsie).

Abb. b. Ulcus rodens: Histologie.
Die oberflächlich ulzerierte Geschwulst dringt in Form von Ausläufern und Verästelungen tief in die darunterliegende Dermis ein.

Abb. c. Basalzellkarzinom, sklerodermieförmiger Typ.
Dünne, innerhalb eines kollagenreichen Stromas verstreute Zellstränge. Die Wucherung geht oft über die Grenzen der klinischen Läsion hinaus.

Abb. d. Basalzellkarzinom, pigmentierter Typ.
Völlig pigmentiertes Knötchenkarzinom. Die Färbung kann von einem mehr oder weniger gesprenkelten Braun bis zu ausgesprochen schwärzlichen Tönen, die sodann ein malignes Melanom zur Diskussion stellen, reichen.

Abb. e. Basalzellkarzinom, pigmentierter Typ.
Das Melaninpigment ist in den damit "tätowierten" epitheliomatösen Strängen ebenso vorhanden wie im Stroma, wo es von den Makrophagen aufgenommen wird.

PLATE 14   PLANCHE 14   TAFEL 14

I.3.2 Squamous cell (epidermoid) carcinoma of the lids

Clinical features. This tumour develops on a precancerous lesion (actinic keratosis, Bowen's disease) or appears on a healthy skin. It is definitely less frequent than basal cell carcinoma and would seem to prefer the upper lid. It may present two main aspects:
- the ulcerative or ulcero-proliferating type, showing a crater surrounded by a hard, elevated border seated on an indurated base. The floor of the crater is granular, irregular, bleeding and sometimes bristling with whitish spots which are beads of keratin;
- the proliferating type which is more exophytic.

Histopathology. The tumour is made of cellular buds which grow towards the deeper layers of the skin. They are made of squamous cells which show a definite evolution towards keratinisation (Horn pearls).
Two types deserve a special description:
- the adenoid type;
- the spindle-cell type.

Adenoid epidermoid carcinoma (adeno-acanthoma of Lever)
The tumour has a lobular arrangement. Among the lobules, some degree of acantholysis (rupture of the intercellular bridges of the squamous cells). The whole structure presents a pseudo-glandular appearance accounting for the term adeno-acanthoma, formerly in use.

Spindle-cell epidermoid carcinoma
This is a poorly differentiated, anaplastic variety; its cells present many mitotic figures and atypical nuclei, become spindle-shaped, with parallel alignment, sometimes mimicking a sarcoma.

Prognosis. It is definitely less favourable than that of basal-cell carcinoma: metastases may occur, principally into the regional lymph nodes; the search for an associated lymph node involvement thus becomes indispensable during clinical examination.

I.3.2 Carcinome spino-cellulaire (épidermoïde) des paupières

Clinique. Il peut succéder à une lésion précancéreuse (kératose actinique, maladie de Bowen) ou apparaître en peau saine. Il est nettement moins fréquent que le carcinome baso-cellulaire et siégerait de préférence à la paupière supérieure. Il se présente sous deux principaux aspects:
- la forme ulcéreuse ou ulcéro-végétante: cratère entouré d'un bourrelet dur et saillant et reposant sur une base indurée. La cavité est bourgeonnante, irrégulière, saignante parfois hérissée de pointillés blanchâtres, qui sont autant de grains de kératine;
- la forme saillante et végétante plus exophytique.

Histopathologie. Le tissu tumoral est constitué de bourgeons s'enfonçant en profondeur, au sein desquels les cellules ont un caractère malpighien et évoluent nettement vers la kératinisation (globes cornés).
Deux types sont un peu particuliers:
- le type adénoïde;
- le type fusiforme.

Carcinome épidermoïde adénoïde (adéno-acanthome de Lever)
La tumeur prend une disposition lobulaire. Au sein des lobules un certain degré d'acantholyse (rupture des ponts d'union entre les cellules malpighiennes) fait que la structure de la prolifération prend une allure pseudo-glandulaire d'où l'ancienne dénomination d'adéno-acanthome.

Carcinome épidermoïde à cellules fusiformes
C'est une forme peu différenciée, anaplasique où les cellules riches en mitoses et monstruosités s'allongent, deviennent fusiformes se disposant côte à côte jusqu'à simuler un sarcome.

Pronostic. Il est nettement moins favorable que celui des carcinomes baso-cellulaires car des métastases sont possibles, au premier chef dans les ganglions satellites. C'est pourquoi la recherche d'une adénopathie associée est indispensable lors de l'examen clinique.

I.3.2 Stachelzellkarzinom (Plattenepithelkarzinom) des Lides

Klinik. Es kann sich aus einer präkanzerösen Erkrankung (aktinische Keratose, Bowensche Krankheit) oder aus gesunder Haut entwickeln. Es ist eindeutig weniger häufig als das Basalzellkarzinom und soll vorzugsweise am oberen Lid anzutreffen sein. Es tritt unter zwei Aspekten auf:
- ulzerös oder ulzerös-wuchernd: von einem harten, vorstehenden Wulst umgebener Krater auf einem verhärteten Grund. Die Vertiefung ist körnig, unregelmäßig, blutend, manchmal mit weißlichen Pünktchen gespickt: diese sind Hornperlen;
- erhaben, wuchernd, mehr exophytisch.

Histopathologie. Das Tumorgewebe besteht aus tief eindringenden Epithelsprossen, in deren Innerem die Zellen einen Malpighi-Charakter haben und sich deutlich zur Keratinisierung hin entwickeln (Hornperlen). Zwei Typen sind etwas eigenartig:
- der adenoide Typ;
- der fusiforme Typ.

Adenoides Plattenepithelkarzinom (Leversches Adenoakanthom)
Die Geschwulst ist lobulär angeordnet. Innerhalb der Läppchen bewirkt ein bestimmter Akantholyse-Grad (fehlende Interzellularbrücken zwischen den Stachelzellen), daß die Struktur der Neubildung eine Pseudo-Drüsengestalt annimmt; daher die frühere Bezeichnung Adenoakanthom.

Plattenepithelkarzinom mit spindelförmigen Zellen (fusiformer Typ)
Dies ist eine wenig differenzierte, anaplastische Form, in der sich die an Mitosen und Entartungen reichen Zellen verlängern, spindelförmig werden und sich so nebeneinander anordnen, daß man ein Sarkom vermuten könnte.

Prognose. Diese ist weit weniger günstig als bei einem Basalzellkarzinom, da Metastasierung, hauptsächlich in die umliegenden Lymphknoten, möglich ist. Deshalb ist bei der klinischen Untersuchung die gleichzeitige Nachforschung nach einer Lymphdrüsenbeteiligung unumgänglich.

PLATE 14 PLANCHE 14 TAFEL 14

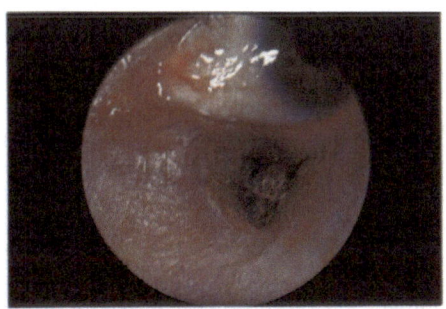

a

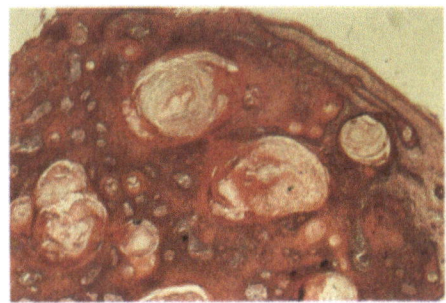

b

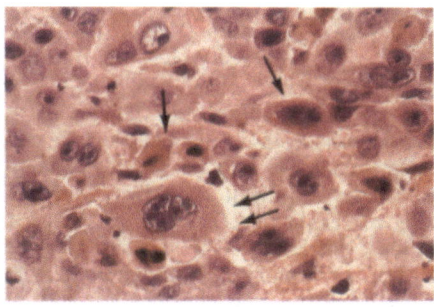

c

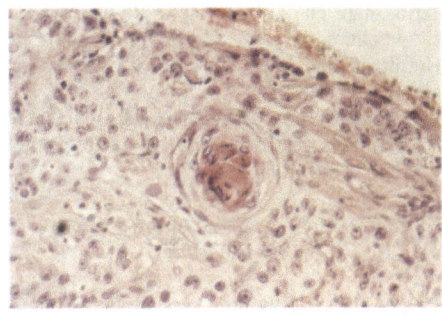

d

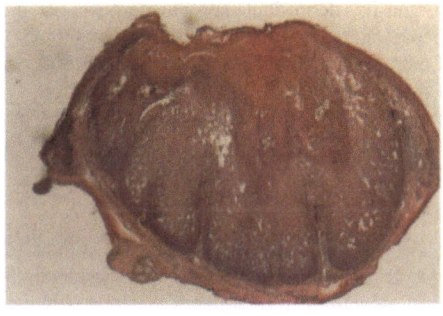

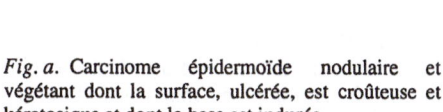

e

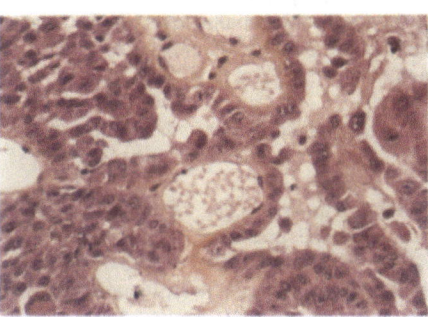

f

Fig. a. Nodular and proliferating epidermoid carcinoma. Its ulcerated surface is scurfy and keratotic; it rests on an indurated base.

Fig. b. Epidermoid carcinoma. It presents foci of keratinization (horn pearls). According to the number of these foci, the tumour is considered as more or less differentiated.

Fig. c. Epidermoid carcinoma, cytological aspect. Polygonal squamous cells, sometimes bound together by prickles (horn cells), but of irregular shape; dyskeratotic cells (→) (monocellular keratinisation) and nuclear monstrosities (⇉) may be found.

Fig. d. Development of a horn pearl. The squamous cells flatten and gather concentrically around a center which becomes progressively keratinized (this is different from the sudden keratinization of the pseudo-cysts of a seborrheic keratosis or of keratinizing basal cell carcinoma).

Fig. e. Epidermoid carcinoma, adenoid type. Lobules surround a crater filled with keratin; some aspects suggest pseudo-glandular cavities.

Fig. f. Epidermoid carcinoma, adenoid type. Cuboid cells gather into strands sometimes surrounding a capillary, or lining fissures or cavities, giving the proliferation a pseudo-glandular appearance. But some cells part from each other (acantholysis) and peel between the strands or into the cavities.

Fig. a. Carcinome épidermoïde nodulaire et végétant dont la surface, ulcérée, est croûteuse et kératosique et dont la base est indurée.

Fig. b. Carcinome épidermoïde proliférant en profondeur, riche en foyers de kératinisation ou globes cornés. Plus ceux-ci sont nombreux, plus la tumeur est considérée comme "différenciée".

Fig. c. Carcinome épidermoïde, aspect cytologique. Cellules malpighiennes polygonales à limites nettes parfois unies par des ponts d'union (cellules à épines), mais de forme irrégulière; il existe des cellules dyskératosiques (→) (kératinisation monocellulaire) et des monstruosités nucléaires (⇉).

Fig. d. Formation d'un globe corné. Les cellules malpighiennes s'aplatissent, se groupent de façon concentrique autour d'un foyer kératinisé de façon progressive et non abrupte (comme dans la verrue séborrhéïque ou le carcinome baso-cellulaire kératinisant).

Fig. e. Carcinome épidermoïde adénoïde. Disposition en lobules bordant un cratère rempli de kératine; on y devine la présence de cavités pseudo-glandulaires.

Fig. f. Carcinome épidermoïde adénoïde. Cellules de forme cubique entourant parfois un capillaire ou bordant des fentes ou des cavités, donnant à la prolifération un aspect pseudo-glandulaire. Mais certaines cellules se séparent de leurs voisines (acantholyse) et desquament entre les travées ou dans les cavités.

Abb. a. Knötchenförmiges, wucherndes Plattenepithelkarzinom. Vorragendes Knötchen, dessen geschwürige Oberfläche krustig und verhornt und dessen Basis verhärtet ist.

Abb. b. In die Tiefe wucherndes Plattenepithelkarzinom. Weniger basophil als ein Basalzellkarzinom und reich an Verhornungszentren oder Hornperlen. Je zahlreicher diese sind, umso mehr wird der Tumor als "differenziert" betrachtet.

Abb. c. Zytologischer Aspekt eines Plattenepithelkarzinoms. Polygonale, deutlich abgegrenzte Basalzellen, manchmal durch Interzellularbrücken (Stachelzellen) verbunden, aber von unregelmäßiger Form; es gibt dyskeratotische Zellen (→) (mit monozellulärer Keratinisierung) und Kernentartungen (⇉).

Abb. d. Bildung einer Hornperle. Die Basalzellen flachen ab, gruppieren sich konzentrisch um ein immer stärker verhornendes Zentrum. (Im Unterschied zu der abrupten Verhornung der Pseudozysten der seborrhoischen Warze oder des keratinisierenden Basalzellkarzinoms.)

Abb. e. Adenoide Form eines Plattenepithelkarzinoms. Läppchenartige Anordnung am Rand eines mit Keratin gefüllten Kraters; das Vorhandensein von drüsenartigen Hohlräumen läßt sich erraten.

Abb. f. Adenoide Form eines Plattenepithelkarzinoms. Kubische, in Strängen angeordnete Zellen, die manchmal eine Kapillare umschließen oder Spalten oder Hohlräume einsäumen, die der Geschwulst ein Pseudodrüsenaussehen verleihen. Manche Zellen trennen sich durch Akantholyse von ihren Nachbarzellen und schilfern sich zwischen den Strängen oder in die Hohlräume ab.

29

PLATE 15 PLANCHE 15 TAFEL 15

I.3.3 Squamous cell (epidermoid) carcinoma of the conjunctiva

Clinical features. This may develop on a precancerous lesion (actinic keratosis or carcinoma in situ) or appear in healthy tissue. It is sometimes difficult clinically to differentiate between a precancerous lesion and a definite carcinoma. The tumour may be nodular or exophytic, papillomatous with many capillaries running along the axes of each papilla. Less often the proliferation develops superficially during a variable period, without nodule formation, mimicking a highly vascularized chronic conjunctivitis: this is the very misleading diffuse type.

Histopathology. The peculiarity of the epidermoid carcinomas of the conjunctiva, which from a cytological point of view are similar to those of the skin, is their tendency to proliferate superficially rather than in depth; thus, when they spread out on the cornea, they never grow beyond the level of Bowman's membrane. Invasion of the eyeball, which is rare, occurs mostly at the limbus.

I.3.4 Muco-epidermoid carcinoma of the conjunctiva

Clinical features. This carcinoma is much rarer than the preceding one, and more invasive: involvement of the eyeball or of the orbit is indeed frequent here. It appears mostly after the age of 70, is located at the limbus and often presents misleading features (Fig. d).

Histopathology. Its peculiarity is the presence of a double component, both epidermoid and mucous, whence its designation. The epidermoid proliferation is usually only slightly differentiated, dyskeratotic but not greatly keratotic and containing also normal mucous cells, similar to those of the conjunctival epithelium; these cells are easily demonstrated by the usual stains for mucus.

Prognosis. The prognosis of these muco-epidermoid carcinomas is extremely poor: on the one hand the recurrences are frequent and appear early; on the other hand the tumour rapidly invades the neighbouring structures, breaking into the eyeball and even into the orbit, where it may represent a threat to life.

I.3.3 Carcinome spino-cellulaire (épidermoïde) de la conjonctive

Clinique. Il peut succéder à une lésion précancéreuse (kératose actinique ou carcinome in situ) ou apparaître d'emblée en tissu sain. D'ailleurs il est parfois difficile cliniquement de différencier une lésion précancéreuse d'un carcinome déclaré. La tumeur peut être nodulaire ou exophytique papillomateuse, très vascularisée par des capillaires parcourant l'axe de chaque papille. Plus rarement la prolifération se fait en surface pendant un temps plus ou moins long sans formation nodulaire, et prenant alors le masque d'une conjonctivite rebelle très vascularisée; c'est la très trompeuse forme diffuse.

Histopathologie. Le caractère particulier des carcinomes épidermoïdes de la conjonctive, qui cytologiquement sont analogues à ceux de la peau, est leur tendance à proliférer plutôt en surface qu'en profondeur si bien que lorsqu'ils débordent sur la cornée, ils ne dépassent pas la membrane de Bowman.
Lorsque, très rarement, ils pénètrent à l'intérieur du globe oculaire l'effraction se produit au limbe.

I.3.4 Carcinome muco-épidermoïde de la conjonctive

Clinique. Ce carcinome beaucoup plus rare que le précédent est beaucoup plus envahissant, pénétrant fréquemment le globe oculaire ou l'orbite. De siège limbique il est surtout fréquent après 70 ans et d'aspect souvent trompeur (Fig. d).

Histopathologie. Son caractère particulier est la présence dans la tumeur d'une double composante épidermoïde et muqueuse d'où le qualificatif de "muco-épidermoïde". La prolifération épidermoïde est généralement peu différenciée, dyskératosique mais peu kératosique et s'y mêlent des cellules muqueuses analogues à celles de l'épithélium conjonctival normal, que mettent bien en évidence les colorants habituels du mucus.

Pronostic. Le pronostic de ces carcinomes muco-épidermoïdes est redoutable car non seulement les récidives sont fréquentes et précoces mais de plus la tumeur envahit rapidement les structures environnantes pénétrant à l'intérieur du globe oculaire et pouvant même gagner l'orbite, comportant alors un risque vital.

I.3.3 Plattenepithelkarzinom der Bindehaut

Klinik. Es kann auf eine präkanzeröse Läsion (aktinische Keratose oder Carcinoma in situ) folgen oder primär im gesunden Gewebe auftreten. Wie dem auch sei, es ist manchmal klinisch schwierig, eine präkanzeröse Läsion von einem eigentlichen Karzinom zu unterscheiden. Die Geschwulst kann knötchenförmig oder papillär nach außen wachsend auftreten, stark vaskularisiert durch Kapillaren, die der Achse jeder Papille folgen. Seltener entwickelt sich die Wucherung während einer mehr oder weniger langen Zeit an der Oberfläche, ohne Knötchenbildung, wobei sie eine stark vaskularisierte, der Behandlung nicht zugängliche Konjunktivitis vortäuscht; dies ist die sehr irreführende diffuse Form.

Histopathologie. Die Besonderheit der Plattenepithelkarzinome der Bindehaut, die zytologisch denen der Haut ähnlich sind, besteht darin, mehr an der Oberfläche als in der Tiefe zu wuchern, so daß sie, wenn sie auf die Hornhaut übergehen, über der Bowmanschen Membran bleiben.
Wenn sie in sehr seltenen Fällen ins Innere des Bulbus vordringen, so erfolgt der Einbruch am Limbus.

I.3.4 Muko-epidermoides Karzinom der Bindehaut

Klinik. Dieses Karzinom, das weitaus seltener ist als das vorausgegangene, breitet sich viel stärker aus und dringt häufig in den Bulbus oder die Augenhöhle ein. Es geht vom Limbus aus und kommt vor allem bei über 70jährigen vor; sein Aussehen ist oft irreführend (Abb. d).

Histopathologie. Sein besonderes Merkmal ist das Vorhandensein einer gleichzeitigen epidermoiden und Schleimkomponente, daher die Bezeichnung "muko-epidermoid". Die epidermoide Wucherung ist im allgemeinen wenig differenziert, dyskeratotisch, aber wenig verhornt; darunter mischen sich Schleimzellen, die denen des normalen Bindehautepithels entsprechen; diese sind mit den üblichen Färbemitteln gut nachzuweisen.

Prognose. Die Prognose für diese muko-epidermoiden Karzinome ist reserviert zu stellen, da nicht nur häufig und frühzeitig Rezidive auftreten, sondern der Tumor außerdem schnell in die umliegenden Strukturen und ins Innere des Bulbus eindringt, sogar auf die Orbita übergreift und damit lebensgefährlich wird.

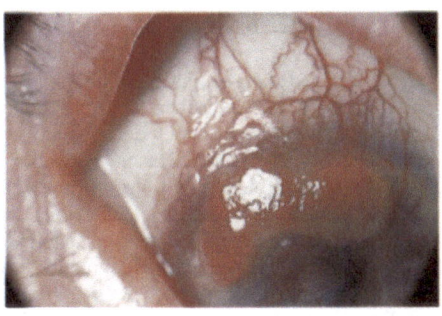

a

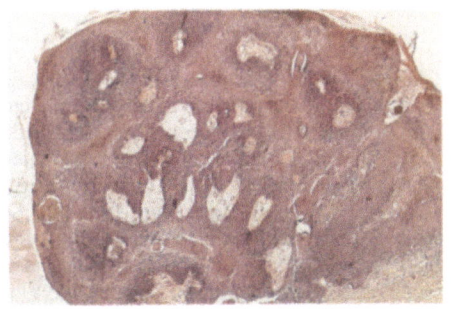

b

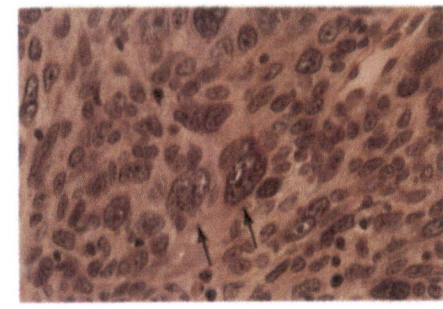

c

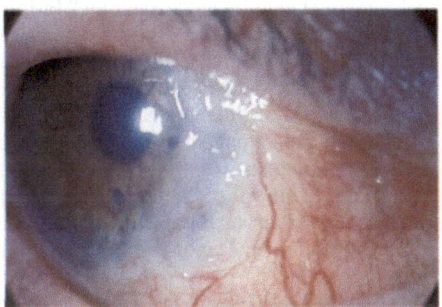

d

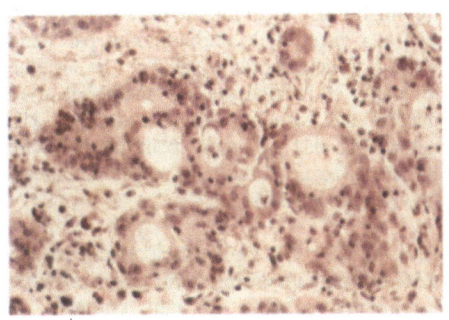

e

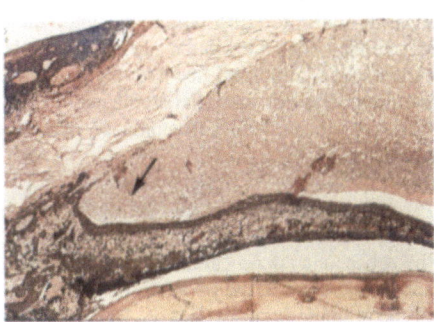

f

Fig. a. Epidermoid carcinoma of the limbus of *nodular type.* Pinkish, highly vascularized with a mamillate surface; sometimes of a whiter shade, when the lesion is superficially keratinized.

Fig. b. Epidermoid carcinoma of the *papillary type,* showing multiple connective-vascular axes, and the papillomatous exophytic pattern of the tumour.

Fig. c. Nuclear monstrosities are obvious here (→). These conjunctival carcinomas are often less differentiated than those of the lids and show less dyskeratosis.

Fig. d. Muco-epidermoid carcinoma of the limbus, mimicking a torpid greyish ulcer, surrounded by a conjunctival swelling, and extending on to the cornea.

Fig. e. Acinouslike clustering of mucous cells, surrounding a cavity which may contain mucus.

Fig. f. Intra-ocular invasion of a muco-epidermoid carcinoma.
A flat sheet of tumour cells covers the anterior surface of the iris (→) and a more massive growth is seen in the stroma of the iris and ciliary body.

Fig. a. Carcinome épidermoïde du limbe de type nodulaire, rosé, très vascularisé mamelonné. Parfois la teinte est plus blanche lorsque la lésion est kératinisée en surface.

Fig. b. Carcinome épidermoïde de type papillaire montrant les multiples axes conjonctivo-vasculaires et la disposition papillomateuse, exophytique de la tumeur.

Fig. c. Les monstruosités nucléaires sont ici évidentes (→). Ces carcinomes conjonctivaux sont souvent moins bien différenciés que les palpébraux et présentent moins de dyskératose.

Fig. d. Carcinome muco-épidermoïde du limbe évoluant sous le masque d'un ulcère torpide grisâtre, bordé d'un bourrelet conjonctival et s'étendant sur la cornée.

Fig. e. Disposition acineuse des cellules muqueuses entourant une cavité qui peut contenir du mucus.

Fig. f. Pénétration intra-oculaire d'un carcinome muco-épidermoïde.
Une lame cellulaire recouvre la face antérieure de l'iris (→) et les boyaux tumoraux envahissent le stroma irien et ciliaire.

Abb. a. Plattenepithelkarzinom am Limbus, knötchenförmiger Typ. Stark vaskularisiert, mit warzenähnlichen Erhebungen, rosa. Die Färbung ist manchmal weißlicher, wenn die Läsion an der Oberfläche verhornt ist.

Abb. b. Plattenepithelkarzinom vom papillären Typ mit den vielfachen Konjunktiva-Gefäßachsen und der papillomatösen, exophytischen Anordnung.

Abb. c. Die Kernmißbildungen sind hier (→) sehr offenkundig. Karzinome der Bindehaut sind oft weniger differenziert als die der Lider und weisen weniger Dyskeratose auf.

Abb. d. Muko-epidermoides Karzinom des Limbus, ein gräuliches, torpides Ulcus vortäuschend, eingesäumt von einem Konjunktiva-Wulst, sich auf die Cornea ausdehnend.

Abb. e. Azinöse Anordnung der Schleimzellen, die eine Vertiefung umgeben, in der sich Schleim befinden kann.

Abb. f. Eindringen eines muko-epidermoiden Karzinoms ins Augeninnere.
Ein Karzinomstrang bedeckt die Vorderseite der Iris (→), Tumorschläuche dringen in das Iris- und Ziliarstroma vor.

I.3.5 Sebaceous carcinomas

Clinical features. They develop mostly from the meibomian glands, which are located in the tarsal plate, but sometimes also from the glands of Zeis, which are associated with the cilia. The meibomian carcinoma often mimics the aspect of a chalazion; but three features make this diagnosis questionable: an extensive infiltrate of the lid margin, a yellowish tinge, and recurrence after surgery. On the contrary the location of the carcinoma of the glands of Zeis is in front of the tarsal plate and the tumour often overlaps the lid margin. In this case it can mimic a chronic blepharoconjunctivitis.

Histopathology. This tumour of lobular structure is formed by clear cells filled with lipids; atypical nuclei and mitotic figures are numerous. Invasion of the overlying epidermis or epithelium is possible ("pagetoïd" aspect). Sometimes this tumour remains without definite differentiation into clear sebaceous cells; the lobular structure and the cyto-nuclear abnormalities are of diagnostic importance in this case. Fat stains may help to rule out a basal cell carcinoma or Merkel's tumour.

Prognosis. The meibomian carcinoma is considered as one of the most agressive among the sebaceous adeno-carcinomas. Recurrences are frequent, as is the invasion of the orbit or of the regional lymph nodes.

I.3.6 Sweat gland carcinomas

Clinical features. These rare tumours mostly present the aspect of a nodule deeply embedded in the eyelid; the skin in front of the lesion is reddish or unaltered. When the lid margin is involved, confusion with blepharitis is possible.

Histopathology. These adeno-carcinomas can present various features: a nodular type, with cubical eosinophilic, sometimes mitotic cells (in the lobules, outlines of sweat gland ducts can be seen); a papillary type; a rare mucinous type with a lesser tendency to metastasize. As well as in meibomian carcinomas, the cells of these tumours can sometimes invade the epidermis ("Extra-mammary Paget's disease").

I.3.5 Carcinomes sébacés

Clinique. Ils intéressent surtout les glandes de Meibomius, situées dans le tarse mais peuvent aussi se développer aux dépens des glandes de Zeis annexées aux cils. Le carcinome meibomien prend le plus souvent l'aspect trompeur d'un chalazion mais il faudra se méfier: d'une infiltration étendue de la marge palpébrale; d'une coloration légèrement jaunâtre; et d'une récidive de la lésion après intervention. Le carcinome des glandes de Zeis est par contre antérieur au plan tarsal et déborde largement sur la marge palpébrale. Dans ces cas la lésion peut simuler une blépharo-conjonctivite traînante.

Histopathologie. C'est une tumeur lobulaire constituée de cellules claires chargées de lipides, riches en atypies cellulaires et en mitoses. Ces cellules peuvent envahir l'épiderme ou l'épithélium conjonctival susjacent (envahissement "pagetoïde" de l'épithélium). Le carcinome sébacé est parfois très peu différencié, n'aboutissant pas nettement à la cellule claire sébacée; la structure lobulaire et la richesse en anomalies cytonucléaires doivent alors attirer l'attention. Une coloration des graisses peut alors éviter l'erreur avec un carcinome baso-cellulaire ou une tumeur de Merkel.

Pronostic. Le carcinome meibomien est considéré comme un des plus agressifs des adénocarcinomes sébacés. Il faut craindre des récidives et l'extension se fait volontiers vers l'orbite ou les ganglions satellites.

I.3.6 Carcinomes sudoraux

Clinique. Tumeurs rares, elles se présentent le plus souvent sous l'aspect d'un nodule enchassé dans l'épaisseur de la paupière et recouvert d'un tégument peu modifié ou rougeâtre. Lorsque la marge palpébrale est intéressée la lésion peut prendre l'allure d'une blépharite.

Histopathologie. Ces adéno-carcinomes peuvent prendre différents aspects: des types nodulaires formés de lobules contenant des cellules cubiques éosinophiles, parfois en mitose (au sein de ces lobules on peut distinguer quelques ébauches canaliculaires); des types papillaires; des types mucineux plus rares mais ayant moins tendance à métastaser. Comme dans les carcinomes sébacés les cellules tumorales peuvent parfois essaimer dans l'épiderme ("Paget extra-mammaire").

I.3.5 Karzinom der Talgdrüsen

Klinik. Sie betreffen hauptsächlich die im Tarsus gelegenen Meibomschen Drüsen, können sich jedoch auch in den Wimpern benachbarten Zeisschen Drüsen entwickeln. Das Meibomsche Karzinom nimmt meist das täuschende Aussehen eines Chalazions an, dabei sollten allerdings folgende Anzeichen mißtrauisch machen: eine ausgedehnte Infiltration des Lidrandes, eine leichte Gelbfärbung, ein Rezidiv der Läsion nach dem Eingriff. Das Karzinom der Zeisschen Drüsen liegt hingegen vor dem Tarsus und dehnt sich weit über den Lidrand aus. In solchen Fällen kann die Läsion eine protrahiert verlaufende Blepharokonjunktivitis vortäuschen.

Histopathologie. Es ist ein gelappter Tumor, bestehend aus hellen, mit Lipiden beladenen, an atypischen Zelleigenschaften und Mitosen reichen Zellen. Diese Zellen können in die Epidermis oder das darüberliegende Bindehautepithel eindringen ("pagetoide" Infiltration des Epithels). Dieses Talgdrüsenkarzinom ist manchmal sehr wenig differenziert, wenn dabei keine deutlich helle Talgzellen auftreten; die gelappte Struktur und die vielfachen Zellkernanomalien müssen dann auf sich aufmerksam machen. Eine Färbung der Fette kann in diesem Fall eine Verwechslung mit einem Basalzellkarzinom oder einem Merkelschen Tumor verhindern.

Prognose. Das Meibomsche Karzinom wird als eines der agressivsten Talgdrüsenkarzinome angesehen. Rezidive sind zu befürchten, und es dringt oft in die Orbita oder in die umliegenden Lymphknoten ein.

I.3.6 Schweißdrüsenkarzinom

Klinik. Diese seltenen Tumoren treten meist als in die Lider eingelassene, mit kaum verändertem oder rötlichem Überzug bedeckte Knötchen auf. Ist der Lidrand betroffen, so kann die Läsion einer Blepharitis ähnlich sein.

Histopathologie. Diese Adenokarzinome können ein unterschiedliches Aussehen annehmen: knötchenbildender Typ, gelappt, kubische, eosinophile, manchmal in Mitose befindliche Zellen enthaltend (innerhalb der Läppchen sind einige kanalförmige Formationen auszumachen); papillärer Typ; muzinöser Typ, der seltener ist, aber weniger zu Metastasen neigt. Wie bei den Talgdrüsenkarzinomen können die Tumorzellen manchmal in die Epidermis ausschwärmen ("extramammärer Paget").

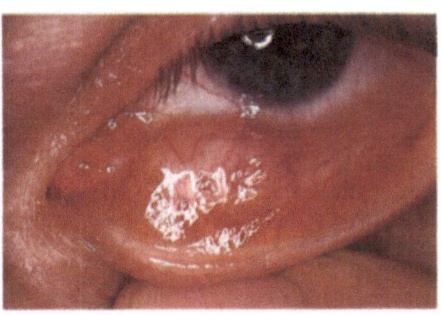

a

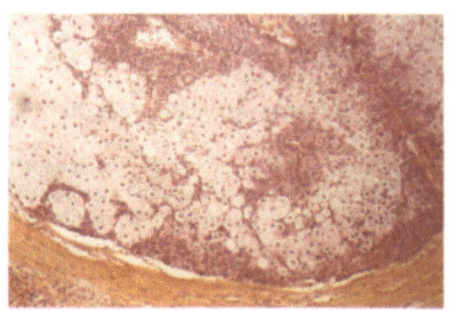

b

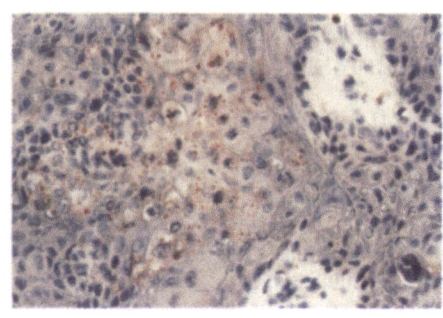

c

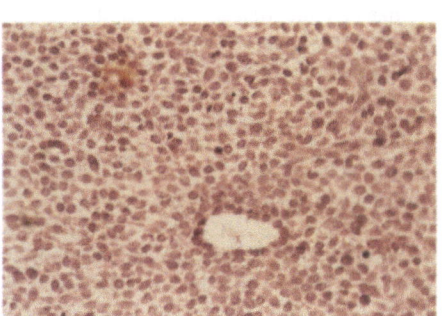

d

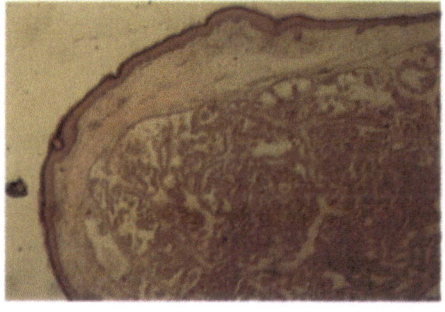

e

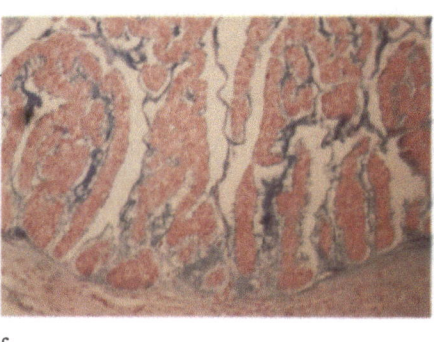

f

Fig. a. Meibomian carcinoma.
Looking like a chalazion of abnormal size, highly vascularized, infiltrating a large part of the eyelid. Its growth may lead to the ulceration of the conjunctiva.

Fig. b. Well differentiated meibomian adeno-carcinoma.
The dark cells at the periphery of the nodule become progressively clear, optically empty cells with small central nuclei (and not peripheral as in fatty tissue).

Fig. c. Sebaceous carcinoma.
The clear cells in the center of the lobule contain fat droplets. The staining with Sudan III (which can be used only on unfixed specimens) is positive.

Fig. d. Sweat gland adeno-carcinoma.
A glandular cavity, lined with cubical cells, is seen in an area of poorly differentiated cells. It sometimes contains an eosinophilic material which takes up MPS stains.

Fig. e. Sweat gland adeno-carcinoma, papillary type.
Intradermal tumour made of papillary structures covered with cubical cells, and presenting a conjunctivo-vascular core.

Fig. f. Sweat gland carcinoma, mucinous type.
Between strands of cubical eosinophilic cells, there are areas containing sialomucin, which is well demonstrated by Alcian Blue.

Fig. a. Carcinome meibomien.
Aspect d'un chalazion de taille anormale, très vascularisé, infiltrant largement la paupière. L'évolution se fait vers la conjonctive qui peut s'ulcérer.

Fig. b. Adéno-carcinome meibomien bien différencié.
Les cellules sombres de la périphérie des lobules se transforment progressivement en cellules claires, optiquement vides, à petit noyau central (et non périphérique comme dans les cellules adipeuses).

Fig. c. Carcinome sébacé.
Les cellules claires centro-lobulaires contiennent des lipides comme le prouve la coloration au Soudan III (praticable uniquement sur pièces non fixées).

Fig. d. Adéno-carcinome sudoral nodulaire.
Présence au sein d'une plage de cellules peu différenciées d'une cavité glandulaire bordée de cellules cubiques. On peut y trouver un matériel éosinophile prenant les colorants des mucopolysaccharides.

Fig. e. Adéno-carcinome sudoral papillaire.
Tumeur intradermique, constituée de papilles ramifiées tapissées de cellules cubiques et soutenues par des axes conjonctivo-vasculaires.

Fig. f. Adéno-carcinome sudoral mucineux.
Travées de cellules cubiques éosinophiles séparées par des plages de mucine (sialomucine) bien mise en évidence par le Bleu Alcian.

Abb. a. Meibomsches Karzinom.
Aussehen eines anormal großen Chalazions, stark vaskularisiert, das Lid weitgehend infiltrierend. Im weiteren Verlauf wird die Konjunktiva erfaßt, die geschwürig werden kann.

Abb. b. Gut differenziertes Karzinom der Meibomschen Drüsen.
Die dunklen Zellen an der Peripherie der Knötchen verwandeln sich nach und nach in helle, optisch leere Zellen mit kleinem zentralem (und nicht wie in adipösen Zellen an der Peripherie gelegenem) Kern.

Abb. c. Karzinom der Talgdrüsen.
Die hellen Zellen im Zentrum des Knötchens enthalten Lipide, wie die mit Soudan III vorgenommene (nur auf nicht fixierten Präparaten durchführbare) Färbung beweist.

Abb. d. Schweißdrüsenkarzinom, knötchenbildender Typ.
Mit kubischen Zellen eingesäumte Drüsenvertiefung innerhalb eines Feldes kaum differenzierter Zellen. Es ist darin ein eosinophiler Stoff, der die Farbstoffe der Mukopolysaccharide annimmt, anzutreffen.

Abb. e. Schweißdrüsenkarzinom, papillarer Typ.
Innerhalb der Haut gelegener Tumor, bestehend aus verästelten Papillen, die mit kubischen Zellen bekleidet und von konjunktivalen und Gefäßachsen gestützt sind.

Abb. f. Schweißdrüsenkarzinom, muzinöser Typ.
Stränge eosinophiler, kubischer Zellen, die durch Muzinfelder getrennt sind. Sialomuzine ist mit Alcian-Blau deutlich nachgewiesen.

33

PLATE 17 PLANCHE 17 TAFEL 17

II. PIGMENTED TUMOURS OF THE LIDS AND THE CONJUNCTIVA

II.1 Benign pigmented tumours

General. Benign melanomas are pigmented naevi or naevo-cellular naevi which are usually simply called naevi. They are sometimes congenital, but more often appear during childhood; they may have sudden bursts of growth or of increasing pigmentation. They are definitely more frequent on the conjunctiva than on the cutaneous surface of the lids. The following varieties are described, according to the depth of the lesion:
- junctional naevi;
- compound naevi (Parinaud's dermo-epithelioma or benign cystic naevus is one of them);
- intradermal or deep naevi;
- deep mesenchymal naevi or blue naevi.

Three other types present special features:
- Spitz's juvenile melanoma;
- the giant pigmented naevus;
- the balloon cell naevus.

II.1.1 Junctional naevus

Clinical features. This is a flat pigmented patch, with well defined borders and a uniform pigmentation.

Histopathology. Its name is derived from the location of the cell nests, at the dermo-epithelial junction.

II.1.2 Compound naevus

Clinical features. Its aspect is similar to that of the junctional naevus, but it is usually more prominent. When localized at the lid margin, it can be found facing a similar lesion on the opposite lid ("kissing naevus").

Histopathology. The naevus cell nests separate progressively from the dermo-epidermal junction.

II. TUMEURS MÉLANIQUES PALPÉBRO-CONJONCTIVALES

II.1 Tumeurs mélaniques bénignes

Généralités. Les tumeurs mélaniques bénignes sont les naevi pigmentés ou naevo-cellulaires qui en pratique sont simplement dénommés naevi. Parfois congénitaux ils apparaissent plutôt dans l'enfance mais peuvent présenter des poussées de croissance ou de pigmentation. Ils sont nettement moins fréquents sur la face cutanée des paupières que sur la conjonctive. On distingue suivant l'étage intéressé dans la profondeur du tissu:
- les naevi jonctionnels;
- les naevi composés (dont le dermo-épithéliome de Parinaud);
- les naevi intradermiques;
- les naevi mésenchymateux profonds ou naevi bleus.

Sont particuliers:
- le mélanome juvénile de Spitz;
- le naevus pigmentaire géant;
- le naevus à cellules ballonisantes.

II.1.1 Naevus jonctionnel

Clinique. Petite tache plane, à limites nettes, de pigmentation uniforme.

Histopathologie. Il est dit jonctionnel du fait de la situation même des groupements cellulaires ou "thèques", à la jonction dermo-épidermique.

II.1.2 Naevus composé

Clinique. D'aspect voisin du naevus jonctionnel il est cependant plus saillant. Parfois, localisé à la marge palpébrale, il peut se trouver en face d'une lésion semblable à l'autre paupière ("kissing naevus").

Histopathologie. Les thèques se séparent progressivement de la jonction dermo-épidermique.

II. PIGMENTIERTE TUMOREN DER LIDER UND BINDEHAUT

II.1 Gutartige pigmentierte Tumoren

Allgemeines. Gutartige pigmentierte Tumoren sind pigmentierte Naevi, die in der Praxis einfach Naevi genannt werden. Sie sind manchmal angeboren, entstehen eher in der Kindheit und können zeitweise an Umfang und Pigmentierung zunehmen. Sie sind auf der Lidhaut eindeutig seltener als auf der Bindehaut. Man unterscheidet je nach der betroffenen Tiefe der Gewebeschicht:
- junctionaler Naevus;
- compound naevus (zusammengesetzter Naevus) (darunter das Dermo-Epitheliom nach Parinaud);
- subepithelialer Naevus (intradermaler Naevus);
- tiefer mesenchymaler Naevus oder Naevus bleu.

Besonderheiten sind:
- das juvenile Melanom nach Spitz;
- der Riesenpigmentfleck;
- der Ballonzellnaevus.

II.1.1 Junctionaler Naevus

Klinik. Kleiner, gut abgegrenzter Fleck mit gleichmäßiger Pigmentierung.

Histopathologie. Die Benennung junctionaler Naevus rührt von der Lokalisation der Zellgruppen oder "Nester" am Übergang zwischen Epidermis/Epithel und Dermis/subepitheliales Stroma her.

II.1.2 Compound naevus

Klinik. Er gleicht im Aussehen dem junctionalen Naevus, tritt jedoch stärker hervor. Wenn er am Lidrand lokalisiert ist, kann sich eine gleiche Läsion am gegenüberliegenden Lid befinden ("kissing naevus").

Histopathologie. Die "Nester" setzen sich nach und nach von der Übergangszone Dermis-Epidermis ab.

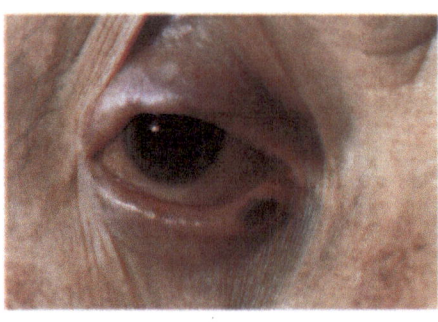

a

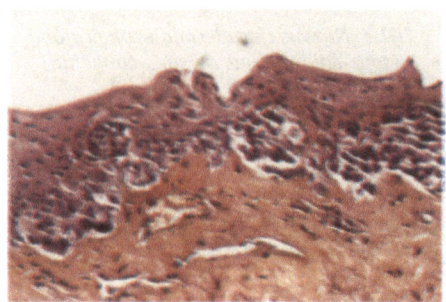

b

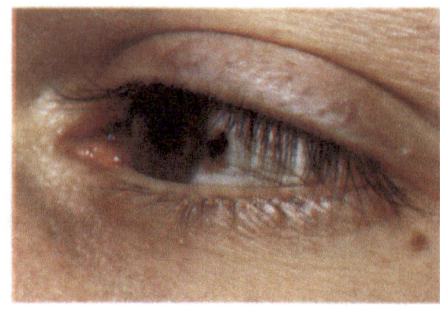

c

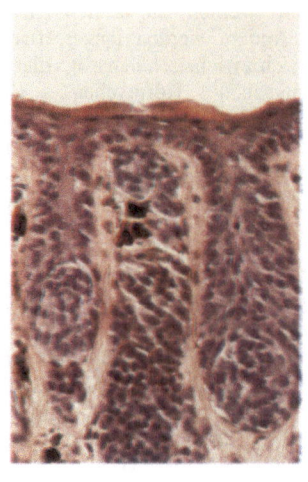

d

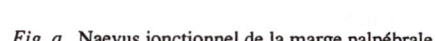

e

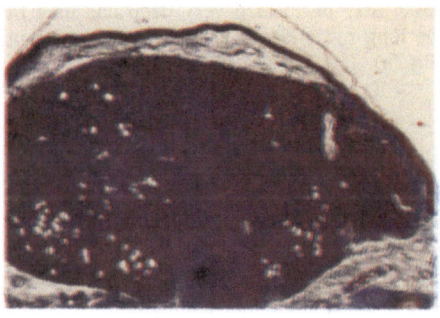

f

Fig. a. Junctional naevus of the lid margin.

Fig. b. Junctional naevus: histopathology.
The naevus cell nests are spherical or ovoid, of a regular shape, devoid of cytological abnormalities; they remain located at the dermo-epidermal junction.

Fig. c. Compound naevus of the conjunctiva.
The lesion shows definite limits, is slightly prominent, more or less pigmented. But sometimes it is a pink unpigmented naevus.

Fig. d. Cutaneous compound naevus of the lid: histopathology.
The naevus cell nests, which make bulge outwards the epidermal rete ridges, tend to migrate towards the papillary portion of the dermis ("Abtropfung").

Fig. e. Intradermal naevus of the lid margin.
Ovoid protrusion thickening the lid margin, without modification of the eyelashes. It is often unpigmented, thus creating possible confusion with a papilloma.

Fig. f. Intradermal naevus: histopathology (Masson's trichromic stain).
The naevus has lost all contact with the epidermis. It sinks deeply into the dermis, and can even reach the hypodermis. The surgical excision must be broad both laterally and in depth.

Fig. a. Naevus jonctionnel de la marge palpébrale.

Fig. b. Naevus jonctionnel palpébral: histopathologie.
Les thèques arrondies ou ovalaires, régulières, sans anomalies cytologiques restent cantonnées à la jonction dermo-épidermique.

Fig. c. Naevus composé de la conjonctive.
Lésion bien limitée mais légèrement saillante, plus ou moins pigmentée, parfois simplement rosée; c'est alors un "naevus achrome".

Fig. d. Naevus composé cutané de la paupière: histopathologie.
Les thèques qui gonflent les crêtes épidermiques ont tendance à migrer dans le derme papillaire ("Abtropfung").

Fig. e. Naevus intradermique de la marge.
Saillie ovalaire épaississant la marge palpébrale sans altération des cils. Souvent achrome il est alors confondu avec un papillome.

Fig. f. Naevus intradermique: histopathologie (Trichrome Masson).
Le naevus, sans contact avec l'épiderme, s'enfonce profondément dans le derme pouvant même atteindre l'hypoderme d'où la nécessité d'exérèses non seulement étendues latéralement mais également en profondeur.

Abb. a. Junctionaler Naevus am Lidrand.

Abb. b. Junctionaler Naevus: Histopathologie.
Die rundlichen oder ovalen, regelmäßigen "Nester" ohne zytologische Anomalien bleiben auf die Dermis-Epidermis-Verbindung beschränkt.

Abb. c. Compound Naevus der Konjunktiva.
Gut abgegrenzte, aber leicht hervorstehende Läsion, mehr oder weniger pigmentiert, manchmal einfach rosa; es ist dann ein "achromer Naevus".

Abb. d. Compound Naevus: Histopathologie.
Die Nester, die die Cristae cutis anschwellen lassen, neigen zur Abtropfung in das Stratum papillare.

Abb. e. Subepithelialer (intradermaler) Naevus am Lidrand.
Ovale, den Lidrand verdickende Erhabenheit ohne Veränderung der Wimpern. Sie ist häufig nicht besonders gefärbt und kann dann mit einem Papillom verwechselt werden.

Abb. f. Subepithelialer Naevus: Histopathologie (Trichromfärbung nach Masson).
Ohne Kontakt mit der Epidermis dringt der Naevus tief in die Dermis ein und kann sogar das Unterhautgewebe erreichen, daher die Notwendigkeit nicht nur seitlich ausgedehnter, sondern auch tief angelegter Exzisionen.

II.1.3 Intradermal naevus (subepidermic or subepithelial)

Clinical features. This lesion is more frequent on the eyelid than on the conjunctiva, often nodular, more or less pigmented, sometimes sprouting a tuft of hair (Plate 17, Fig. e). At the lid margin it can sometimes be confused with a papilloma.

Histopathology. The cell nests have lost all contact with the epithelial basement membrane. At the surface of the lesion the naevocytes present a pseudo-epithelial aspect, with large, round, sometimes multinucleated cells but without any signs of malignancy. At a deeper level most of the round cells become smaller. Some of them become long and flat and take on an onion bulb arrangement: Neuro-naevus of Masson, with "Meissnerian bodies" or "lames foliacées". If the hair follicle is included in the naevus cell proliferation, the term naevus pilosus is used. These naevi may be located very deep and may in the long run undergo a process of involution (Fig. b).

II.1.4 Cystic benign naevus (Parinaud's dermo-epithelioma)

Clinical features. This is a type of compound naevus of the conjunctiva with a preferential location at the limbus. It is mostly observed in children or adolescents. Small cysts are visible under slit lamp examination.

Histopathology. All the characteristic features of a benign compound naevus are present. The pseudocysts are due to invaginations from the epithelial surface.

II.1.5 Balloon cell naevus

This histological variety of compound naevus is characterized by the presence of large cells in close contact with each other, with definite limits, with a clear, finely vesicular cytoplasm. These cytological features can also be found sometimes in a melanoma.

II.1.3 Naevus intradermique ou profond (sous-épidermique ou sous-épithélial)

Clinique. Plus fréquent à la paupière qu'à la conjonctive il est volontiers hémisphérique ou nodulaire plus ou moins pigmenté, parfois surmonté d'une touffe de poils. A la marge palpébrale (Planche 17, Fig. e) il peut être confondu avec un papillome.

Histopathologie. Les thèques n'ont plus aucun rapport avec la basale épithéliale. Dans les plans superficiels les naevocytes ont une morphologie pseudo-épithéliale avec de grandes cellules arrondies multinucléées sans caractère péjoratif. En profondeur les cellules deviennent plus petites et arrondies. D'autres s'allongent, s'aplatissent et se disposent en bulbes d'oignon, c'est le neuro-naevus de Masson, avec les "corps Meissneriens" ou "lames foliacées". Lorsque des follicules pilaires se mêlent à la prolifération naevique on parle de naevus pileux (et non pilaire). Souvent très étendus en profondeur ces naevi peuvent à la longue subir des phénomènes d'involution (Fig. b).

II.1.4 Naevus kystique bénin (dermo-épithéliome de Parinaud)

Clinique. C'est un type de naevus composé particulier à la conjonctive, où il se localise en général. Il est surtout fréquent chez l'enfant et l'adolescent. De petits kystes sont visibles à la lampe à fente.

Histopathologie. Ce sont des naevi composés bénins creusés de cavités pseudo-kystiques. Ces dernières sont dues à des invaginations de l'épithélium de surface.

II.1.5 Naevus à cellules ballonisantes

C'est une simple variante histologique de naevus composé caractérisée par la présence de grandes cellules jointives, à limites nettes, à cytoplasme clair finement vésiculeux. Cet aspect cytologique peut parfois se rencontrer aussi dans un mélanome.

II.1.3 Intradermaler Naevus (subepidermal oder subepithelial)

Klinik. Er tritt häufiger am Lid als an der Bindehaut auf und ist gerne halbkugelig oder knötchenförmig und mehr oder weniger pigmentiert, manchmal sitzt ein Haarbüschel darauf. Am Lidrand kann er mitunter mit einem Papillom verwechselt werden (Tafel 17, Abb. e).

Histopathologie. Die Zellverbände haben keinerlei Zusammenhang mit der epithelialen Basalschicht mehr. An der Oberfläche haben die Naevozyten eine pseudo-epitheliale Morphologie mit großen, abgerundeten, multinukleären Zellen ohne Malignitätszeichen. In der Tiefe werden die Zellen kleiner und runder. Andere werden länger, flacher und ordnen sich zwiebelschalenartig: dies sind die "Meissnerschen Körperchen" (Masson). Wenn sich Haarbälge unter die Naevusproliferation mischen, spricht man von einem Naevus pili. Dieser reicht oft sehr tief und kann sich auf die Dauer zurückbilden (Abb. b).

II.1.4 Gutartiger zystischer Naevus (Dermo-epitheliom nach Parinaud)

Klinik. Dieser spezielle compound naevus der Konjunktiva sitzt zumeist am Limbus. Er kommt vor allem bei Kindern und Jugendlichen häufig vor. An der Spaltlampe beobachtet man kleine Zysten.

Histopathologie. Es sind gutartige compound naevi, durchsetzt von Pseudozysten, daher der von der WHO vorgeschlagene Name gutartiger zystischer Naevus.

II.1.5 Ballonzellnaevus

Er ist eine einfache histologische Variante des compound naevus. Bezeichnend sind die großen, deutlich abgegrenzten, eng aneinanderliegenden Zellen mit hellem, fein vesikulärem Plasma. Deren Vorhandensein gibt jedoch keine absolute Gewähr für Gutartigkeit.

PLATE 18 PLANCHE 18 TAFEL 18

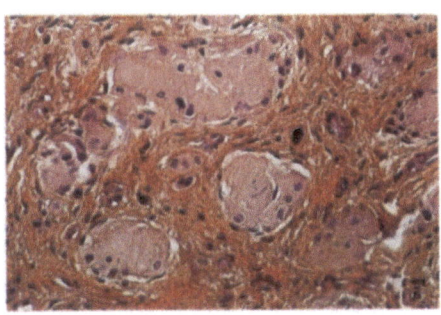

a

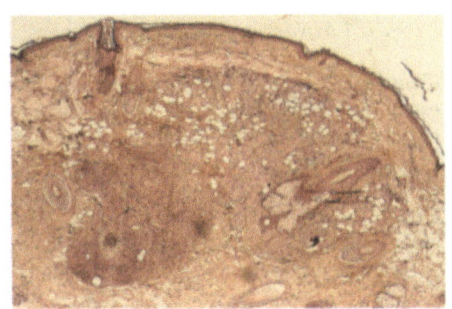

b

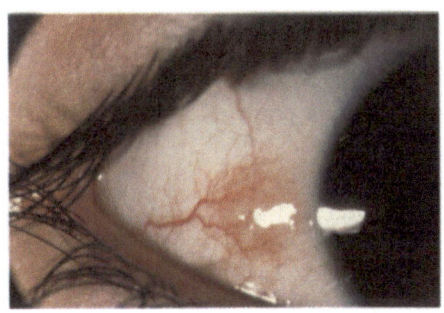

c

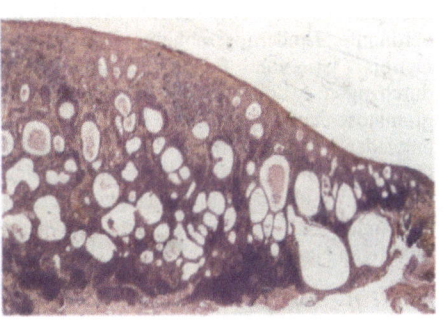

d

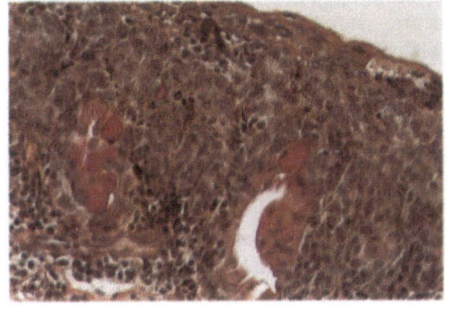

e

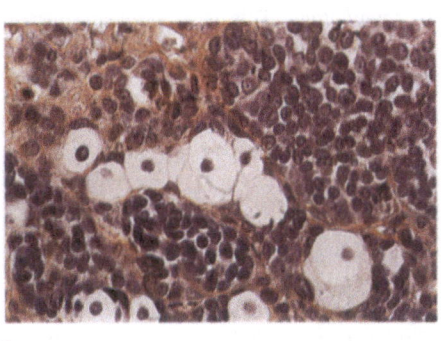

f

Fig. a. Intradermal naevus: "Meissnerian bodies".
These are deeply located, often close to the hair follicles. They are characteristic of the "neuro-naevi" of Masson who considered them to be of Schwannian origin.

Fig. b. Naevus naevo-cellularis partim lipomatodes.
Involution process of an intradermal naevus with fat lobules in the superficial portion of the dermis.

Fig. c. Cystic benign naevus of the limbal conjunctiva.
Pink unpigmented naevus sometimes presenting a stippling of pigment. Slit lamp examination reveals microcysts at the epithelial level.

Fig. d. Cystic benign naevus.
Pseudocystic cavities (invaginations of the conjunctival epithelium) are intermingled with the naevus cell nests.

Fig. e. Cystic benign naevus.
The mucous cells in the epithelium lining the microcysts are here stained with muci-carmin.

Fig. f. Balloon cell naevus.
These clear cells do not contain lipids. They would seem to be naevus cells showing an arrest of melanin biosynthesis.

Fig. a. Naevus intradermique: "corps Meissnériens".
Profonds, souvent au voisinage des follicules pilaires. Ils sont caractéristiques des "neuro-naevi" de Masson qui les considérait comme d'origine schwannienne.

Fig. b. Naevus naevo-cellularis partim lipomatodes.
Processus d'involution d'un naevus intradermique avec lobules adipeux dans le derme superficiel.

Fig. c. Dermo-épithéliome de la conjonctive limbique.
Naevus achrome, rose chair ponctué parfois d'un piqueté pigmenté. L'examen au biomicroscope découvrira dans l'étage épithélial des microkystes.

Fig. d. Naevus kystique bénin.
Des cavités pseudokystiques (épithélium conjonctival invaginé) se mêlent aux thèques naeviques.

Fig. e. Naevus kystique bénin.
Le muci carmin colore des cellules à mucus dans l'épithélium bordant les pseudokystes.

Fig. f. Naevus à cellules ballonisantes.
Les cellules claires ne contiennent pas de lipides. Il s'agirait de cellules naeviques présentant un arrêt de la biosynthèse de la mélanine.

Abb. a. Intradermaler Naevus: "Meissnersche Körperchen".
Tiefgelegen, häufig in der Nachbarschaft von Haarbälgen. Sie sind charakteristisch für die "Neuro-Naevi" nach Masson, der sie als von der Schwann-Scheide ausgehend betrachtete.

Abb. b. Naevus naevo-cellularis partim lipomatodes.
Rückbildung eines intradermalen Naevus mit adipösen Läppchen in der oberflächlichen Dermis.

Abb. c. Gutartiger zystischer Naevus der Conjunctiva am Limbus.
Nicht besonders gefärbter Naevus, fleischrosa, manchmal pigmentiert gesprenkelt. Die Untersuchung unter dem Biomikroskop zeigt Mikrozysten im Epithel.

Abb. d. Gutartiger zystischer Naevus.
Pseudozysten (eingestülptes Bindehautepithel) mischen sich unter Naevus-Zellnester.

Abb. e. Gutartiger zystischer Naevus.
Karmin färbt die Schleimzellen im die Pseudozysten auskleidenden Epithel.

Abb. f. Ballonzellnaevus.
Die hellen Zellen enthalten keine Lipide. Es soll sich um Naevuszellen handeln, bei denen die Melanin-Biosynthese sistiert.

37

II.1.6 Giant pigmented naevus

Clinical features. This large congenital naevus is rare, and its prognosis is uncertain; indeed, this tumour is the main source of malignant melanoma in childhood (1/3 of the cases).

Histopathology. This heavily pigmented naevus, with many hair follicles, can be associated with melanocytosis of the central nervous system.

II.1.7 Juvenile melanoma of S. Spitz (naevus with epithelioid and/or spindle-shaped cells)

Clinical features. It is mostly located on the face of a child before puberty, rarely in an adult. Prominent, hemispherical, sessile, or polypoid and pediculated, it is painless. Its surface is smooth, its colour pink, sometimes red, with patches of pigment.

Histopathology. This is a compound naevus producing bulging and thinning of the epidermis; the superficial layers of the dermis present small telangiectases, whence sometimes an aspect mimicking an angioma. The cells are spindle-shaped or pseudo-epithelial. Certain bizarre cells may arouse suspicion of malignancy but this lesion is always benign.

II.1.8 Blue naevus of Tièche (mesenchymal naevus)

Clinical features. Either flat or prominent, it is of a slate blue colour, sometimes very dark, whence its name.

Histopathology. The tumour consists of spindle-shaped melanocytes overlaid by melanin granules and located deep within the dermis, without any contact with the epithelium. Sometimes the cells are round, globular and rich in melanin: this is the pattern of the "cellular" blue naevus. The association of a blue naevus with an overlying compound naevus is called a "combined" naevus.

II.1.6 Naevus pigmentaire géant

Clinique. Ce naevus congénital étendu, rare, est de pronostic réservé car il reste la principale source de mélanome malin chez l'enfant (1/3 des cas).

Histopathologie. Naevus très pigmenté et riche en annexes pilaires, il peut être associé à une mélanocytose du système nerveux central.

II.1.7 Mélanome juvénile de Spitz (naevus à cellules épithélioïdes et/ou fusiformes)

Clinique. Il siège de préférence à la face chez l'enfant d'âge prépubertaire, rarement chez l'adulte. En dôme ou polypoïde, pédiculé, il est indolore, lisse, de couleur rosée parfois rouge mais tacheté de quelques macules pigmentées.

Histopathologie. C'est un naevus composé soulevant l'épiderme qui est aminci et dont le derme superficiel est parcouru de fines télangiectasies, d'où un aspect parfois angiomateux. Les cellules sont soit fusiformes, soit épithélioïdes. Certaines bizarreries cellulaires ont pu égarer le diagnostic vers la malignité alors qu'il s'agit d'un naevus entièrement bénin.

II.1.8 Naevus bleu de Tièche (naevus mésenchymateux)

Clinique. Plat ou en dôme il doit son nom à sa teinte bleu ardoisé parfois très sombre.

Histopathologie. La tumeur est faite de mélanocytes fusiformes surchargés de mélanine, situés dans le derme profond, sans contact avec l'épithélium de surface. Parfois les cellules sont globuleuses arrondies, riches en mélanine: c'est le naevus bleu "cellulaire". Lorsqu'un naevus bleu se trouve associé à un naevus composé sus-jacent c'est un naevus "combiné".

II.1.6 Riesenpigmental

Klinik. Kongenitaler, großflächiger Naevus, selten, jedoch mit reservierter Prognose, da er nach wie vor beim Kind häufig zum Melanokarzinom führt (1/3 der Fälle).

Histopathologie. Stark pigmentierter, reichlich mit Haaradnexen durchsetzter Naevus. Er kann mit einer Melanozytose des zentralen Nervensystems einhergehen.

II.1.7 Juveniles Spitz Melanom (Naevus mit epitheloiden und/oder spindelförmigen Zellen)

Klinik. Es tritt gewöhnlich im Gesicht des vorpubertären Kindes, selten beim Erwachsenen auf. Es ist vorgewölbt oder polypoid, gestielt, glatt und schmerzlos, rosafarben, manchmal rot, aber durch einige Pigmentflecken gesprenkelt.

Histopathologie. Compound Naevus, der die verdünnte Epidermis anhebt. Die vordere Dermis ist von feinen Telangiektasien durchzogen, woraus sich das bisweilen angiomatöse Aussehen erklärt. Die Zellen sind entweder spindelförmig oder epitheloid. Gewisse bizarre Zellbilder haben in der Diagnose zur Annahme von Bösartigkeit geführt; es handelt sich jedoch um einen durchwegs gutartigen Naevus.

II.1.8 Naevus bleu nach Tièche (Mesenchymaler Naevus)

Klinik. Es ist flach oder leicht vorgewölbt und hat seinen Namen von der manchmal sehr dunklen schieferblauen Färbung.

Histopathologie. Der Tumor besteht aus spindelförmigen, mit Melanin überladenen Pigmentzellen, die tief in der Dermis eingelagert sind und keine Berührung mit dem oberflächlichen Epithel haben. Manchmal sind diese Zellen rundlich, aber melaninreich, dies ist der "zelluläre" blaue Naevus. Tritt ein Naevus bleu zusammen mit einem darüberliegenden Compound naevus auf, so ist dies ein "zusammengesetzter" Naevus.

PLATE 19   PLANCHE 19   TAFEL 19

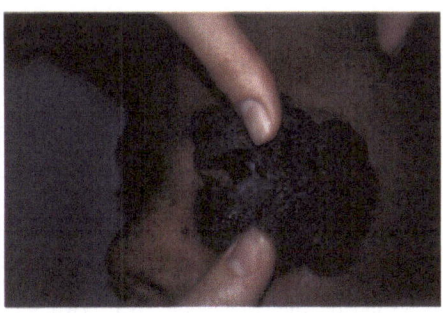

a

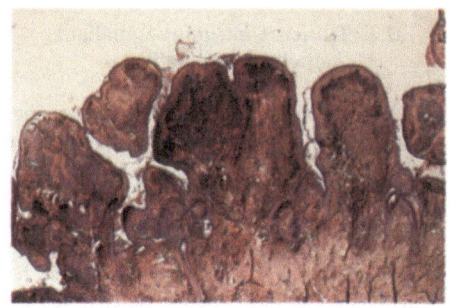

b

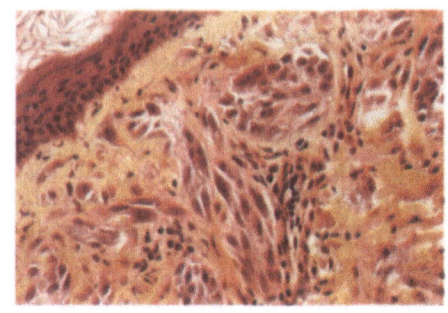

c

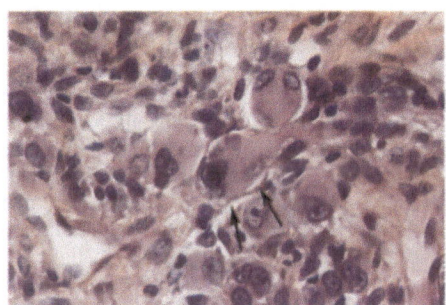

d

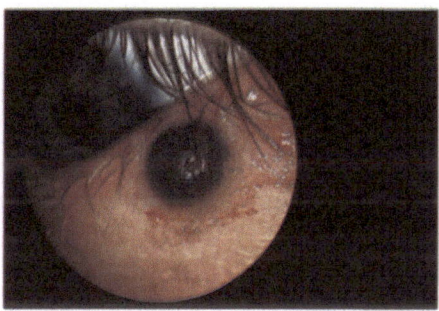

e

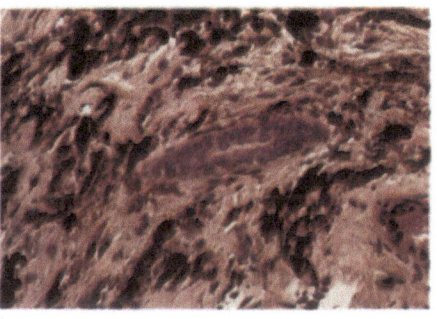

f

Fig. a. Giant pigmented naevus of the eyelid.
Heavily pigmented verrucous naevus involving both lids and inducing their occlusion.

Fig. b. Giant pigmented naevus.
Papillomatous, pigmented compound naevus involving the deeper layers of the skin, where it can present a neuroid structure.

Fig. c. Juvenile melanoma of S. Spitz with spindle cells.
In the upper dermis, the cell nests contain spindle cells with elongated nuclei and their arrangement is perpendicular to the skin surface ("rain drops").

Fig. d. Juvenile melanoma of Spitz with epithelioid cells.
Presence of polygonal eosinophilic cells sometimes presenting abnormal aspects: certain cells are globular, with two nuclei, others are larger at one end with an irregular nucleus ("racket-cell") (➔).

Fig. e. Blue naevus of the eyelid.
Hemispherical, with a smooth surface, and a slate grey colour.

Fig. f. Blue naevus: histopathology.
The deeper layers of the dermis contain heavily pigmented star-shaped or spindle-shaped melanocytes.

Fig. a. Naevus pigmentaire géant des paupières.
Naevus verruqueux très pigmenté envahissant les deux paupières et entraînant leur occlusion.

Fig. b. Naevus pigmentaire géant.
Naevus composé très papillomateux et pigmenté gagnant les plans profonds où il prend souvent un aspect neuroïde.

Fig. c. Mélanome juvénile de Spitz à cellules fusiformes.
Dans le derme superficiel les thèques contiennent des cellules fusiformes à noyau allongé se disposant perpendiculairement à la surface "en gouttes de pluie".

Fig. d. Mélanome juvénile de Spitz à cellules épithélioïdes.
Cellules polygonales éosinophiles à morphologie parfois anormale: certaines cellules sont arrondies, binucléées; d'autres ont une extrémité renflée contenant un noyau irrégulier (cellule "en raquette") (➔).

Fig. e. Naevus bleu de la paupière.
En dôme, lisse, de teinte ardoisée.

Fig. f. Naevus bleu: histopathologie.
Le derme profond est occupé par des mélanocytes rameux ou fusiformes surchargés de pigment mélanique.

Abb. a. Riesenpigmentmal der Lider.
Stark pigmentierter "Warzennaevus", der beide Lider befällt und ihren Verschluß zur Folge hat.

Abb. b. Riesenpigmentmal.
Stark papillomatöser und pigmentierter Compound Naevus, der in die tiefen Schichten eindringt, wo er oft ein neuroides Aussehen annimmt.

Abb. c. Juveniles Spitz Melanom mit spindelförmigen Zellen.
In der vorderen Dermis enthalten die Nester spindelförmige Zellen mit länglichem Kern, die "wie Regentropfen" senkrecht zur Oberfläche angeordnet sind.

Abb. d. Juveniles Spitz Melanom mit epithcloiden Zellen.
Eosinophile polygonale Zellen mit manchmal anormaler Morphologie: manche Zellen sind abgerundet, binukleär, andere haben ein bauchiges Ende mit einem unregelmäßigen Kern ("Tennisschläger-Zellen") (➔).

Abb. e. Blauer Naevus am Lid.
Flach vorgewölbt, glatt, von schieferblauer Farbe.

Abb. f. Naevus bleu: Histopathologie.
Verästelte oder spindelförmige, mit Melaninpigment überladene Melanozyten besetzen die tiefere Dermis.

PLATE 20　　　　　　　　　　　PLANCHE 20　　　　　　　　　　　TAFEL 20

II.2 Malignant melanomas of the eyelids and the conjunctiva

General. It was accepted until recently that malignant melanomas develop either on a preexisting naevus, of the junctional variety particularly, or directly, on a normal skin. It seems now that actually most melanomas, particularly the melanomas on acquired melanosis and the superficial spreading melanomas, present an evolution in two stages:
- the first stage is superficial, along the dermo-epidermal junction: the *extension* is *radial*, and there are no metastases during that stage;
- the second stage is that of the invasion of the underlying dermis: the *extension* is *vertical*, and malignancy certain.

Other melanomas invade the underlying dermis straightaway, without any radial extension beforehand: these are the *nodular melanomas* or melanomas *"de novo"*.

There are however melanomas arising from a preexisting naevus, but they are less frequent than was previously thought. On the other hand, naevi of a certain type (the so called "dysplastic naevi"), which appear in the adult and are sometimes hereditary, are apt to become malignant.

II.2.1 Precancerous Hutchinson-Dubreuilh melanosis, Reese melanosis (melanoma developed on acquired melanosis) or lentigo maligna melanoma

Clinical features. This variety of melanosis appears usually after the age of 60. Brownish spots progressively invade the conjunctiva, the eyelids, and sometimes the cornea. The growth of black nodules is a sign of malignancy.

Histopathology. In Hutchinson-Dubreuilh melanosis, atypical melanocytes proliferate along the basement membrane. Their pigment is partly taken up either by the epithelial cells, or by macrophages of the dermis, which are mixed with inflammatory cells. The invasion of the dermis by large spindle-shaped cells with cyto-nuclear abnormalities and mitotic figures is the sign of malignant transformation (vertical extension stage).

II.2. Tumeurs mélaniques malignes palpébro-conjonctivales

Généralités. Classiquement les mélanomes malins se développaient soit à partir d'un naevus préexistant (jonctionnel notamment); soit d'emblée, en peau saine (mélanome malin d'emblée). Actuellement on admet que la plupart des mélanomes malins, en particulier les mélanomes sur mélanose acquise et les mélanomes à extension superficielle, suivent une évolution biphasique:
- un premier stade superficiel le long de la jonction dermo-épidermique: *extension radiale* au cours de laquelle il n'y aurait pas de métastases;
- un second stade d'envahissement du derme sous-jacent: *extension verticale*, de malignité confirmée.

Enfin d'autres mélanomes envahissent le derme d'emblée sans précession d'extension radiale ce sont les mélanomes *nodulaires* ou *de novo*.

Il reste néanmoins quelques mélanomes naissant d'un naevus préexistant mais leur nombre semble très réduit. Cependant, certains naevi, dits "dysplasiques", qui semblent survenir sur un terrain familial particulier et apparaissent à l'âge adulte, sont susceptibles de dégénérer.

II.2.1 Mélanome sur mélanose précancéreuse de Hutchinson-Dubreuilh, mélanose de Reese (mélanose acquise) encore appelé mélanome sur lentigo malin

Clinique. Cette mélanose apparaît en général après 60 ans sous forme de taches brunes envahissant très progressivement la conjonctive, les paupières, la cornée parfois. L'apparition de nodules noirâtres est signe de dégénérescence.

Histopathologie. Dans la mélanose acquise des mélanocytes atypiques se multiplient le long de la basale. Ils vont rejeter leur pigment d'une part dans les cellules épithéliales, d'autre part dans le chorion où il est repris par des macrophages mêlés à des cellules inflammatoires. L'envahissement du derme par de grandes cellules fusiformes riches en anomalies cyto-nucléaires et en mitoses signe le passage à la malignité (stade d'extension verticale).

II.2 Maligne pigmentierte Tumoren (Melanome) der Lider und Bindehaut

Allgemeines. Nach klassischer, herkömmlicher Auffassung nimmt man an, daß sich bösartige Melanome entweder von einem bereits vorhandenen (vor allem Compound Naevus), oder de novo in gesunder Haut entwickeln. Heute ist man der Auffassung, daß die meisten der bösartigen Melanome, insbesondere die Melanome bei erworbener Melanose und die sich oberflächlich ausbreitenden Melanome, einer Zweiphasenentwicklung unterliegen:
- ein erstes, oberflächliches Stadium entlang der Verbindung zwischen Dermis und Epidermis: seitliche, *radiale Ausbreitung*, in deren Verlauf es nicht zu Metastasen kommen soll;
- ein zweites Stadium des Übergreifens in die darunterliegende Dermis: *vertikale Ausbreitung*, nachweislich bösartig.

Andere Melanome treten direkt, ohne vorherige oberflächliche Ausbreitung, in der Dermis auf; dies sind die *knötchenförmigen Melanome*.

Es bleiben doch noch einige aus einem zuvor vorhandenen Naevus entstehende Melanome, ihre Zahl scheint indes geringer als man glaubte. Die sogenannten "dysplastischen" Naevi, die anscheinend bei bestimmter familiärer Anlage anzutreffen sind und im Erwachsenenalter auftreten, können maligne entarten.

II.2.1 Melanom auf prekanzeröser erworbener Melanose nach Hutchinson-Dubreuilh, Reesescher Melanose, auch Melanom auf Lentigo maligna genannt

Klinik. Die Melanose tritt im allgemeinen nach 60 in Form brauner Flecken, die nach und nach die Bindehaut, die Lider, manchmal die Hornhaut überwuchern, in Erscheinung. Das Auftauchen schwärzlicher Knötchen ist ein Degenerationsanzeichen.

Histopathologie. Im Stadium der oberflächlichen Ausbreitung vermehren sich die atypischen Melanozyten entlang der Basalschicht. Sie geben ihr Pigment einerseits an die Epithelzellen, andererseits an das Stroma ab, wo es von den die entzündlichen Zellen begleitenden Makrophagen aufgenommen wird. Die Infiltration der Dermis mit großen, spindelförmigen Zellen, die vielerlei Zellkernanomalien aufweisen und sich in Mitose befinden, zeigt den vollzogenen Übergang zur Bösartigkeit (vertikale Ausbreitung).

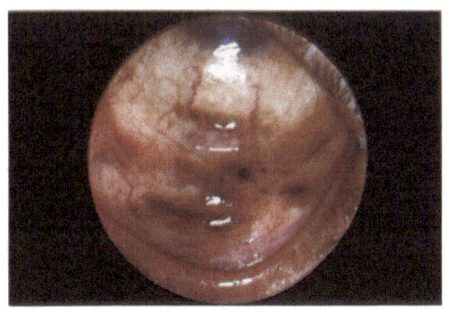

a

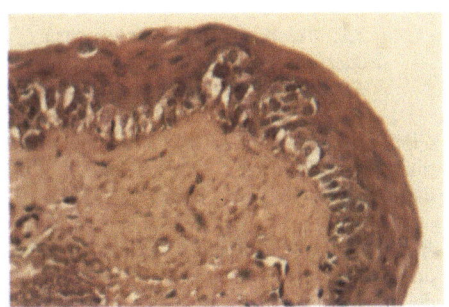

b

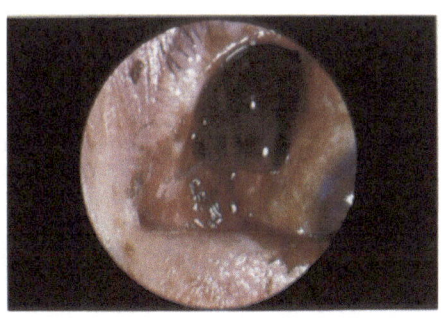

c

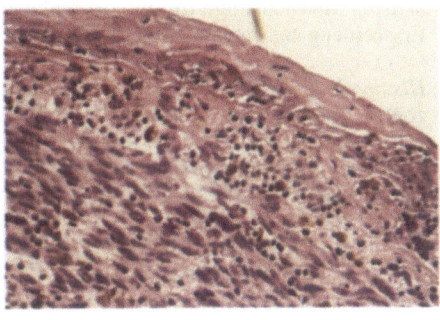

d

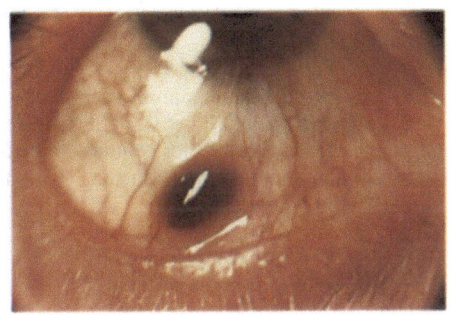

e

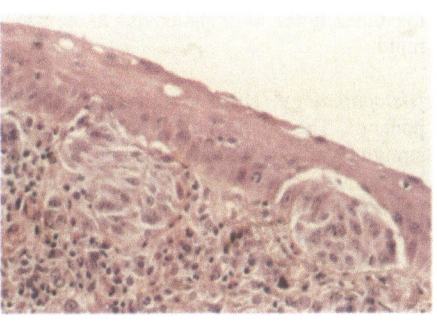

f

Fig. a. Precancerous melanosis of the conjunctiva. Spots of brownish, non-homogeneous colour, of a "dirty" appearance, with ill defined limits, and spreading slowly.

Fig. b. Precancerous melanosis of the conjunctiva. Along the epithelial basement membrane, some spindle-shaped melanocytes present a vertical orientation ("palisade-like"); sometimes they form cell clusters. Their ovoid nuclei are often dystrophic.

Fig. c. Malignant melanoma on a precancerous melanosis. Presence in the fornix of a large black nodule which spreads over the brownish bulbar conjunctiva.

Fig. d. Malignant melanoma on a precancerous melanosis. Proliferation of spindle-shaped cells, surrounded by an infiltrate of inflammatory cells in the subepithelial connective tissue.

Fig. e. SSM of the conjunctiva. Dome shaped lesion with uneven pigmentation, indistinct limits, irregular outlines.

Fig. f. SSM of the conjunctiva: histopathology. Junctional clusters of cells, made up of epithelioid or spindle-shaped cells, and presenting sharp outlines. An inflammatory infiltrate is already noticeable, a preliminary step towards malignancy.

Fig. a. Mélanose précancéreuse de la conjonctive. Plages brunâtres inhomogènes, d'aspect "sale", à limites floues, irrégulières, s'étendant lentement "en tache d'huile".

Fig. b. Mélanose précancéreuse de la conjonctive. Le long de la basale épithéliale des mélanocytes allongés se disposent verticalement "en palissade", parfois groupés en thèques. Leur noyau ovalaire est souvent dystrophique.

Fig. c. Dégénérescence d'une mélanose précancéreuse. Apparition d'un gros nodule noirâtre dans le cul-de-sac s'étalant sur la conjonctive bulbaire brunâtre.

Fig. d. Mélanome sur mélanose précancéreuse. Le chorion est envahi par une prolifération de cellules fusiformes au sein d'un infiltrat inflammatoire.

Fig. e. Mélanome à extension superficielle de la conjonctive. Lésion en dôme, à pigmentation inhomogène, à limites peu nettes.

Fig. f. Mélanome à extension superficielle de la conjonctive: histopathologie. Thèques jonctionnelles à limites nettes composées de cellules fusiformes ou épithélioïdes. Un infiltrat inflammatoire, prélude à la malignité, est déjà présent.

Abb. a. Präkanzeröse Melanose der Bindehaut. Bräunliche, unebenmäßige Felder von "schmutzigem" Aussehen, mit unscharfen Grenzen, unregelmäßig, die sich langsam "ölfleckartig" ausweiten.

Abb. b. Präkanzeröse Melanose der Bindehaut. Entlang der epithelialen Basalschicht ordnen sich längliche Melanozyten senkrecht, "palissadenartig", manchmal zu Nestern zusammengeschlossen an. Ihr ovaler Kern ist oft dystrophisch.

Abb. c. Degeneration einer präkanzerösen Melanose. In der Umschlagsfalte taucht ein dickes, schwärzliches Knötchen auf, das sich auf der bräunlichen Bindehaut des Bulbus ausdehnt.

Abb. d. Melanom auf präkanzeröser Melanose. Das Stroma ist von proliferierenden spindelförmigen Zellen inmitten eines entzündlichen Infiltrats durchsetzt.

Abb. e. Sich oberflächlich ausbreitendes Melanom der Bindehaut. Vorgewölbte Läsion mit ungleichmäßiger Pigmentierung und unscharfen Grenzen (Superficial Spreading Melanoma oder SSM).

Abb. f. Sich oberflächlich ausbreitendes Melanom der Bindehaut: Histopathologie. In der Epithel-Dermis-Übergangszone findet man scharf begrenzte Zellnester mit spindelförmigen oder epitheloiden Zellen. Ein entzündliches Infiltrat, erstes Anzeichen für Bösartigkeit, ist bereits vorhanden.

41

II.2.2 Superficial spreading melanoma (SSM)

Clinical features. It appears in middle aged patients and its diameter rarely exceeds a few centimeters (Plate 20, Fig. e).

Histopathology. During the radial spreading stage the spheroid nests of cells remain located along the epithelial basement membrane; some cells migrate individually into the overlying epithelium (pagetoid invasion) but there is no pigment in the chorion. Formerly this type of melanoma was sometimes mistaken for a junctional naevus. The presence of a vertical proliferation is the sign of malignancy (vertical extension stage).

II.2.3 Nodular melanoma

Clinical features. It appears around the fifth decade and is fortunately less frequent than the other types of melanomas. Its course is rapid.

Histopathology. There is no horizontal component. The dermis is deeply invaded straightaway. The cells present numerous monstrosities and are surrounded by an inflammatory reaction.

Prognosis of the palpebro-conjunctival melanomas

Prognosis depends on:
- the histogenetical type;
- the depth of the invasion;
- the location of the tumour on the conjunctiva.

Histogenetical type. The nodular melanoma soon produces metastases; its prognosis is poor. The SSM presents only radial extension for 2 to 5 years before invading the dermis. The death rate after 5 years is from 30% to 50%. The melanoma on lentigo maligna has a better prognosis:
- its period of radial extension is long (sometimes up to 15 years);
- regional lymph nodes are less often invaded;
- the death rate after 5 years is from 15% to 20%.

Vertical extension. The classification into 5 levels according to Clark is in fact not applicable in ophthalmology. Breslow's criteria are more useful: the prognosis is excellent as long as the maximal thickness of the tumour, as measured with a micrometic eyepiece, does not exceed 0.75 mm; it becomes uncertain above 1.5 mm.

Localization of the lesion in the conjunctiva. The prognosis of melanomas is much worse if they are located in a fornix or at the caruncle rather than on the bulbus, where the dense, almost avascular sclera is an obstacle to invasion.

II.2.2 Mélanome superficiel extensif (Superficial spreading melanoma ou SSM des auteurs anglo-saxons)

Clinique. Dépassant rarement quelques centimètres de diamètre il survient chez l'adulte d'âge moyen (Planche 20, Fig. e.).

Histopathologie. Au stade d'extension radiale des thèques arrondies restent situées le long de la basale épithéliale; certaines cellules émigrent individuellement dans l'épithélium sus-jacent (envahissement pagétoïde) mais il n'y a pas de pigment dans le chorion. Ce mélanome a pu être confondu dans le passé avec un naevus jonctionnel. L'extension en profondeur de la prolifération affirme sa malignité (stade d'extension verticale).

II.2.3 Mélanome nodulaire

Clinique. Heureusement plus rare que les autres types de mélanome, il apparaît aux environs de la cinquantième année et évolue rapidement.

Histopathologie. Il ne comporte aucune composante horizontale. Il envahit d'emblée, profondément le derme et les cellules contiennent de nombreuses monstruosités au sein d'une réaction inflammatoire.

Pronostic des mélanomes palpébro-conjonctivaux

Il dépend:
- du type histogénétique;
- du degré d'extension en profondeur;
- du siège de la tumeur sur la conjonctive.

Type histogénétique. Le mélanome nodulaire est le plus redoutable: il métastase précocement. Le SSM évolue pendant 2 à 5 ans avant d'envahir le derme. Le pourcentage de décès à 5 ans est de 30 à 50%. Le mélanome sur mélanose de Dubreuilh a le moins mauvais pronostic:
- sa période d'évolution radiale non métastasiante est souvent très longue (15 ans parfois);
- il essaimerait moins dans les aires ganglionnaires;
- son pourcentage de décès à 5 ans serait de 15 à 20%.

Extension en profondeur. La classification en cinq niveaux de Clark est en fait inapplicable dans le domaine oculaire. On utilisera plutôt les critères de Breslow basés sur l'évaluation à l'oculaire micrométrique de la plus grande épaisseur de la tumeur: au-dessous de 0,75 mm le pronostic serait excellent alors qu'au-delà de 1,5 mm il devient beaucoup plus réservé.

Localisation topographique. A la conjonctive, les mélanomes des culs-de-sac ou de la caroncule sont de pronostic beaucoup plus grave que ceux de la conjonctive bulbaire où la sclère, dense et peu vasculaire, forme une barrière à l'invasion.

II.2.2 Sich oberflächlich ausbreitendes Melanom (Superficial Spreading Melanoma (SSM))

Klinik. Es hat selten mehr als ein paar Zentimeter Durchmesser und tritt beim Erwachsenen mittleren Alters auf (Tafel 20, Abb. e).

Histopathologie. Im Stadium der oberflächlichen Ausbreitung bleiben rundliche Nester entlang der epithelialen Basalschicht bestehen; manche Zellen wandern einzeln in das darübergelegene Epithel ein (Pagetoide Wucherung), aber im Chorion findet sich kein Pigment. Dieses Melanom konnte früher mit einem junktionalen Naevus verwechselt werden. Bezeichnend für die Bösartigkeit ist das Tiefenwachstum der Proliferation (vertikale Ausbreitung)

II.2.3 Noduläres Melanom

Klinik. Es ist glücklicherweise seltener als die anderen Melanomarten, tritt um die fünfzig in Erscheinung und entwickelt sich rasch.

Histopathologie. Es enthält keinerlei horizontale Komponente. Es dringt sofort tief in die Dermis ein, und die Zellen weisen zahlreiche Abnormitäten innerhalb eines Gebietes mit entzündlicher Reaktion auf.

Prognose der Melanome der Lider und Bindehaut

Sie hängt vom:
- histogenetischen Typ;
- vom Grad der Tiefendurchsetzung;
- von der Lokalisation in der Bindehaut ab.

Histogenetischer Typ. Das noduläre Melanom ist das gefährlichste: es bildet frühzeitig Metastasen. Das SSM entwickelt sich über 2 bis 5 Jahre, bevor es in die Dermis eindringt. Die Mortalität nach 5 Jahren liegt bei 30 bis 50%. Das Melanom bei einer Melanose nach Dubreuilh hat die am wenigsten schlechte Prognose:
- die Dauer der oberflächlichen Ausbreitung ohne Metastasenbildung ist oft recht lang (manchmal 15 Jahre);
- es soll sich seltener in den Lymphknoten ausbreiten;
- die Mortalität nach 5 Jahren soll bei 15 bis 20% liegen.

Eindringen in die Tiefe. Die Clarksche Fünfstufeneinteilung ist am Auge nicht anwendbar. Es sind eher die Breslowschen Kriterien anzuwenden, die auf der mit dem Mikrometerokular festgehaltenen größten Tumordicke beruhen: unter 0,75 mm soll die Prognose ausgezeichnet sein, während sie bei über 1,5 mm viel schlechter wird.

Lokalisation in der Bindehaut. Die Prognose ist bedeutend schlechter bei Lokalisationen im Fornix oder in der Karunkel als in der Bulbusbindehaut. Die dicke und wenig gefäßführende Sklera ist hier ein Hindernis für die Ausbreitung.

PLATE 21 PLANCHE 21 TAFEL 21

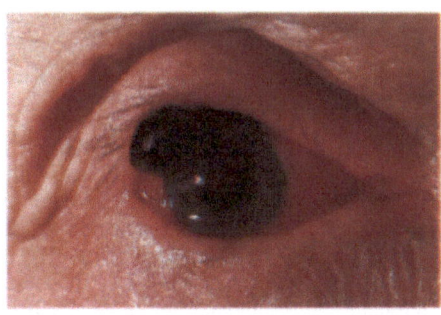

a

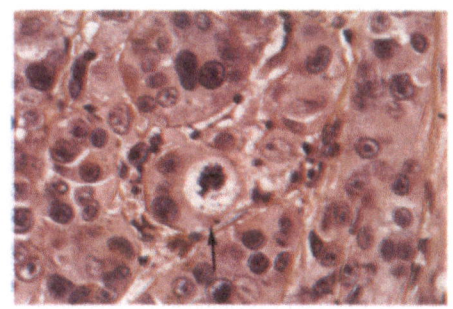

b

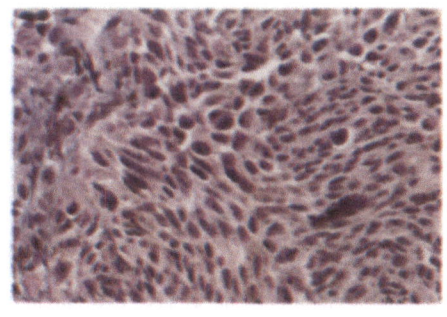

c

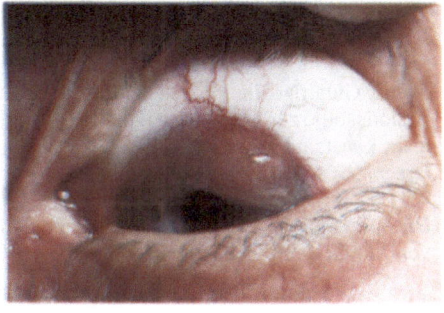

d

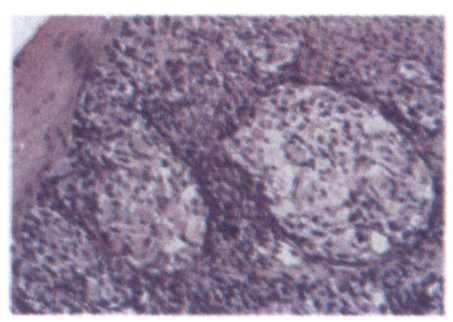

e

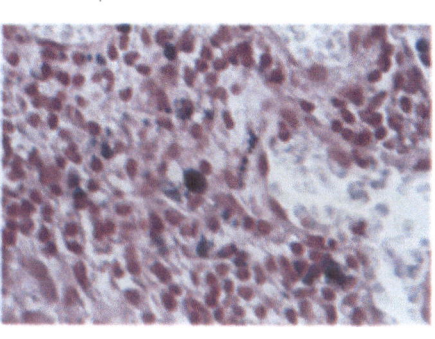

f

Fig. a. Nodular melanoma of the conjunctiva.
Blackish pediculate mass bulging under the eyelid; conjunctival hyperhaemia provides evidence of a simultaneous inflammatory reaction. This type of tumour can rapidly become ulcerated.

Fig. b. Nodular melanoma of the conjunctiva with "epithelioid" cell-type.
Clusters of large cells with eosinophilic cytoplasm, almost no melanin, hypertrophic nucleus, with a large nucleolus, numerous mitotic figures (→).

Fig. c. Nodular melanoma of the conjunctiva presenting a mixed, spindle-shaped – epithelioid structure.

Fig. d. Clinically unpigmented melanoma of the limbus.
Surgical excision has been followed by recurrences after one year, and after four years. At that time an acquired melanosis was seen, partly .pigmented, partly sine pigmento.

Fig. e. Naevo-carcinoma with slight pigmentation; histopathology of case showed in Fig. d.

Fig. f. The presence of melanin becomes obvious with Fontana's silver stain.

Fig. a. Mélanome nodulaire de la conjonctive.
Masse noirâtre, pendulaire, saillante sous la paupière et accompagnée d'une réaction inflammatoire dont témoigne l'hyperhémie conjonctivale. Une telle tumeur peut rapidement s'ulcérer.

Fig. b. Mélanome nodulaire de la conjonctive de type "épithélioïde".
Grandes cellules groupées en thèques, à cytoplasme éosinophile contenant peu de mélanine, à noyau hypertrophique, à gros nucléole et souvent en mitose (→).

Fig. c. Mélanome nodulaire de la conjonctive à cytologie mixte fusiforme et épithélioïde.

Fig. d. Mélanome cliniquement achrome du limbe.
L'exérèse chirurgicale a été suivie d'une récidive locale après un an, puis après 4 ans. A ce moment on a noté une mélanose acquise récente, en partie pigmentée, en partie sine pigmento.

Fig. e. Aspect de naevo-carcinome à pigmentation discrète; histopathologie du cas de la Fig. d.

Fig. f. Cette pigmentation apparait évidente après coloration de Fontana.

Abb. a. Noduläres Melanom der Bindehaut.
Schwärzliche, bewegliche, vorstehende Masse, unter dem Lid vortretend, begleitet von einer entzündlichen Reaktion, auf welche die Bindehauthyperämie hinweist. Ein solcher Tumor kann rasch geschwürig aufbrechen.

Abb. b. Noduläres Melanom der Bindehaut vom "epitheloiden" Typ.
Große, zu Nestern gruppierte Zellen mit eosinophilem Plasma, wenig Melanin enthaltend. Hypertrophische Kerne mit großen Nukleolen, häufig in Mitose (→).

Abb. c. Noduläres Melanom der Bindehaut, gemischtzellig aus spindelförmigen und epithelartigen Zellen.

Abb. d. Klinisch unpigmentiertes Melanom des Limbus.
Rezidive wurden 1 Jahr und 4 Jahre nach der Exzision beobachtet.

Abb. e. Naevo-Karzinom mit leichtem Pigmentgehalt: Histopathologie des Falles von Abb. d.

Abb. f. Die Silberfärbung nach Fontana zeigt eindeutig diese Pigmentation.

III. XANTHOMATOUS TUMOURS

III.1 Tuberous xanthoma of the lid

Clinical features. When the condition is one of the signs of a hypercholesterolemic hereditary, or of a secondary, xanthomatosis, it can be found in association with other cutaneous or tendinous localizations. If there is no hyperlipemia it is a normocholesterolemic xanthomatosis. The exceptionally rare normolipemic xanthomatosis of Montgomery-Polano, a variety of the latter, may present with corneo-conjunctival involvement. (For clinical description see legend Fig. a.)

Histopathology. The epidermis is normal. The abnormal histiocytes proliferate in the superficial and middle dermis.

III.2 Xanthelasma

Clinical features. This benign skin lesion is usually located near the inner canthus. It is advisable to check serum cholesterol, though it is usually normal. (For clinical description see legend Fig. c).

Histopathology. Areas of lipidized cells are located in the dermis.

III.3 Juvenile xanthogranuloma of the eyelid and conjunctiva (Naevo-xantho-endothelioma)

Clinical features. Involvement of eyelids and conjunctiva is rare as compared with that of the iris (Plate 45, Chapter XXII.4). It may be observed in nurslings during the first year and disappear spontaneously after some months. It is usually found together with other similar skin lesions. On the eyelid it is a small yellow or brownish, oval, well limited, papular lesion. When the conjunctiva is involved it is usually at the limbus.

Histopathology. This motley lesion is characterized by the simultaneous presence in the dermis, often in its deeper layers, of both xanthoma and inflammatory cells. In the early stages numerous thin-walled vessels with large endothelial cells are present. Later on, fibrosis will appear and finally become predominant.

III. TUMEURS XANTHOMATEUSES

III.1. Xanthome tubéreux palpébral

Clinique. Il peut faire partie du tableau d'une xanthomatose hypercholestérolémique familiale ou secondaire et être alors associé à d'autres éléments cutanés ou tendineux. Lorsqu'il n'existe pas d'hyperlipémie il s'agit de xanthomatose normocholestérolémique dont fait partie l'exceptionnelle xanthomatose normolipidémique de Montgomery-Polano où on peut rencontrer des localisations conjonctivo-cornéennes. (Description clinique cf légende Fig. a.)

Histopathologie. L'épiderme est normal et la prolifération d'histiocytes pathologiques se situe dans le derme superficiel et moyen.

III.2. Xanthélasma (ou xanthome plan)

Clinique. Lésion bénigne localisée à l'angle interne des paupières, elle doit faire rechercher une hypercholestérolémie qui est loin d'être constante (Description clinique cf. légende Fig. c).

Histopathologie. Le derme est occupé par des plages de cellules xanthélasmisées.

III.3 Xanthogranulome juvénile de la paupière et de la conjonctive (Naevo-xantho-endotheliome)

Clinique. Les localisations palpébro-conjonctivales du xanthogranulome juvénile sont plus rares que celles de l'uvée (Planche 45, Chapitre XXII.4). Elles sont le fait de nourrissons dans la première année de la vie et s'effacent spontanément en quelques mois ou années. Elles peuvent être solitaires mais en fait elles sont souvent associées à d'autres localisations cutanées. A la paupière c'est une petite papule circonscrite ovalaire, indolore, jaunâtre ou jaune brun. La conjonctive peut être intéressée surtout dans la région du limbe.

Histopathologie. Lésion bigarrée caractérisée par la présence dans le derme d'un amas cellulaire dense souvent étendu en profondeur, à la fois xanthomateux et inflammatoire. Au début, des vaisseaux nombreux, à parois fines, à endothélium turgescent, parcourent la lésion mais plus tard apparaît une fibrose qui finit par dominer.

III. XANTHOMATÖSE TUMOREN

III.1 Tuberöses Xanthom des Lides

Klinik. Es kann Teil einer familiären, durch Hypercholesterinämie verursachten oder sekundären Xanthomatose sein und dann mit anderen Haut- oder Sehnenveränderungen einhergehen. Bei nicht vorhandener Hyperlipämie handelt es sich um die normocholesterolämische Xanthomatose, zu der auch die nur ausnahmsweise auftretende normolipidämische Xanthomatose nach Montgomery-Polano gehört, bei der es zu conjunktiva-cornealer Beteiligung kommen kann. (Beschreibung unter Legende zu Abb. a.)

Histopathologie. Die Epidermis ist normal, und die Vermehrung der pathologischen Histiozyten erfolgt in der oberen und mittleren Dermis.

III.2 Xanthelasma des Lides (oder flaches Xanthom)

Klinik. Gutartige, im inneren Winkel gelegene Läsion, sollte zur Suche nach einer bei weitem nicht konstanten Hypercholesterinämie veranlassen. (Beschreibung unter Legende Abb. c).

Histopathologie. Die Dermis ist mit Feldern von Xanthelasma-Zellen belegt.

III.3 Juveniles Xanthogranulom des Lides und der Konjunktiva (Naevo-xantho-endotheliom)

Klinik. Das juvenile Xanthogranulom tritt seltener am Lid und an der Bindehaut auf als in der Uvea (Tafel 45, Kapitel XXII.4). Es ist bei Säuglingen im ersten Lebensjahr anzutreffen und verschwindet spontan in einigen Monaten oder Jahren. Es kann einzeln auftreten, kommt aber häufig zusammen mit anderen Hautlokalisationen vor. Auf dem Lid ist es eine kleine, kreisförmig umschriebene oder ovale, schmerzlose, gelbliche oder gelblich-braune Papel. Die Bindehaut kann davon vor allem im Limbusbereich betroffen sein.

Histopathologie. Uneinheitliche Läsion, gekennzeichnet durch eine dichte, häufig in die Tiefe reichende, gleichzeitig xanthomathöse und entzündliche Zellanhäufung. Zu Beginn durchsetzen zahlreiche feinwandige Gefäße mit geschwollenem Endothelium die Läsion, aber später tritt eine Fibrose auf, die schließlich dominiert.

PLATE 22 PLANCHE 22 TAFEL 22

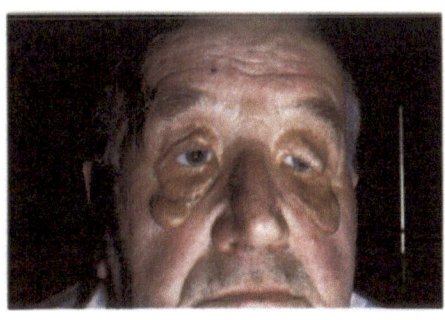

a

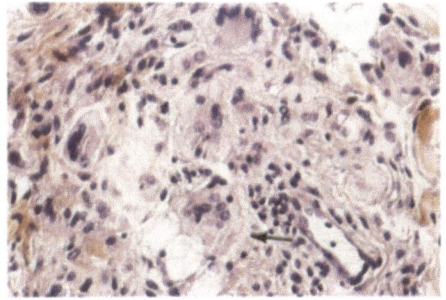

b

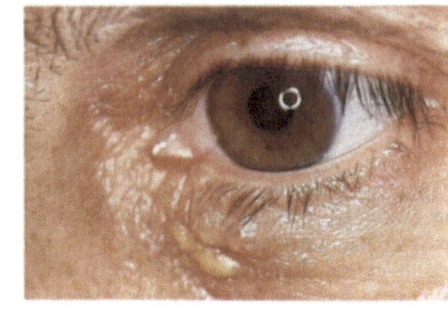
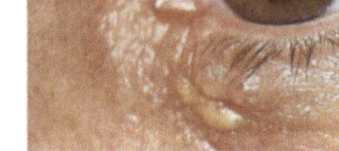

c

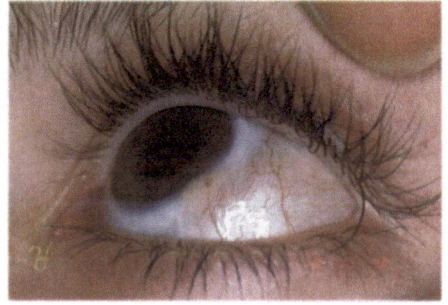

d

e

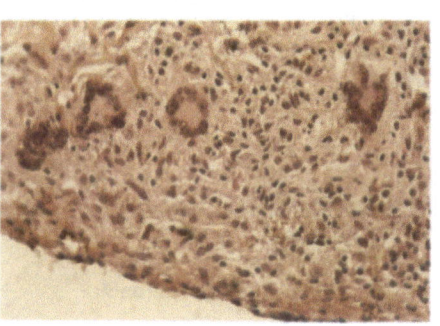

f

Fig. a. Tuberous xanthoma.
Nodular, sometimes pediculate, yellowish, painless lesions of soft consistency, which deform the eyelids.

Fig. b. Infiltrate made of histiocytes with foamy cytoplasm, filled with lipid droplets (xanthoma cells).
Presence of Touton multinucleated cells in which the nuclei are arranged in a circle; the cytoplasm is homogeneous in the center, foamy at the periphery (→).

Fig. c. Xanthelasma.
Small flat yellowish papules near the medial canthus.

Fig. d. Xanthelasma: histopathology.
In the dermis, presence of lipidized cells with their nuclei in the center (and not peripheral as in the adipocyte). These cells are chiefly grouped around the vessels and epidermal appendages. Touton cells are exceptional here.

Fig. e. Juvenile xanthogranuloma of the limbus.
Prominent, well vascularized lesion. Photophobia and epiphora are common symptoms.

Fig. f. Juvenile xanthogranuloma of the conjunctiva: histopathology.
Proliferation of histiocytes, some of which are lipidized. Presence of many Touton cells, and mononucleated leucocytes.

Fig. a. Xanthomes tubéreux.
Formations nodulaires et pendulaires molles indolores et jaunâtres alourdissant les paupières.

Fig. b. Infiltrat fait d'histiocytes à cytoplasme spumeux remplis de gouttelettes lipidiques (cellules "xanthélasmisées").
Présence de quelques cellules de Touton: plasmodes multinucléées dont les noyaux en couronne entourent une zone cytoplasmique centrale homogène cependant que la périphérie est finement vacuolaire (→).

Fig. c. Xanthélasma.
Petites papules jaunâtres aplaties de l'angle interne des paupières.

Fig. d. Xanthélasma: histopathologie.
Présence dans le derme de plages de cellules xanthélasmisées à petit noyau central (et non périphérique comme dans les adipocytes). Elles se groupent plus volontiers au voisinage des vaisseaux et des annexes et contiennent des cholestérides. Les cellules de Touton y sont rares.

Fig. e. Xanthogranulome juvénile du limbe.
Lésion saillante, bien vascularisée. Elle peut entraîner photophobie et larmoiement.

Fig. f. Xanthogranulome juvénile de la conjonctive: histopathologie.
Prolifération d'histiocytes dont certains sont xanthélasmisés. Nombreuses cellules de Touton, nombreux leucocytes mononucléés.

Abb. a. Tuberöses Xanthom.
Knötchenförmige und gestielte, weiche, schmerzlose und gelbliche, die Lider beschwerende Gebilde.

Abb. b. Infiltrat aus Histiozyten mit schaumigem Zytoplasma, die mit Lipidtröpfchen gefüllt sind (sogenannte Xanthelasma-Zellen).
Anwesenheit einiger Touton-Zellen: mehrkernige Plasmodien, deren kranzförmig angeordnete Kerne eine zentrale, gleichmäßige Zytoplasmazone umgeben, während die Zytoplasmaperipherie fein vakuolisiert ist (→).

Abb. c. Xanthelasma.
Kleine gelbliche, abgeflachte Papeln im inneren Augenwinkel.

Abb. d. Xanthelasma: Histopathologie.
In der Dermis befinden sich deutlich abgegrenzte Felder von hellen Zellen mit schaumigem Zytoplasma ("xanthelasmaartige Zellen") mit kleinem zentralem (und nicht wie bei den Fettzellen peripherem) Kern. Sie liegen mit Vorliebe in Gefäß- und Hautadnexenhöhe und enthalten Cholesteride. Touton-Zellen sind darin selten.

Abb. e. Juveniles Xanthogranulom am Limbus.
Erhabene Läsion, gut vaskularisiert. Sie kann Photophobie und Tränen zur Folge haben.

Abb. f. Juveniles Xanthogranulom der Konjunktiva: Histopathologie.
Vermehrung von Histiozyten, von denen manche xanthelasmaartig sind. Zahlreiche Touton-Zellen, zahlreiche mononukleäre Leukozyten.

45

PLATE 23 PLANCHE 23 TAFEL 23

IV. VASCULAR BENIGN TUMOURS

IV.1 Palpebro-conjunctival lymphangiomas

Clinical features. Lymphangiomas are usually present at birth, but owing to their very slow progression, they are often noticed only in childhood or adolescence. In the eyelid they are pink, fluctuant subcutaneous masses; in the conjunctiva they are more obvious. Their limits are mostly imprecise, and they can extend into the orbit or to the face. Their evolution occurs in haemorrhagic episodes, with palpebral ecchymoses, and attacks of inflammation with local pain.

Histopathology. These lymphangiomas are of the cavernous type: their cavities contain a seroproteic liquid and lymphocytes, rarely red blood cells. Because they extend diffusely into the adjacent tissues, their surgical excision is difficult and can be followed by bouts of inflammation which alter their histological aspect.

V. VASCULAR MALIGNANT TUMOURS

V.1 Kaposi's sarcoma

Clinical features. Formerly exceptionally observed in the ocular area – except in central Africa – Kaposi's sarcoma has been recognized recently as one of the signs of AIDS and as such its palpebro-conjunctival involvement must be considered here. On the eyelid it presents as a red, richly vascularized nodule, sometimes mimicking a chalazion. On the lid margin it recalls a telangiectasic granuloma. It is not rare in the conjunctiva (Fig. c).

Histopathology. Cells of vascular type and spindle-shaped pseudosarcomatous cells are mixed in variable proportions. Modern techniques of immuno-labelling and ultrastructure tend to favour a vascular origin from mesenchymal vasoformative cells.

VI. TUMOURS OF ADIPOSE TISSUE

VI.1 Lipoma of the conjunctiva

Clinical features. This benign tumour appears mostly in a male patient after fifty, and can be bilateral; its preferential location is the supero-temporal conjunctiva.

Histopathology. A thin layer of connective tissue separates the tumour from the epithelium. Owing to its indistinct limits, it is often difficult to differentiate a true lipoma from herniated orbital fat through a dehiscent septum.

IV. TUMEURS VASCULAIRES BÉNIGNES

IV.1 Lymphangiomes palpébro-conjonctivaux

Clinique. Tumeurs d'ordinaire congénitales, les lymphangiomes sont d'évolution lente si bien qu'ils ne sont souvent perceptibles qu'au cours de l'enfance ou de l'adolescence. A la paupière ce sont des masses sous-cutanées fluctuantes de couleur rosée; lorsqu'elles atteignent la conjonctive elles deviennent plus visibles. Ils sont en règle diffus, pouvant gagner l'orbite ou déborder sur la face. Ils évoluent par poussées émaillées d'hémorragies, d'ecchymoses palpébrales et de poussées inflammatoires accompagnées de douleurs.

Histopathologie. Ce sont des lymphangiomes de type caverneux dont les cavités contiennent un liquide séro-albumineux et des lymphocytes, rarement quelques hématies. Ils infiltrent de façon diffuse les tissus voisins si bien que leur exérèse chirurgicale est très délicate, pouvant être suivie de lymphoedème et de poussées inflammatoires qui remanient la lésion.

V. TUMEURS VASCULAIRES MALIGNES

V.1 Sarcome de Kaposi

Clinique. Auparavant exceptionnel dans la sphère oculaire sauf en Afrique centrale, le sarcome de Kaposi s'est révélé être ces dernières années une des manifestations du SIDA et sa localisation palpébro-conjonctivale doit être connue. Sur la paupière c'est un nodule rouge, angiomateux pouvant simuler un chalazion vascularisé. Sur la marge palpébrale il simule un bourgeon charnu. Enfin il n'est pas rare à la conjonctive (Fig. c).

Histopathologie. Prolifération faite d'éléments vasculaires et de cellules fusiformes d'allure sarcomateuse en proportions variables comprises dans un réseau de réticuline. Les techniques modernes d'immuno-marquage et l'ultrastructure plaident en faveur d'une origine vasculaire à partir d'éléments mésenchymateux à pouvoir vasoformateur.

VI. TUMEURS DU TISSU ADIPEUX

VI.1 Lipome de la conjonctive

Clinique. Tumeur bénigne rencontrée le plus souvent dans le sexe masculin après 50 ans, elle siège en général dans la partie supérotemporale de la conjonctive bulbaire et peut être bilatérale.

Histopathologie. La tumeur, séparée de l'épithélium par une mince lame de tissu conjonctif, est souvent mal limitée en profondeur si bien qu'il est difficile de dire s'il s'agit d'un lipome vrai ou d'une hernie de la graisse orbitaire à travers une déhiscence du septum.

IV. GUTARTIGE GEFÄßTUMOREN

IV.1 Palpebral-konjunktivale Lymphangiome

Klinik. Lymphangiome sind gewöhnlich kongenitale Tumoren und entwickeln sich langsam, so daß sie sich in vielen Fällen erst im Lauf der Kindheit oder Jugend bemerkbar machen. Am Lid sind es subkutane, fluktuirende, rosafarbene Massen; wenn sie die Bindehaut erreichen, werden sie deutlicher sichtbar. Sie sind im allgemeinen diffus, können auf die Orbita übergreifen oder sich auf das Gesicht ausdehnen. Sie entwickeln sich schubweise mit Blutungen, flächenhaften Ecchymosen an den Lidern oder als mit Schmerzen einhergehende Entzündungen.

Histopathologie. Es sind Lymphangiome vom kavernösen Typ, deren Hohlräume eine serösalbuminöse Flüssigkeit und Lymphozyten, selten einige Erythrozyten, enthalten. Sie infiltrieren diffus das umliegende Gewebe, so daß ihre operative Entfernung sehr heikel ist, da sie Lymphödeme und entzündliche Schübe nach sich ziehen können, welche das Bild der Läsion wieder ändern.

V. MALIGNE GEFÄßTUMOREN

V.1 Kaposi Sarkom

Klinik. Das früher außer in Zentralafrika nur ausnahmsweise im Augenbereich aufgetretene Kaposi-Sarkom erwies sich in den letzten Jahren als eines der AIDS-Anzeichen, und seine Lokalisation am Lid und an der Bindehaut muß bekannt sein. Am Lid ist es ein rotes, angiomatöses Knötchen, das für ein vaskularisiertes Chalazion gehalten werden kann. Am Lidrand täuscht es ein fleischiges Wärzchen vor. Nicht selten kommt es an der Bindehaut vor (Abb. c).

Histopathologie. Wucherung aus Gefäßelementen und spindelförmigen, sarkomartigen Zellen in unterschiedlichen Anteilen. Die modernen Immun-Markierungstechniken und die Ultrastruktur plädieren für eine vaskuläre Ursache, ausgehend von mesenchymalen Elementen mit der Fähigkeit, Gefäße zu bilden.

VI. TUMORE DES FETTGEWEBES

VI.1 Lipom der Bindehaut

Klinik. Gutartiger, zumeist bei über fünfzigjährigen Männern anzutreffender Tumor, der im allgemeinen im oberen temporalen Teil der Conjunctiva bulbi auftritt, bisweilen beidseitig.

Histopathologie. Der vom Epithel durch eine dünne Bindegewebslamelle getrennte Tumor ist gegen die Tiefe zu schlecht abgegrenzt, so daß schwer zu sagen ist, ob es sich um ein echtes Lipom oder um einen Prolaps des Orbitalfettes durch eine Septumdehiszenz handelt.

46

PLATE 23 PLANCHE 23 TAFEL 23

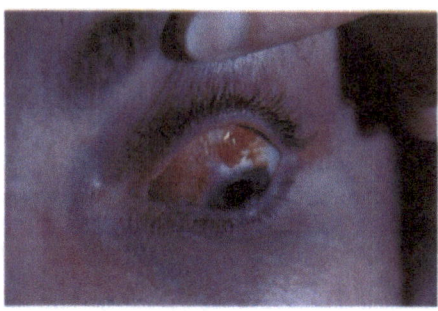

a

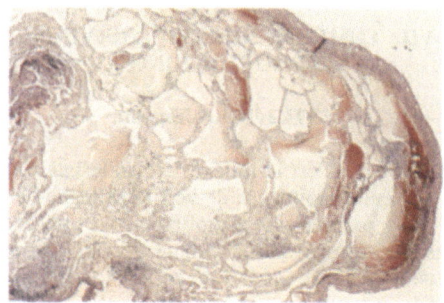

b

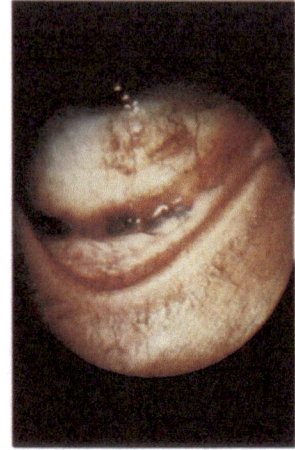

c

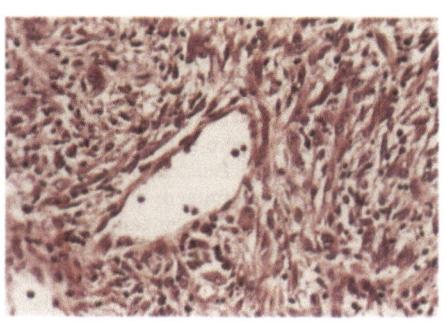

d

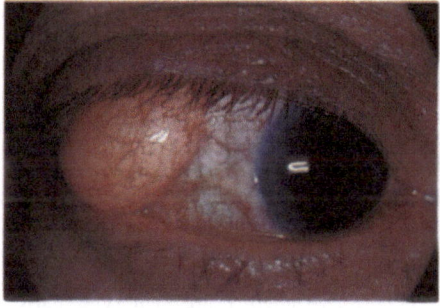

e

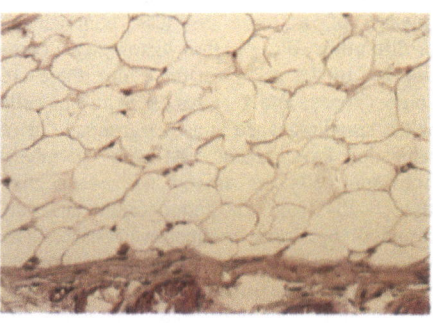

f

Fig. a. Lymphangioma of the conjunctiva.
Irregular subconjunctival lymphatic dilatations, some of them containing red blood cells.

Fig. b. Cavernous lymphangioma made of vascular type cavities with irregular walls and a flattened endothelium. They contain a more or less strongly eosinophilic liquid, but no blood.

Fig. c. Kaposi's sarcoma of the conjunctiva.
Moniliform vascular dilatations surrounded by haemorrhages in the inferior fornix. A superficial examination could lead to the diagnosis of subconjunctival haemorrhage.

Fig. d. Kaposi's sarcoma: histopathology.
Compact area of spindle-shaped cells, some of which have definitely dystrophic nuclei. A vessel with a well-defined wall is seen. Sometimes simple vascular cavities lined by tumour cells are present. A more or less important reactive inflammation and diffuse haemorrhages accompany this tumour cell proliferation.

Fig. e. Lipoma of the conjunctiva.
In the supero-temporal quadrant there is a yellowish-pink prominent nodule with a smooth surface. The conjunctiva is freely mobile on it.

Fig. f. Lipoma of the conjunctiva: histopathology.
The tumour is made of fatty tissue: the cells present an optically empty cytoplasm and a flat peripheral nucleus.

Fig. a. Lymphangiome conjonctival.
Dilatations lymphatiques boudinées courant sous la conjonctive et dont certaines contiennent du sang.

Fig. b. Lymphangiome caverneux constitué de cavités de type vasculaire, à limites irrégulières et à endothélium aplati mais ne contenant qu'une sérosité plus ou moins éosinophile et non du sang.

Fig. c. Sarcome de Kaposi de la conjonctive.
Dilatations vasculaires moniliformes occupant le cul-de-sac inférieur et accompagnées de plages hémorragiques. Un examen superficiel pourrait conclure à une hémorragie sous-conjonctivale.

Fig. d. Sarcome de Kaposi: histopathologie.
Au sein d'une plage dense de cellules fusiformes dont certaines possèdent des noyaux nettement dystrophiques circule un vaisseau à paroi nette; mais parfois il ne s'agit que de fentes vasculaires bordées de cellules tumorales. A cette prolifération s'associe une réaction inflammatoire plus ou moins importante et des suffusions hémorragiques.

Fig. e. Lipome de la conjonctive.
Présence dans le quadrant supéro-temporal d'un nodule saillant d'un jaune rosé à surface lisse. La conjonctive qui le recouvre glisse facilement sur lui sans aucune adhérence.

Fig. f. Lipome de la conjonctive: histopathologie.
La prolifération est faite de tissu cellulo-adipeux avec des cellules à cytoplasme optiquement vide et à noyau périphérique aplati.

Abb. a. Lymphangiom der Konjunktiva.
Wulstige lymphatische Erweiterungen, die unter der Bindehaut verlaufen und von denen manche Blut enthalten.

Abb. b. Kavernöses Lymphangiom, bestehend aus gefäßartigen Erweiterungen, unregelmäßig abgegrenzt, mit einem abgeflachten Endothel. Sie enthalten eine mehr oder weniger eosinophile seröse Flüssigkeit und kein Blut.

Abb. c. Kaposi-Sarkom der Konjunktiva.
Längliche Gefäßdilatationen, die den unteren Fornix einnehmen und mit Hämorragiefeldern einhergehen. Eine oberflächliche Untersuchung könnte auf eine subkonjunktivale Blutung schließen lassen.

Abb. d. Kaposi-Sarkom: Histopathologie.
Inmitten eines dichten Feldes spindelförmiger Zellen, von denen manche einen eindeutig dystrophischen Kern haben, befindet sich ein Gefäß mit glatter Wand oder manchmal nur ein einfacher, von Tumorzellen umgebener Gefäßspalt. Zu dieser Proliferation kommen eine mehr oder weniger starke entzündliche Reaktion und Blutaustritte hinzu.

Abb. e. Lipom der Bindehaut.
Im oberen, temporalen Viertel befindet sich eine gelblich-rosafarbene "Kugel" mit glatter Oberfläche. Die Bindehaut, die sie überdeckt, läßt sich leicht darüber verschieben.

Abb. f. Lipom der Konjunktiva: Histopathologie.
Die Wucherung besteht aus Zell- und Fettgewebe, dessen Zellen ein optisch leeres Zytoplasma und einen peripher gelegenen, abgeflachten Kern haben.

47

PLATE 24 PLANCHE 24 TAFEL 24

VII. PALPEBRO-CONJUNCTIVAL TUMOURS OF NERVE TISSUE

VII.1 Neurofibroma

Clinical features. This tumour is the main clinical expression of von Recklinghausen's neurofibromatosis. In the eyelid it presents the features of a plexiform neuroma which may extend to the face in parallel folds, "draped" under a thickened skin ("Pachydermatocele" or "neuromatous elephantiasis"). The conjunctiva may be involved and also the orbit. In this case there is also an enlargement of the orbital bony frame, often a dehiscence of the bone, and an enlargement of the superior orbital fissure. A pulsating non-expanding proptosis may result, but without bruit and without alteration of the episcleral vessels. J. François' triad is an association of palpebral, orbital and uveal neuro-fibromatosis.

Histopathology. A neurofibroma is the consequence of a more or less homogenous proliferation of all the histological components of the nerve: in the centre there are some axones, and bundles of Schwann cells with spindle-shaped nuclei grouped in a palisade arrangement. At the periphery Schwann cells are mixed with connective tissue cells from the endoneurium and surrounded by loose connective tissue. The whole tumour remains inside the perineural sheath. These lesions are highly vascularized, and therefore surgery may sometimes be risky.

VII.2 Schwannoma

This tumour is very rare in the eyelid. It can form small intradermal nodules along the course of a nerve. These firm nodules are sometimes very painful, or can mimic a chalazion. The usual location of schwannoma in the ocular area is the orbit (Plate 35, Chapter XVI.1).

VII.3 Merkel cell tumour (Trabecular carcinoma)

Clinical features. This tumour has been described recently and is relatively frequent in the eyelid. It develops chiefly in elderly people, on the margin of the upper lid. It has a characteristic clinical aspect. Despite its slow progression, local recurrences are frequent, and it can invade the regional lymph nodes or metastasize to other organs.

Histopathology. The microscopical aspect of this infiltrating, poorly differentiated tumour is suggestive of Merkel cell tumour. The cells are cuboidal or globular, with ill-defined limits, but present a homogeneous morphology. In the round nuclei the chromatin is evenly distributed; mitotic figures are frequent. Specific stains demonstrate the neurosecretory function of these cells (Fig. f).

VII. TUMEURS DU TISSU NERVEUX PALPÉBRO-CONJONCTIVAL

VII.1 Neurofibrome

Clinique. C'est la principale manifestation de la Neurofibromatose de von Recklinghausen. A la paupière le neurofibrome se présente sous l'aspect d'un névrome plexiforme qui peut déborder sur la face en replis étagés, en "drapé" sous une peau épaisse et plissée, c'est le "pachydermatocèle" ou "éléphantiasis névromateux". La conjonctive peut également être intéressée. Lorsque l'orbite est envahie il existe en outre un élargissement du cadre orbitaire avec souvent perte de substance osseuse et élargissement de la fente sphénoïdale. Il s'ensuit une exophtalmie pulsatile, mais non expansive, sans souffle ni modification des vaisseaux conjonctivaux. L'association d'une neurofibromatose de la paupière de l'orbite et de l'uvée constitue la triade de J. François.

Histopathologie. Le neurofibrome est la conséquence d'une prolifération de tous les éléments constitutifs du nerf périphérique: axones, cellules de Schwann, endonèvre et périnèvre. En effet la partie centrale est occupée par quelques axones et des faisceaux de cellules de Schwann à noyaux fusiformes juxtaposés en palissade. A la périphérie les cellules de Schwann sont mêlées aux cellules conjonctives de l'endonèvre au sein d'un collagène peu dense. Le tout reste contenu dans la gaine du périnèvre. L'abondante vascularisation de ces lésions risque de rendre très hémorragique toute intervention.

VII.2 Schwannome

Le schwannome est très rare à la paupière où il peut se manifester par de petites nodosités intradermiques sur le trajet d'un nerf, nodosités fermes parfois très douloureuses ou simulant un chalazion. Sa localisation oculaire la plus habituelle reste l'orbite (Planche 35, Chapitre XVI.1).

VII.3 Tumeur à cellules de Merkel (Carcinome trabéculaire)

Clinique. Tumeur d'individualisation récente, relativement fréquente aux paupières, elle est l'apanage du sujet âgé. La paupière supérieure particulièrement la marge, paraît plus souvent atteinte que l'inférieure. Son aspect est assez caractéristique. Bien que de croissance lente elle récidive souvent localement et peut essaimer dans les ganglions satellites et à distance.

Histopathologie. C'est une tumeur infiltrante, indifférenciée, dont l'aspect est néanmoins très évocateur. Les cellules sont de morphologie uniforme, cubiques ou globuleuses, à limites imprécises. Le noyau arrondi à chromatine régulière est très souvent en mitose. Les colorations signalétiques révèlent leur nature neurosécrétoire (Fig. f).

VII. PALPEBRO-KONJUNKTIVALE NERVENTUMOREN

VII.1 Neurofibrom

Klinik. Dies ist die Hauptmanifestation der Neurofibromatose von Recklinghausen. Am Lid erscheint das Neurofibrom wie ein plexiformes Neurom, das in gestuften Falten, mit verdickter und gefälteter Haut auf das Gesicht übergreifen kann. Es ist dies die "neuromatöse Elefantiasis". Die Konjunktiva kann ebenfalls davon betroffen sein. Wenn die Augenhöhle befallen ist, tritt häufig eine Erweiterung der Orbita mit Verlust von Knochensubstanz und Erweiterung der Sphenoidalspalte auf. Dies hat einen pulsierenden, dem Puls synchronen aber nicht expansiven Exophtalmus, ohne Geräusch und ohne Veränderung der Bindehautgefäße, zur Folge. Die gleichzeitige Neurofibromatose von Lidern, Augenhöhle und Uvea stellt die Trias von J. François dar.

Histopathologie. Das Neurofibrom ist die Folge einer mehr oder weniger gleichmäßigen Wucherung aller Bestandteile des peripheren Nervs: Axon, Schwannzellen, Endo- und Perineurium. Der innere axiale Teil wird von einigen Axonen und Bündeln von Schwann-Zellen mit spindelförmigen, palissadenartig aneinandergereihten Kernen eingenommen. Peripher sind die Schwann-Zellen mit endoneuralen Bindegewebszellen in einem wenig dichten Kollagen gemischt. Das Ganze ist von der Perineuriumsscheide umschlossen. Der reichliche Gefäßgehalt dieser Gewebe erhöht für jeglichen operativen Eingriff das Risiko starker Hämorrhagien.

VII.2 Schwannom

Das Schwannom ist am Lid sehr selten; es kann dort als kleines, intradermales, knötchenartiges Gebilde im Verlauf eines Nerven in Erscheinung treten. Diese derben Knötchen sind manchmal sehr schmerzhaft oder können ein Chalazion vortäuschen. Jedoch ist die Augenhöhle die häufigste Lokalisationsform (Tafel 35, Kapitel XVI.1).

VII.3 Merkel-Zell-Tumor (Trabekel-Karzinom)

Klinik. Dieser erst in jüngerer Zeit beschriebene, an den Lidern verhältnismäßig häufige Tumor ist den älteren Menschen vorbehalten. Das obere Lid und insbesondere der Rand scheint öfter als das untere daran zu erkranken. Das Aussehen ist recht charakteristisch. Wenngleich von langsamen Wuchs rezidiviert er oft lokal und kann sich auf die umliegenden Lymphknoten ausdehnen oder in die Ferne metastasieren.

Histopathologie. Es ist dies ein infiltrierender, undifferenzierter Tumor, im Aussehen indessen charakteristisch. Die Zellen sind gleichartig, würfel- oder kugelförmig, mit ungenauen Grenzen. Der rundliche Kern mit regelmäßigem Chromatin befindet sich sehr oft in Mitose. Die entsprechenden Färbungen erbringen den Nachweis einer Neurosekretion (Abb. f).

PLATE 24 PLANCHE 24 TAFEL 24

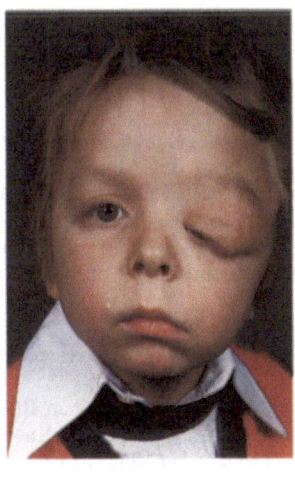

a

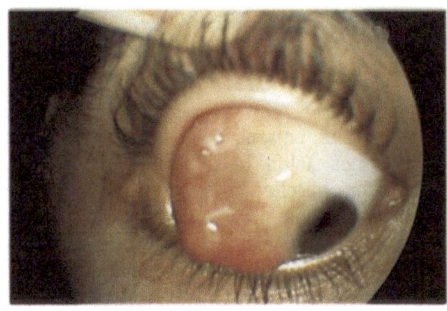

b

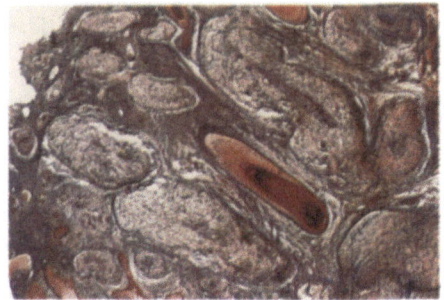

c

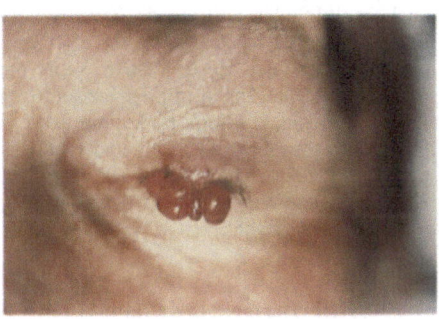

d

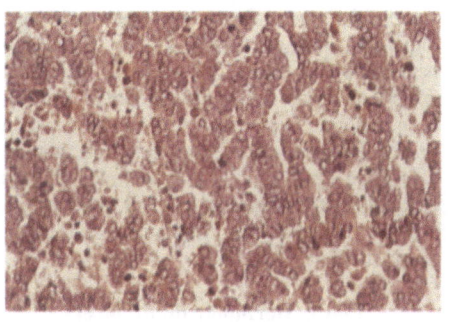

e

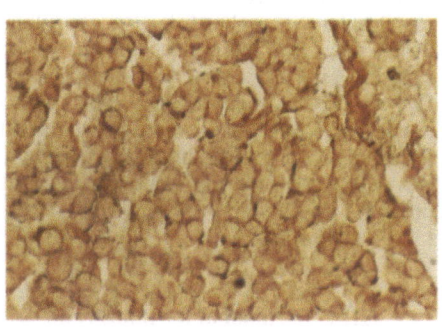

f

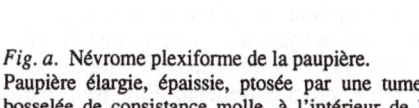

Fig. a. Plexiform neuroma of the eyelid.
The eyelid is enlarged, thickened, pushed down by an irregular tumour of soft consistency. By palpation, nodosities and fibrous bundles may be felt.

Fig. b. Subconjunctival neurofibroma of the lateral canthus.
In this rare location the tumour is made up of pink, firm nodules which adhere to the episclera, but are covered by a normal conjunctiva.

Fig. c. Plexiform neuroma of the eyelid (Masson's trichome).
Under low power the intermingling of thickened nerves is easily seen. They are often bent, and sectioned accordingly at variable angles.

Fig. d. Merkel cell tumour of the lid margin.
Reddish juxtaposed pediculate nodules with a smooth surface, without ulceration, painless and leaving the eyelashes intact.

Fig. e. Merkel cell tumour.
The tumour is located in the dermis. It is made up of lobules and anastomosed strands of cells (trabecular carcinoma), which are separated by layers of connective tissue containing lymphoplasmacytic cells.

Fig. f. Grimelius's staining.
This technique shows (as a brown stippling) intracytoplasmic argyrophilic granulations, similar to those of the neurosecretory endocrine cells.

Fig. a. Névrome plexiforme de la paupière.
Paupière élargie, épaissie, ptosée par une tumeur bosselée de consistance molle, à l'intérieur de laquelle on perçoit des nodosités et des cordons fibreux en "pelotons de ficelle".

Fig. b. Neurofibrome sous-conjonctival de l'angle externe.
Cette localisation rare est constituée de nodules, rosés, fermes, adhérents à l'épisclère mais recouverts d'une muqueuse normale.

Fig. c. Névrome plexiforme de la paupière (Trichrome Masson).
Le faible grossissement montre bien l'enchevêtrement de troncs nerveux dilatés, repliés sur eux-mêmes et sectionnés sous diverses incidences.

Fig. d. Tumeur à cellules de Merkel de la marge palpébrale.
Nodules juxtaposés pédiculés, à surface lisse non ulcérée, rougeâtres, indolores et épargnant les cils.

Fig. e. Tumeur à cellules de Merkel.
La tumeur siège dans le derme. Elle est constituée de lobules et de travées anastomosées (carcinome trabéculaire), séparées par des lames de tissu conjonctif contenant des cellules lymphoplasmocytaires.

Fig. f. Coloration de Grimelius.
Cette coloration met en évidence, sous forme d'un piqueté brun, des granulations argyrophiles intracytoplasmiques analogues à celles des cellules endocrines neuro-sécrétoires.

Abb. a. Plexiformes Neurom des Lides.
Vergrößertes, verdicktes Lid, ptotisch durch eine höckrige Geschwulst von weicher Konsistenz, in deren Innerem Knötchen und faserige Schnüre wie "Knäuel" zu sehen sind.

Abb. b. Subkonjunctivales Neurofibrom, im äußeren Augenwinkel.
Bei dieser seltenen Lokalisation treten rosafarbene, derbe, auf der Episklera haftende Knötchen auf, die aber von einer normalen Schleimhaut bedeckt sind.

Abb. c. Plexiformes Neurom des Lids (Masson's Trichromfärbung).
Die Trichromfärbung nach Masson (schwache Vergrößerung) zeigt deutlich die Windungen der erweiterten, auf sich zurückgebogenen und in verschiedenen Richtungen geschnittenen Nerven.

Abb. d. Merkel-Zell-Tumor am Lidrand.
Gestielte, aneinandergereihte Knötchen mit glatter, nicht geschwüriger Oberfläche, rötlich, schmerzlos, die Wimpern aussparend.

Abb. e. Merkel-Zell-Tumor.
Die in der Dermis sitzende Geschwulst besteht aus Läppchen und anastomisierenden Strängen (Trabekel-Karzinom), die durch Bindegewebssepten mit lymphoplasmatischen Zellen getrennt sind.

Abb. f. Grimelius-Färbung.
Diese Färbung weist argyrophile Granulationen im Zytoplasma nach, vergleichbar mit denen der endokrinen neurosekretorischen Zellen.

49

VIII. DYSGENETIC TUMOURS OF THE CONJUNCTIVA, LIDS AND ORBIT

These tumours fit into the category of choristomas, as defined by Albrecht, i.e. they are made up of tissues of normal structure but which do not normally occur in the region in question. It is normal tissue abnormally situated.

VIII.1 Dermoid cyst

Clinical features. Most often situated in the outer part of the upper lid, this cyst can leave its mark on the underlying bone and even erode it. It can also be dumbbell-shaped, and extend into the orbit. It evolves progressively, sometimes marked by inflammatory bouts or even suppurations which can open to the skin.

Histopathology. Unilocular more often than multilocular, it is lined by an epithelium which may open during the growth of the cyst. Its lipid-rich content then comes in contact with the adjacent dermis, resulting in a lipophagic foreign body reaction with giant and lipidized cells. This process may destroy the wall of the cyst and make the diagnosis difficult.

VIII.2 Dermoid of the limbus and dermis-like choristoma

Clinical features. A small full tumour without any cystic characteristics and which one must be careful not to include in the same category as the eyebrow dermoid cyst. It is present at birth but can grow progressively. It can be part of a first arch syndrome and be linked for example to accessory auricular appendages (Goldenhar syndrome). Certain dermoids can completely cover the surface of the cornea and even be bilateral and hereditary. American studies refer to them as *"dermis-like choristomas"*.

Histopathology. It is a veritable little dermo-epidermic islet which replaces a sector of the limbal conjunctivo-corneal mucous membrane. The underlying sclera and cornea are often thin, a fact which calls for prudence during surgical excision of the lesion.

VIII. TUMEURS DYSGÉNÉTIQUES DE LA CONJONCTIVE, DES PAUPIÈRES ET DE L'ORBITE

Ces tumeurs entrent dans la catégorie des choristomes selon la définition d'Albrecht, c'est-à-dire qu'elles comportent des tissus de structure normale mais qui n'existent pas normalement dans la région considérée. Ce sont des tissus normaux anormalement situés.

VIII.1 Kyste dermoïde

Clinique. Situé le plus souvent à la queue du sourcil il peut marquer de son empreinte la paroi osseuse sous-jacente et même l'éroder. Il peut également se prolonger à l'intérieur de l'orbite, en bissac. Son évolution est progressive parfois émaillée de poussées inflammatoires ou même de suppurations avec ouverture à la peau.

Histopathologie. Plus souvent uni que pluriloculaire il est tapissé d'un épiderme qui peut lors de la croissance du kyste, présenter des solutions de continuité mettant en contact avec le derme avoisinant son contenu riche en lipides. Il peut en résulter une réaction de résorption lipophagique avec cellules géantes et xanthélasmisées; celle-ci peut aboutir à la destruction de la paroi, rendant alors le diagnostic difficile.

VIII.2 Dermoïde du limbe et "dermis-like choristoma"

Clinique. Petite tumeur pleine sans aucun caractère kystique et qu'il faut donc se garder d'assimiler au kyste dermoïde du sourcil. Elle est présente dès la naissance mais peut s'accroître progressivement. Elle peut faire partie d'un syndrome du 1er arc et s'associer par exemple à un appendice prétragien (syndrome de Goldenhar). Certains dermoïdes peuvent recouvrir totalement la surface de la cornée, être même bilatéraux et héréditaires; ils sont connus dans la littérature américaine sous le nom de *"dermis-like choristomas"*.

Histopathologie. C'est un véritable petit îlot dermo-épidermique en lieu et place de la muqueuse conjonctivo-limbique. La sclère et la cornée sous-jacentes sont souvent amincies ce qui commande la prudence lors de l'exérèse de la lésion.

VIII. DYSGENETISCHE TUMOREN DER LIDER UND ORBITA

Diese Tumoren gehören zur Kategorie der Choristome nach der Albrechtschen Definition, das heißt sie enthalten Gewebe mit normaler Struktur, die normalerweise in dem betreffenden Bereich aber nicht vorhanden sind. Es sind normale Gewebe an der falschen Stelle.

VIII.1 Dermoidzyste

Klinik. Sie sitzt meist am feinen Brauenende und kann den darunterliegenden Knochen eindellen und sogar erodieren. Sie kann sich auch sanduhrartig ins Innere der Orbita erstrecken. Sie wächst zunehmend, manchmal mit entzündlichen Schüben oder sogar Eiterung und Aufbrechen der Haut.

Histopathologie. Die eher einzeln, seltener auch multilokulär auftretende Zyste ist mit einer Epidermis ausgekleidet, die sich beim Größerwerden der Zyste öffnen kann und ihren lipidreichen Inhalt mit der benachbarten Dermis in Kontakt bringt. Es kommt dabei zu einer Fettresorption mit Riesen- und xanthelasmaartigen Zellen und mitunter sogar zur Zerstörung der Wandung, was dann die Diagnose schwierig macht.

VIII.2 Dermoid des Limbus und "dermis-like choristoma"

Klinik. Kleiner, voller Tumor ohne jedes Zystenmerkmal, bei dem man sich also davor hüten muß, ihn mit der Dermoidzyste der Braue gleichzusetzen. Er ist bereits bei der Geburt vorhanden, kann aber mit der Zeit größer werden. Er kann Teil eines 1. Kiemenbogensyndroms sein und sich beispielsweise einem präaurikularen Anhange anschließen (Goldenhar-Syndrom). Manche Dermoide können die Hornhaut auf der ganzen Fläche überdecken, sogar beidseitig und erblich sein; in der amerikanischen Literatur sind sie unter dem Namen *"dermis-like choristomas"* bekannt.

Histopathologie. Eine richtige Dermis-Epidermis-Insel befindet sich an der Stelle der Konjunktiva-Limbus-Schleimhaut. Die darunterliegende Sklera und Kornea sind oft sehr dünn, weshalb bei der operativen Entfernung der Läsion Vorsicht geboten ist.

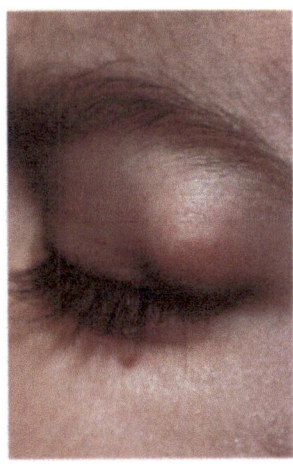

a

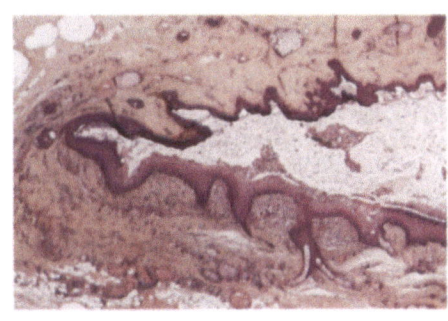

b

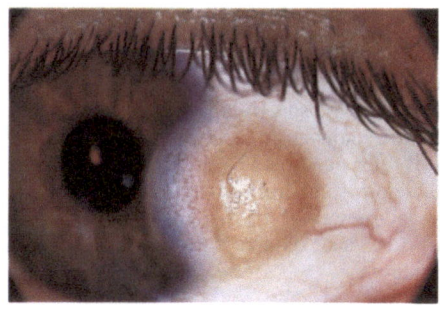

c

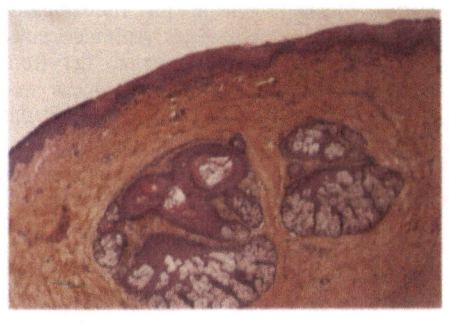

d

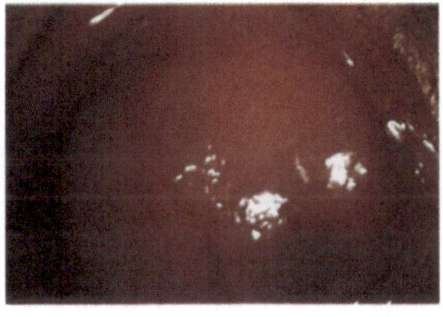

e

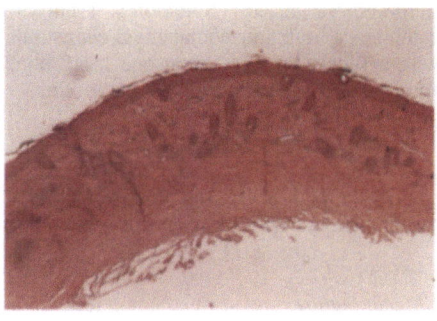

f

Fig. a. Dermoid cyst in the outer part of the upper lid.
Tumour with the following characteristics: ovoid, firm, painless, mobile under the skin, which does not undergo any alteration.

Fig. b. Dermoid cyst of eyebrow: histopathology.
The cystic cavity is lined by an epidermis with sebaceous and sudoral adnexa. Its content consists of hair and lamellae of keratin with lipidic debris.

Fig. c. Limbal dermoid.
Yellowish nodular lesion encroaching upon the cornea, which is opaque in the area of contact. The smooth surface sometimes bristles with fine downy hair.

Fig. d. Limbal dermoid: histopathology.
The conjunctival mucous epithelium is replaced by a keratinized epidermis covering a dense connective tissue in which pilo-sebaceous adnexa are present. Fat lobules can be found deeper down.

Fig. e. Dermis-like choristoma.
The whole surface of the cornea is covered by a sheet of epiderm.

Fig. f. Dermis-like choristoma: histopathology.
Beneath the epidermis, there is a compact connective tissue with some hair follicles.

Fig. a. Kyste dermoïde de la queue du sourcil.
Tumeur ovoïde, ferme, indolore. La peau, normale, est mobile à sa surface.

Fig. b. Kyste dermoïde du sourcil: histopathologie.
La cavité kystique est bordée d'un épiderme avec ses annexes aussi bien sébacées que sudorales. Son contenu, de consistance pâteuse est fait de poils et de lamelles de kératine auxquelles se mêlent des débris lipidiques.

Fig. c. Dermoïde du limbe.
Lésion nodulaire jaunâtre débordant sur la cornée, qui est opaque à son contact; la surface est parfois hérissée de fins duvets.

Fig. d. Dermoïde du limbe: histopathologie.
Muqueuse conjonctivale remplacée par un épiderme kératinisé recouvrant un tissu conjonctif dense au sein duquel on trouve des annexes pilo-sébacées. En profondeur on peut trouver des lobules adipeux.

Fig. e. Dermis-like choristoma.
Toute la surface cornéenne est recouverte d'une lame d'épiderme.

Fig. f. Dermis-like choristoma: histopathologie.
Cet épiderme repose sur un tissu conjonctif dense au sein duquel on reconnaît des follicules pilaires.

Abb. a. Dermoidzyste am Brauenende.
Ovoïder, fester, schmerzloser Tumor. Die unveränderte Haut ist auf der Zyste beweglich.

Abb. b. Dermoidzyste an der Braue: Histopathologie.
Das Zystenlumen ist von Epidermis mit Talg- und Schweißadnexen ausgekleidet. Es enthält manchmal Härchen und ist mit Keratinlamellen gefüllt, unter die sich Fetteile mischen, was ihr die teigige Konsistenz verleiht.

Abb. c. Dermoid am Limbus.
Knötchenförmige, gelbliche Läsion, die auf die bei ihrem Kontakt trübe Hornhaut übergreift; die Oberfläche bedeckt manchmal ein feiner Flaum.

Abb. d. Dermoid am Limbus: Histopathologie.
Konjunktivale Schleimhaut durch eine verhornende Epidermis ersetzt, die ein dichtes Bindegewebe bedeckt, in dem Haar- und Talgadnexen anzutreffen sind. In der Tiefe sind Fettläppchen zu finden.

Abb. e. Dermis-like choristoma.
Die Hornhaut ist auf ihrer gesamten Fläche mit einer Epidermislamelle überzogen.

Abb. f. Dermis-like choristoma: Histopathologie.
Diese Epidermis liegt auf einem dichten Bindegewebe, in dem Haarfollikel zu erkennen sind.

51

PLATE 26 PLANCHE 26 TAFEL 26

VIII.3 Dermolipoma

Clinical features. The usual location of this tumour is the supero-temporal quadrant of the bulbar conjunctiva, rarely the lateral canthus. It is often concealed by the eyelid at birth, and therefore sometimes noticed only after some years. As well as the dermoid of the limbus, it can be one of the signs of a first arch syndrom.

Histopathology. As is suggested by its name, this tumour combines characteristic features of epidermis, dermis and fatty tissue.

VIII.4 Complex choristoma

Clinical features. Its clinical features are identical to those of a dermoid or a dermolipoma.

Histopathology. Histopathology is characterized by the presence of islets of cartilage, lacrymal gland or even smooth muscle in the fibro-adipose tissue. Solomon's syndrome combines a limbal or conjunctival choristoma with a sebaceous naevus on one hand, bone and neurological abnormalities on the other.

VIII.5 Epibulbar osteoma (osseous epibulbar choristoma, episcleral osteoma)

Clinical features. Its most common location is the supero-temporal quadrant of the bulbus. It has the aspect of a small, oval, more or less prominent nodule. It is fixed in the episclera, but the overlying conjunctiva is usually freely mobile over the lesion.

Histopathology. Histopathology is explicit enough, making confusion impossible (Fig. d).

IX. INFLAMMATORY AND DEGENERATIVE PSEUDO-TUMORAL LESIONS

IX.1 Chalazion

Clinical features. A chalazion is at first a small intra-palpebral nodule which sometimes is only detectable by palpation. At that stage it can be prominent under the hypervascularized palpebral conjunctiva. In cases of inflammation it becomes more obvious, and can provoke a telangiectatic granuloma. Later it presents the well known aspect of a prominent palpebral nodule under a normal skin. The latter can be moved over it except in case of superadded inflammation.

Histopathology. It is a lipogranuloma which develops upon the glands of Meibomius and destroys the sebaceous acini. Where there is superadded inflammation and suppuration, a small abcess forms in the center of the granuloma and may open to the skin or to the conjunctiva.

VIII.3 Dermolipome

Clinique. Le dermolipome siège en général dans le secteur supérotemporal de la conjonctive bulbaire, plus rarement dans le canthus externe. Souvent caché par la paupière à la naissance il peut n'être découvert que tardivement. Comme le dermoïde du limbe il peut être associé à des éléments d'un syndrome du 1er arc.

Histopathologie. Comme son nom l'indique il associe des formations dermo-épidermiques à du tissu adipeux.

VIII.4 Choristome complexe

Clinique. Son aspect est identique à celui d'un dermoïde ou d'un dermolipome.

Histopathologie. C'est l'histopathologie qui le différencie par la présence dans le tissu fibro-adipeux d'îlots de cartilage ou de glande lacrymale voire de muscle lisse. L'association d'un choristome limbique ou conjonctival à un naevus sébacé, des anomalies osseuses et neurologiques réalise le syndrome de Solomon.

VIII.5 Ostéome épibulbaire (choristome épibulbaire osseux, ostéome épiscléral)

Clinique. Il siège le plus souvent dans le secteur supéro-temporal du globe oculaire et prend l'aspect d'un petit nodule ovalaire plus ou moins saillant, enchâssé dans l'épisclère. La conjonctive peut être mobilisée à son contact.

Histopathologie. L'histopathologie, explicite, ne prête guère à confusion (Fig. d).

IX. LÉSIONS INFLAMMATOIRES ET DÉGÉNÉRATIVES PSEUDO-TUMORALES

IX.1 Chalazion

Clinique. Au début de son évolution le chalazion ne se manifeste que par un nodule intra-palpébral qui peut n'être retrouvé qu'à la palpation dans l'épaisseur du tarse mais qui peut faire saillie sous la conjonctive palpébrale hyperhémiée en regard. En cas d'inflammation il est plus manifeste. Ultérieurement il prend l'aspect bien connu d'un nodule sous-cutané adhérant au tarse, la peau restant mobile à sa surface sauf inflammation surajoutée.

Histopathologie. C'est un lipogranulome développé aux dépens des glandes de Meibomius et détruisant les acini sébacés. Dans les lésions surinfectées et suppurées le granulome est centré par un micro-abcès qui peut s'étendre et venir s'ouvrir à la conjonctive ou à la peau.

VIII.3 Dermolipom

Klinik. Das Dermolipom sitzt im allgemeinen im oberen temporalen Quadranten der Konjunctiva bulbi, seltener im äußeren Kanthus. Es ist bei der Geburt oft unter dem Lid verborgen und wird erst spät entdeckt werden. Wie das Dermoid des Limbus kann es mit Elementen eines 1. Kiemenbogen-Syndroms einhergehen.

Histopathologie. Wie aus dem Namen hervorgeht, besteht es aus Elementen der Dermis-Epidermis und des Fettgewebes.

VIII.4 Komplexes Choristom

Klinik. Im Aussehen ist es identisch mit einem Dermoid oder Dermolipom.

Histopathologie. Histopathologisch unterscheidet es sich durch das Vorhandensein vereinzelter Knorpel-, Tränendrüsen- oder gar glatter Muskelfragmente im fibroadipösen Gewebe. Ein gleichzeitiges Auftreten eines Choristoms am Limbus oder an der Konjunktiva mit einem Naevus sebaceus und Knochen- und Nervenanomalien bildet das Solomonsche Syndrom.

VIII.5 Epibulbäres Osteom (epibulbäres ossöses Choristom, episklerales Osteom)

Klinik. Es sitzt meist am oberen temporalen Teil des Augapfels und hat das Aussehen eines kleinen ovalen, mehr oder weniger erhabenen Knötchens. Die Konjunktiva ist über der in die Episclera eingelassenen Läsion beweglich.

Histopathologie. Die Histopathologie ist eindeutig und läßt kaum Verwechslungen zu (Abb. d).

IX. ENTZÜNDLICHE UND DEGENERATIVE PSEUDOTUMOREN

IX.1 Chalazion

Klinik. Zu Beginn macht sich das Chalazion nur durch ein Knötchen innerhalb des Lides bemerkbar, das erst bei der Palpation des Tarsus gefunden wird, aber auf der darunter befindlichen Conjunctiva palpebralis eine Vorwölbung bildet. Bei Entzündung ist es auffälliger. Später nimmt es das bekannte Aussehen eines subkutanen Knötchens an, das am Tarsus haftet, wobei die Haut an dessen Oberfläche beweglich bleibt, es sei denn, es kommt eine Entzündung hinzu.

Histopathologie. Es ist ein von den Meibomschen Drüsen ausgehendes Lipogranulom, das die Talg-Acini zerstört. Bei reinfizierten und eitrigen Läsionen liegt in der Mitte des Granuloms ein Mikro-Abszeß, der sich ausdehnen und durch die Konjunktiva oder durch die Haut öffnen kann.

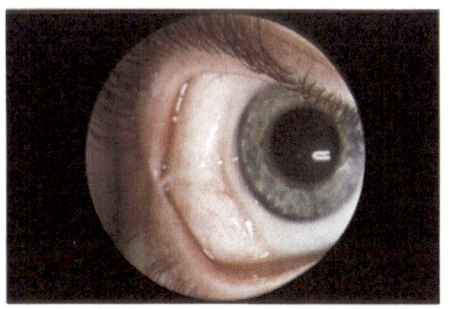

a

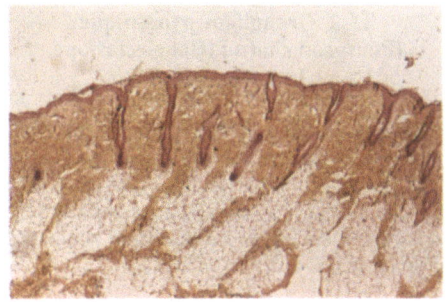

b

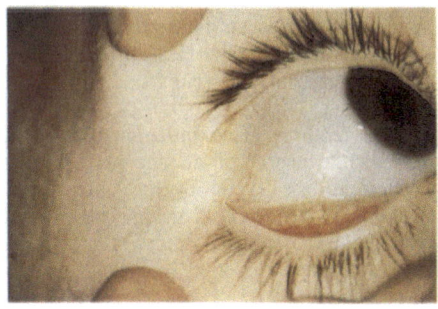

c

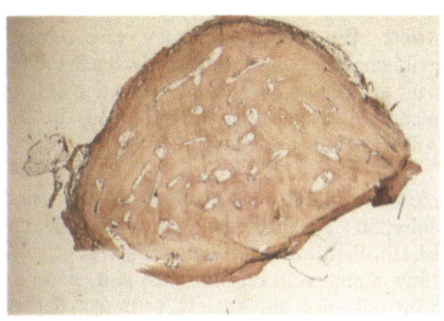

d

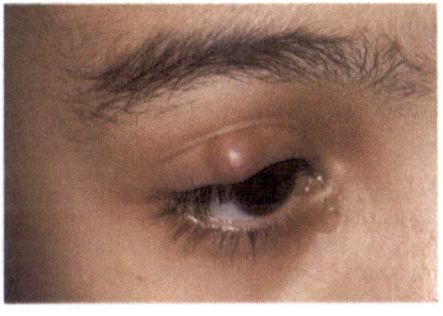

e

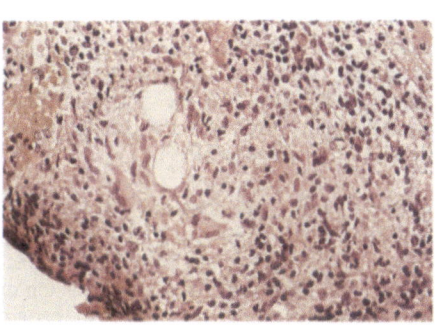

f

Fig. a. Dermolipoma of the lateral canthus.
Whitish swelling with horizontal constriction in the centre. It is fixed to the conjunctiva which cannot be moved over it.

Fig. b. Dermolipoma of the conjunctiva. The conjunctival epithelium is replaced by an epidermis with its appendages, covering a compact connective tissue, and a layer of fatty tissue deeper. The adhesion between epidermis and dermis makes cleavage difficult and may provoke too extensive surgical excisions.

Fig. c. Episcleral osseous choristoma of the lateral canthus, slightly prominent, with presence of a coloboma of the eyelids.

Fig. d. Episcleral osseous choristoma: histopathology.
Lamella of compact bone with membraneous bone formation.

Fig. e. Chalazion of the upper lid with superadded inflammation. Prominent nodule covered by a hyperhaemic skin. If this type of chalazion opens spontaneously through the conjunctiva, it may evolve into a pyogenic granuloma.

Fig. f. Chalazion: histopathology. Area of epithelioid and giant cells surrounding droplets of lipids, which are a good guide for the diagnosis. In the periphery a lymphoplasmacytic or polymorphonuclear inflammatory reaction is usual.

Fig. a. Dermolipome du canthus latéral.
Tuméfaction blanchâtre étranglée à sa partie moyenne par une bride horizontale. Elle fait corps avec la muqueuse conjonctivale qu'on ne peut mobiliser à sa surface.

Fig. b. Dermolipome de la conjonctive. Epithélium conjonctival remplacé par un épiderme muni de ses annexes et reposant sur un tissu conjonctif dense se continuant en profondeur par un pannicule adipeux. L'adhérence entre épiderme et derme supprime tout plan de clivage et peut entraîner des résections trop étendues.

Fig. c. Ostéome épiscléral de l'angle externe.
Saillie jaunâtre discrète occupant le canthus latéral et ayant entraîné un colobome.

Fig. d. Ostéome épiscléral: histopathologie.
Lamelle d'os compact à ossification membraneuse.

Fig. e. Chalazion enflammé de la paupière supérieure. Nodule saillant recouvert d'une peau hyperhémique. Lorsqu'un tel chalazion s'ouvre spontanément à la conjonctive il peut être à l'origine d'un granulome télangiectasique.

Fig. f. Chalazion: histopathologie. Placard de cellules épithélioïdes et de cellules géantes centré par des gouttelettes lipidiques ce qui oriente le diagnostic. Plus en périphérie réaction inflammatoire lympho-plasmocytaire ou à polynucléaires selon les cas.

Abb. a. Dermolipom des äußeren Augenwinkels. Weißliche Anschwellung, die an ihrem mittleren Teil von einer horizontalen Einziehung abgeschnürt ist. Sie ist mit der Konjunktiva verwachsen, die darüber (im Gegensatz zum Lipom) nicht verschoben werden kann.

Abb. b. Dermolipom der Konjunktiva. An der Stelle des Bindehaut-Epithels eine Epidermis mit ihren Adnexen, die auf straffem Bindegewebe liegt, das sich in der Tiefe als Unterhautfettgewebe fortsetzt. Das enge Zusammenhaften von Epidermis und darunterliegender Dermis läßt keinerlei Spaltung zu, so daß es zu einer zu großflächigen Resektion kommen kann.

Abb. c. Episklerales Osteom des äußeren Augenwinkels. Das Osteom bildet eine diskrete gelbliche Erhebung, die den äußeren Kanthus einnimmt und ein Kolobom dieses letzteren bewirkt hat.

Abb. d. Episklerales Osteom: Histopathologie. Kompakte Knochenlamelle mit membranöser Ossifizierung.

Abb. e. Chalazion des Oberlids. Erhabenes Knötchen, von einer hyperämischen Haut bedeckt. Wenn sich ein solches Chalazion spontan an der Bindehaut öffnet, kann es ein teleangiektatisches Granulom verursachen.

Abb. f. Chalazion: Histopathologie. Zellgewebe mit epitheloiden und einigen tuberkuloid wirkenden Riesenzellen, jedoch mit Lipidtröpchen in der Mitte, die die Diagnose erlauben. Weiter an der Peripherie lympho-plasmozytäre oder je nach Fall auch polynukleäre entzündliche Reaktion.

PLATE 27 PLANCHE 27 TAFEL 27

IX.2 Pyogenic granuloma (granuloma telangiectaticum, botryomycoma)

Clinical features. This inflammatory lesion presents the aspect of an angioma. It may develop on the eyelid or the conjunctiva, mostly in connection with an abnormal wound healing, the loosening of sutures after surgery, or the spontaneous opening of a chalazion into the conjunctiva.

Histopathology. It is a granuloma presenting a large number of capillaries converging towards the feeding vessels in the pedicle of the lesion, the only location where the epithelium is preserved, forming a "collarette". These vessels have to be cauterized after excision in order to prevent a recurrence.

IX.3 Pinguecula

Clinical features. This is a small, slightly prominent lesion of the paralimbal conjunctiva, movable on the sclera, without encroachment on the cornea, and located in the axis of the palpebral fissure.

Histopathology. The presence in the subepithelial connective tissue of amorphous deposits taking up the elastin stains is characteristic. But these deposits resist the action of the enzyme elastase. According to certain authors this could be an elastotic degeneration of the collagen fibers, similar to the one observed in senile elastosis of the skin. For others, they are actually abnormal "dysplastic" elastin fibers.

IX.4 Pterygium

Clinical features. Situated at the limbus, in the horizontal axis, more often nasally than temporally, this lesion encroaches more or less upon the cornea.

Histopathology. It can be considered as a "glove-finger"-like fold of the conjunctiva, (epithelium and chorion) at the surface of the limbal cornea. The epithelium which often contains numerous mucous cells, forms a cul-de-sac and becomes progressively atrophic; thus, between Bowman's membrane and the surface there is only a more or less vascularized connective tissue left, which sometimes contains a small epithelial cyst. In the paralimbal subepithelial tissue the same degenerative lesions are present as in pinguecula.

IX.2 Granulome pyogénique (Bourgeon charnu télangiectasique, botryomycome)

Clinique. Lésion inflammatoire d'aspect angiomateux siégeant sur la paupière ou la conjonctive et succédant le plus souvent à une plaie mal cicatrisée, un relâchement de sutures après intervention ou à l'ouverture spontanée d'un chalazion à la conjonctive.

Histopathologie. C'est un bourgeon charnu particulièrement riche en capillaires qui convergent vers des vaisseaux nourriciers situés dans le pédicule de la lésion qui reste seul entouré d'épithélium ("collerette"). Il faudra prendre soin de détruire ces vaisseaux si l'on veut éviter toute récidive.

IX.3 Pinguécula

Clinique. C'est une petite surélévation jaunâtre de la muqueuse conjonctivale limbique, mobile sur la sclère, n'empiétant pas sur la cornée, et sise dans l'axe de la fente palpébrale.

Histopathologie. Il se caractérise par la présence dans le chorion de dépôts amorphes prenant les colorants de l'élastine mais résistant à l'action de l'élastase. Pour certains il s'agirait plutôt d'une dégénérescence élacinique du collagène comme on en voit dans l'élastose sénile cutanée; pour d'autres il s'agirait bien de fibres élastiques mais anormales, "dysplasiques".

IX.4 Ptérygion

Clinique. Il siège au limbe plus souvent nasal que temporal et empiète plus ou moins sur la cornée.

Histopathologie. Il peut être considéré comme un repli "en doigt de gant" de toute l'épaisseur de la muqueuse conjonctivale en avant de la cornée. L'épithélium conjonctival souvent riche en cellules muqueuses forme un cul-de-sac, puis va s'atrophier progressivement, si bien que la membrane de Bowman n'est plus séparée de la surface que par un tissu conjonctif plus ou moins vascularisé au sein duquel on trouve parfois un petit kyste épithélial inclus. Le stroma conjonctival présente quant à lui les mêmes lésions dégénératives que dans le pinguécula.

IX.2 Granuloma pyogenicum (Granuloma telangiectaticum, Botryomycom)

Klinik. Entzündliche Läsion von angiomatösem Aussehen, auf dem Lid oder der Bindehaut auftretend, zumeist infolge einer schlecht geheilten Wunde, Lockerung der Naht nach einer Operation oder spontanen Durchbruchs eines Chalazions durch die Bindehaut.

Histopathologie. Dieses Granulationsgewebe ist besonders reich an Kapillaren, die zu den im Stiel der Läsion sitzenden versorgenden Gefäßen zusammenlaufen. Man wird also auf die Zerstörung dieser letzteren achten müssen, um jegliches Rezidiv zu verhindern. Das Epithel bleibt nur um den Stiel herum weiterbestehen und bildet den "Kragen".

IX.3 Pinguecula (Lidspaltenfleck)

Klinik. Es handelt sich um eine kleine, gelbliche Erhebung der konjuntivalen Schleimhaut am Limbus, beweglich über der Sklera, nicht auf die Kornea übergreifend, in der Achse der Lidspalte liegend.

Histopathologie. Charakteristisch sind amorphe Ablagerungen im Stroma, die Elastin-Farbstoffe annehmen, aber gegen die Einwirkung von Elastase resistent sind. Es wird teilweise die Ansicht vertreten, daß es sich dabei eher um eine elazinische Degeneration des Kollagens handelt, wie das bei der senilen Hautelastose vorkommt. Andere sind hingegen der Meinung, es handle sich wohl um elastische, aber anormal "dysplastische" Fasern.

IX.4 Pterygium (Flügelfell)

Klinik. Es tritt am Limbus häufiger nasal als temporal auf und schiebt sich mehr oder weniger auf die Hornhaut vor.

Histopathologie. Es kann als eine "handschuhfingerartige" Falte der gesamten Dicke der Bindehaut vor der Hornhaut betrachtet werden. Das häufig an Schleimzellen reiche Bindehautepithel bildet über der Hornhaut eine Tasche, atrophiert dann nach und nach, so daß die Bowmansche Membran von der Oberfläche nur noch durch ein mehr oder weniger vaskularisiertes Bindegewebe getrennt ist, in dem manchmal eine kleine Epithelzyste eingeschlossen bleibt. Das Bindehautstroma weist seinerseits dieselben degenerativen Veränderungen wie bei einer Pinguecula auf.

54

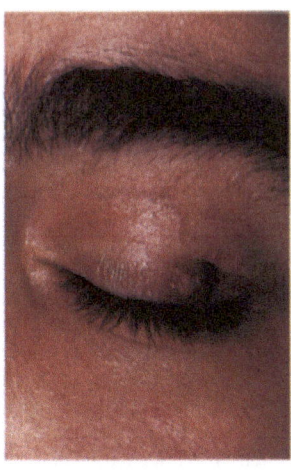

a

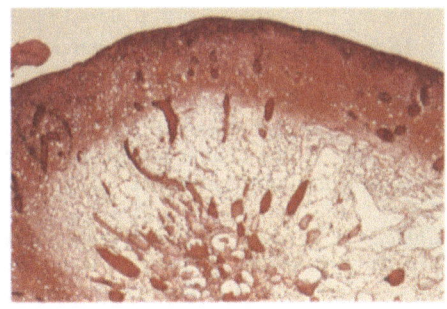

b

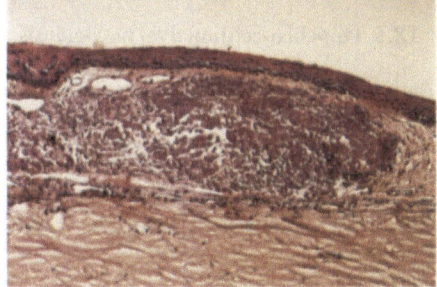

c

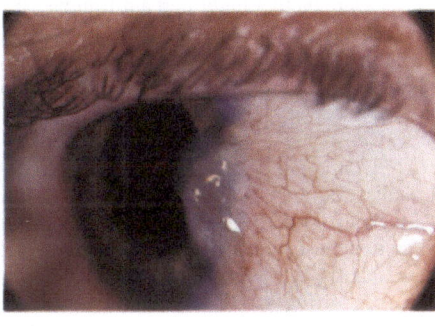

d

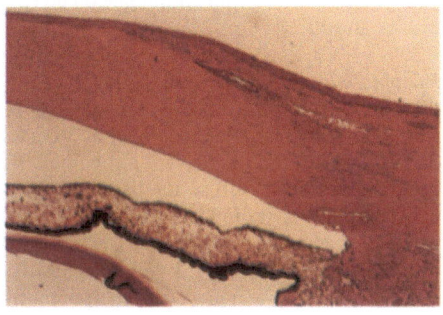

e

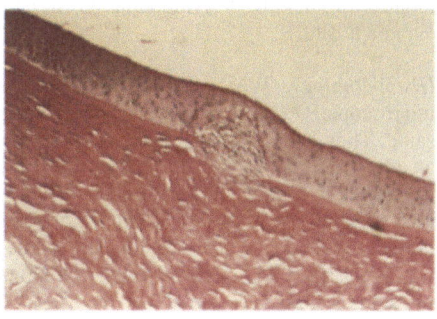

f

Fig. a. Pyogenic granuloma of the upper lid.
Pediculated angiomatous nodule. It is purplish-red and covered with a scab, the removal of which provokes bleeding.

Fig. b. Pyogenic granuloma.
Oedematous and inflammatory connective tissue with numerous vessels; its surface is devoid of epithelium and presents an exudate with fibrin and leukocytes.

Fig. c. Pinguecula: histopathology.
The chorion is characterized by a scarcity of cells and bundles of basophilic fibers, which may in the long run contain deposits of calcium.

Fig. d. Pterygium.
Triangular lesion, the tip of which or "head" encroaches upon the cornea and adheres to it. At the limbus the conjunctiva shows a slight stricture the "collar", and then becomes larger, forming the "body" of the, pterygium which spreads out towards the plica semi-lunaris.

Fig. e. Pterygium.
The epithelium of the conjunctiva grows upon the cornea and then folds back towards the limbus.

Fig. f. Islet of Fuchs.
Small rupture in Bowman's membrane, with some underlying collagen fibers passing through and bulging beneath the corneal epithelium, in front of the head of the pterygium. These "islets", which can be clinically detected, are a sign of progression of the lesion.

Fig. a. Granulome pyogénique de la paupière supérieure.
Nodule angiomateux, rouge pourpre recouvert d'une croûte cruorique dont l'ablation est suivie de saignement.

Fig. b. Granulome pyogénique.
Tissu conjonctif oedémateux et inflammatoire présentant de multiples cavités vasculaires; à sa surface dépourvue d'épithélium, on trouve un exsudat fibrino-leucocytaire.

Fig. c. Pinguécula: histopathologie.
Le chorion pauvre en cellules présente des trousseaux de fibres basophiles pouvant à la longue se surcharger de calcaire.

Fig. d. Ptérygion.
Lésion triangulaire dont la pointe ou "tête" s'avance sur la cornée à laquelle elle adhère. Au limbe la conjonctive forme un léger rétrécissement le "collet" puis s'élargit pour constituer le "corps" du ptérygion qui s'étale en direction du pli semilunaire.

Fig. e. Ptérygion.
L'épithélium conjonctival s'avance sur la cornée et se replie sur lui-même pour regagner le limbe.

Fig. f. Ilots de Fuchs.
En avant de la tête du ptérygion la membrane de Bowman présente de fines ruptures livrant passage à quelques faisceaux collagènes sous-jacents qui viennent soulever l'épithélium cornéen. Ces "îlots", détectables cliniquement, témoignent de la progression de la lésion.

Abb. a. Granuloma pyogenicum des Oberlides.
Gestieltes, angiomatöses Knötchen, purpurrot, bedeckt mit einer Blutkruste, deren Entfernung eine Blutung verursacht.

Abb. b. Granuloma pyogenicum.
Geschwollenes und entzündliches Bindegewebe mit zahlreichen Gefäßlumina; an seiner epithellosen Oberfläche findet sich ein fibrino-leukozytäres Exsudat.

Abb. c. Pinguecula: Histopathologie.
Das an Zellen arme Stroma weist Bündel basophiler Fasern auf, die mit der Zeit Kalk aufnehmen können.

Abb. d. Pterygium.
Dreieckige Läsion, deren Spitze oder "Kopf" sich auf die Hornhaut zuschiebt, wo sie haftet. Am Limbus verengt sich die Bindehaut leicht, "Hals" genannt, und wird dann breiter, um den "Körper" des Flügelfells, das sich in Richtung Plica semilunaris ausdehnt, zu bilden.

Abb. e. Pterygium.
Das Bindehautepithel schiebt sich zwischen Hornhaut und Konjunktiva vor, schlägt sich zurück und erreicht wieder den Limbus.

Abb. f. Fuchssche Inseln.
Vor dem Pterygiumkopf weist die Bowmansche Membran feine Risse auf, die einigen darunterliegenden Kollagenlamellen, die das Hornhautepithel anheben, den Weg frei machen. Diese "Inseln" sind Nachweis für die Progression der Läsion.

IX.5 Palpebro-conjunctival amyloidosis

Amyloidosis is due to the infiltration of connective tissue by an amorphous acellular substance, the physico-chemical characteristics of which are now better known.

Clinical features. Amyloidosis can develop beneath the palpebral epidermis, along the margin or beneath the conjunctiva. Palpebral subcutaneous amyloidosis forms small pink or orange confluent papules which appear studded with purplish dots. It is part of the clinical picture of the immunocytic types of amyloidosis, amyloidosis of the gammopathies or "atypical primitive".
Amyloidosis of the palpebral conjunctiva is the most common of these; it can be apparently solitary, or secondary to a chronic inflammation of the eyelid, especially trachoma. In the bulbar or limbal conjunctiva deposits of amyloid are yellowish or pink lobules mimicking a lymphoma or a carcinoma in situ.

Histopathology. Whatever the location, the microscopical aspect of the deposits is the same. They are usually in direct contact with an often atrophic epithelium. They infiltrate the adjacent deeper situated tissues diffusely and surround vessels which are sometimes closed. At their contact a foreign body reaction is possible. Many characteristic stainings make the diagnosis easier:
- purple metachromasia with cristal violet;
- more or less pronounced staining with PAS;
- green fluorescence under ultraviolet light after treatment of the sections with Thioflavin T;
- red orange staining with Congo red in alcaline solution and birefringence under polarized light.

We know nowadays that the amyloid deposits, with their fibrillary ultrastructure, present a characteristic beta pleated sheath and arise either from fragments of light chains of immunoglobulins or from other proteins of similar structure.

IX.5 Amylose palpébro-conjonctivale

L'amylose est due à une infiltration des tissus de soutien par une substance amorphe, acellulaire dont la constitution physico-chimique est actuellement mieux identifiée.

Clinique. L'amylose peut se localiser sous l'épiderme palpébral, le long de la marge, dans le chorion de la conjonctive ou dans le stroma cornéen. L'amylose palpébrale sous-cutanée forme des micropapules roses ou orangées, confluentes, parsemées de points purpuriques; elle est l'apanage des amyloses immunocytaires, amyloses des gammapathies ou "primitives atypiques".
L'amylose de la conjonctive palpébrale est la plus fréquente, elle est soit d'apparence isolée soit secondaire à une inflammation palpébrale chronique notamment un trachome. Dans la conjonctive bulbaire et au limbe les dépôts amyloïdes sont lobulés, jaunâtres ou rosés, pouvant faire discuter un lymphome ou un carcinome in situ.

Histopathologie. Quelle que soit la localisation, l'aspect des dépôts est identique. Ils se situent en général immédiatement au contact de l'épithélium qui est souvent atrophique. Ils infiltrent de façon diffuse les tissus environnants gagnant la profondeur et engainant des vaisseaux parfois sténosés. Ces dépôts peuvent enfin déterminer à leur contact des réactions macrophagiques de résorption; ils possèdent de nombreuses caractéristiques tinctoriales qui permettent leur identification:
- métachromasie pourpre en présence de Violet de Paris;
- positivité plus ou moins nette au PAS;
- fluorescence verte en lumière ultraviolette après traitement des coupes par la Thioflavine T;
- coloration en rouge orangé par le rouge congo en solution alcaline et biréfringence en lumière polarisée.

On sait maintenant que le matériel amyloïde qui apparaît micro-fibrillaire en ultra-structure est constitué de chaînes protidiques en structure β plissée et provient soit de fragments de chaînes légères d'immunoglobulines soit d'autres protéines de structure voisine.

IX.5 Amyloidose der Lider und Bindehaut

Ursache der Amyloidose ist die Infiltration der Stützgewebe durch eine amorphe, azelluläre Substanz, deren physikalisch-chemische Zusammensetzung inzwischen besser bekannt ist.

Klinik. Die Amyloidose kann unter der palpebralen Epidermis, entlang dem Lidrand, in dem Chorion der Konjunktiva oder im Hornhautstroma lokalisiert sein. Die subkutane Lidamyloidose bildet rosa- oder orangefarbene konfluierende Mikropapeln, die mit Purpura-Punkten übersät sind; sie ist den Immunzellen-Amyloidosen, den Gammapathie-Amyloidosen oder "atypischen Primäramyloidosen" vorbehalten.
Die Amyloidose der Lidbindehaut ist die häufigste; sie tritt entweder isoliert oder sekundär infolge einer chronischen Lidentzündung, insbesondere eines Trachoms, auf. In der Conjunctiva bulbi und am Limbus sind die amyloiden Ablagerungen knötchenförmig, gelblich oder rosa und können an ein Lymphom oder an ein Carcinoma in situ denken lassen.

Histopathologie. Ganz unabhängig von der Lokalisation sind die Ablagerungen in ihrem Aussehen immer identisch. Sie stehen im allgemeinen in unmittelbarem Kontakt mit dem häufig atrophischen Epithel. Sie infiltrieren diffus in das umliegende Gewebe, dringen in die Tiefe ein und umhüllen manchmal verengte Gefäße. Diese Ablagerungen können schließlich im Kontakt mit der Umgebung makrophage Resorptionsreaktionen auslösen; sie besitzen vor allem zahlreiche Färbungseigenschaften, die ihre Identifizierung erlauben:
- purpurne Metachromasie bei Kristallviolett;
- mehr oder weniger eindeutige Positivreaktion bei PAS;
- grüne Fluoreszenz im ultravioletten Licht nach Behandlung der Schnitte mit Thioflavin T;
- Rot-orangefärbung durch Kongo-Rot in alkaliner Lösung und Doppelbrechung im polarisierten Licht.

Man weiß heute, daß der amyloide Stoff, der in Ultrastruktur mikrofibrillär erscheint, aus Proteidketten in gefälteter β-Struktur besteht und entweder von Fragmenten leichter Immunglobulinketten oder anderen Proteinen mit benachbarter Struktur herstammt.

PLATE 28 PLANCHE 28 TAFEL 28

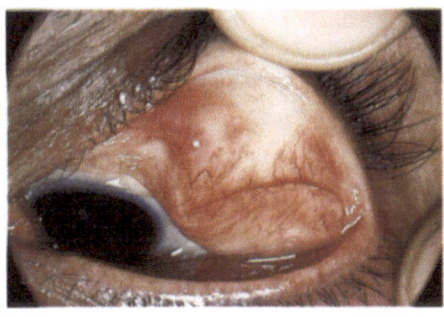

a

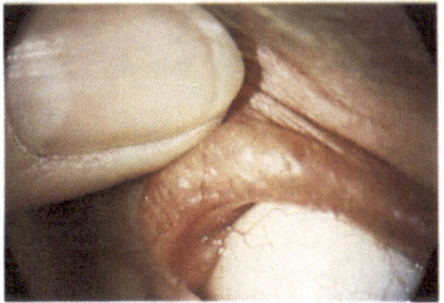

b

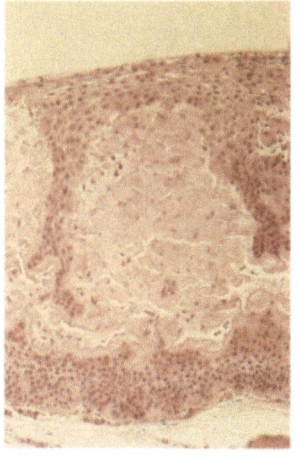

c

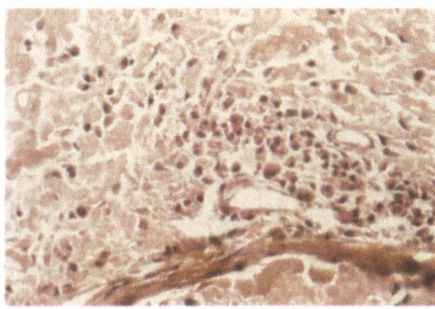

d

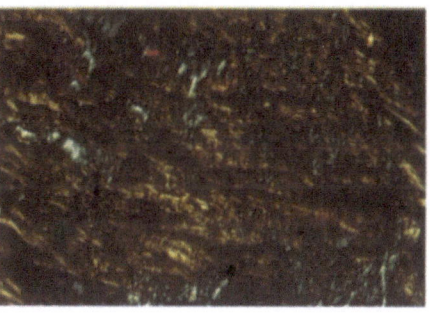

e

f

Fig. a. Amyloidosis of the superior palpebral conjunctiva.
The mucosa is thickened, indurated, and the eyelid can be everted as a single mass.

Fig. b. Amyloidosis of the lid margin.
The latter is yellowish, thickened, smooth and uneven.

Fig. c. Amyloidosis of the limbal conjunctiva: histopathology.
The amyloid deposits are in direct contact with the epithelium. They are amorphous, eosinophilic, homogeneous, sometimes striated, with scanty cells.

Fig. d. Amyloidosis of the palpebral conjunctiva.
Presence of plasma cells between and in direct contact with the amyloid deposits. (This reaction is characteristic of secondary amyloidosis, in particular when post-trachomatous.)

Fig. e. Green fluorescence of a limbal amyloidosis after staining with Thioflavin T.

Fig. f. Yellow-green dichroism of the amyloid substance under polarized light after staining with Congo red (birefringence linked to the β-pleated structure of this substance).

Fig. a. Amylose de la conjonctive palpébrale supérieure.
La muqueuse conjonctivale est épaissie, cartonnée, la paupière s'éversant en bloc.

Fig. b. Amylose de la marge palpébrale.
La marge palpébrale est épaissie, boudinée, lisse, jaunâtre.

Fig. c. Amylose conjonctivale limbique: histopathologie.
Les dépôts amyloïdes, au contact de l'épithélium sont amorphes, peu cellulaires, éosinophiles, homogènes, parfois striés, comme "moirés".

Fig. d. Amylose de la conjonctive palpébrale.
Présence au contact et entre les dépôts amyloïdes de nombreux plasmocytes (réaction particulière aux amyloses secondaires et notamment aux amyloses post-trachomateuses).

Fig. e. Fluorescence verte d'une amylose du limbe après coloration par la Thioflavine T.

Fig. f. Dichroïsme jaune-vert de la matière amyloïde à l'examen en polarisation après coloration par le rouge Congo (biréfringence liée à la structure β plissée de la substance amyloïde).

Abb. a. Amyloidose der Bindehaut des Oberlids.
Die Bindehaut ist verdickt, pappartig. Das Augenlid läßt sich in seiner Ganzheit umstülpen.

Abb. b. Amyloidose des Lidrandes.
Der Lidrand ist verdickt, wulstig, glatt, gelblich.

Abb. c. Amyloidose der Bindehaut am Limbus: Histopathologie.
Die amyloiden Ablagerungen in Epithelkontakt sind amorph, kaum zellulär, eosinophil, homogen, manchmal gerifelt mit "Moiré-Effekt".

Abb. d. Amyloidose der Bindehaut des Lids.
An und zwischen den amyloiden Ablagerungen befinden sich zahlreiche Plasmozyten (typische Reaktion der Sekundäramyloidosen und insbesondere der post-trachomatösen Amyloidosen).

Abb. e. Grüne Fluoreszenz einer Amyloidose des Limbus nach Färbung mit Thioflavin T.

Abb. f. Gelb-grüne Dichromasie der amyloiden Substanz bei Untersuchung mit polarisiertem Licht nach Färbung mit Kongo-Rot (mit der gefältelten β-Struktur der amyloiden Substanz zusammenhängende Doppelbrechung).

57

B

Orbital and orbito-palpebral tumours

*

Tumeurs de l'orbite et orbito-palpébrales

*

Orbitale und orbito-palpebrale Geschwülste

PLATE 29 PLANCHE 29 TAFEL 29

X. FIBROHISTIOCYTIC TUMOURS

X.1 Benign fibrohistiocytoma

These tumours are composed of fibroblasts and histiocytes; the latter, endowed with macrophagic functions, are also able to synthesize collagen.

Clinical features. The orbit, in its superior and medial sectors, seems to be the site in which these tumours occur most frequently; they produce proptosis, sometimes with diplopia and/or lowering of visual acuity. The palpebral or conjunctival localizations, particularly at the limbus (fibroxanthoma), are rare.

Histopathology. Histopathology shows a well defined tumour made up of fascicles of spindle-shaped cells, and a collagen network. When abundantly vascularized with capillaries this tumour may mimic a haemangiopericytoma. It is benign but can recur however, especially if excision is incomplete. *Atypical fibrohistiocytoma* occurs mostly in the elderly. Owing to some cellular abnormalities and to the presence of mitotic figures, it may be difficult to differentiate it from a malignant type. As a rule, however, although it frequently recurs, it does not metastasize.

X.2 Malignant fibrohistiocytoma

Clinical features. It is not possible to distinguish between the benign and the malignant forms, except that the latter grow faster and are likely to metastazise.

Histopathology. The tumour invades the surrounding tissues and presents disseminated areas of necrosis. There are many cytonuclear abnormalities. As radiotherapy and chemotherapy are not particularly effective, surgical treatment is essential. The prognosis is poor.

X.3 Nodular fasciitis

Clinical features. A pseudo-tumorous proliferation arising from the fascia and the connective septa, it is a specifically adult condition. It occurs in the eyelid-eyebrow region, under the conjunctiva, inside Tenon's capsule, or inside the muscle sheaths of the orbit.

Histopathology. This fibroblastic proliferation is reasonably well defined, but an invasion of the surrounding tissues may occur. The lesion, dense at the periphery, becomes looser in the centre where the cells, dissociated by a ground substance with a high content of hyaluronic acid (Alcian Blue positive), become star-shaped. Due to the sometimes irregularly shaped and large nuclei, the possibility of mitotic figures, and the rapid tumour growth, it has sometimes been referred to as pseudo-sarcoma.

X. TUMEURS FIBROHISTIOCYTAIRES

X.1 Fibrohistiocytome bénin

Cette tumeur est composée de fibroblastes et d'histiocytes; ces derniers, doués de fonctions macrophagiques, sont également capables de synthétiser du collagène.

Clinique. L'orbite dans ses secteurs supérieur et nasal paraît être le siège de prédilection de ces tumeurs; elles provoquent une exophtalmie avec parfois diplopie et/ou baisse de l'acuité visuelle. Les localisations palpébrales ou conjonctivales, particulièrement au limbe (fibroxanthome) sont rares.

Histopathologie. C'est une tumeur bien limitée constituée de cellules fusiformes disposées en faisceaux et comportant une trame collagène. Lorsqu'elle est abondamment vascularisée par des capillaires, elle peut simuler un hémangio-péricytome. C'est une tumeur bénigne; mais elle peut récidiver, surtout en cas d'exérèse incomplète.
Le *fibrohistiocytome atypique* se rencontre principalement chez les sujets âgés. Du fait de certaines anomalies cellulaires et de la présence de mitoses il peut être difficile à distinguer d'une forme maligne. Cependant, en règle, il ne métastase pas, bien qu'il récidive souvent.

X.2 Fibrohistiocytome malin

Clinique. Rien ne distingue la forme maligne de la bénigne si ce n'est une croissance plus rapide et la possibilité de métastases.

Histopathologie. La tumeur infiltre les tissus voisins et est parsemée de plages de nécrose. Les anomalies cytonucléaires sont nombreuses. Elle relève de la seule chirurgie car la radiothérapie et la chimiothérapie sont peu efficaces et son pronostic est redoutable.

X.3 Fasciite nodulaire

Clinique. Prolifération pseudo-tumorale se développant aux dépens des fascia et des septa conjonctifs, elle est l'apanage de l'adulte. On la rencontre dans la région palpébro-sourcilière, sous la conjonctive au sein de la capsule de Tenon, ou dans l'orbite dans les gaines musculaires.

Histopathologie. C'est une prolifération fibroblastique assez bien délimitée mais pouvant infiltrer les tissus voisins. La lésion dense en périphérie est plus lâche au centre où les cellules dissociées par une substance fondamentale riche en acide hyaluronique (Bleu Alcian positif) prennent un aspect stellaire. Les noyaux parfois irréguliers, de grande taille, les mitoses possibles, sa croissance rapide, ont pu la faire qualifier de pseudo-sarcomateuse.

X. FIBROHISTIOZYTÄRE TUMOREN

X.1 Gutartiges Fibrohistiozytom

Diese Tumoren bestehen aus Fibroblasten und Histiozyten; diese letzteren haben die Funktionen von Makrophagen und sind außerdem fähig, Kollagen zu synthetisieren.

Klinik. Die oberen und nasalen Bereiche der Orbita scheinen von diesen Tumoren bevorzugt zu werden; sie bewirken einen Exophthalmus, manchmal mit Diplopie und/oder Beeinträchtigung der Sehschärfe. Lokalisationen in den Lidern oder in der Konjunktiva, insbesondere am Limbus (Fibroxanthom) sind selten.

Histopathologie. Es handelt sich um einen gut abgegrenzten Tumor, der aus bündelartig geordneten, spindelförmigen Zellen mit einem Kollagen-Raster besteht. Wenn er stark mit Kapillaren vaskularisiert ist, kann er ein Hämangioperizytom vortäuschen. Es ist ein gutartiger Tumor, der jedoch besonders bei unvollständiger Entfernung rezidivieren kann.
Das *atypische Fibrohistiozytom* ist insbesondere bei älteren Menschen anzutreffen. Auf Grund des Vorhandenseins gewisser Zellanomalien und von Mitosen kann es vorkommen, daß es schwer von einer bösartigen Form zu unterscheiden ist. In der Regel bildet es indessen keine Metastasen, obwohl es häufig rezidiviert.

X.2 Bösartiges Fibrohistiozytom

Klinik. Abgesehen vom schnellerem Wachstum und der möglichen Metastasenbildung unterscheidet nichts die bösartige von der gutartigen Form.

Histopathologie. Der Tumor infiltriert die umliegenden Gewebe und ist mit Nekrosefeldern übersät. Die Zellkernanomalien sind zahlreich. Es kommt allein die Chirurgie in Frage, denn Radiotherapie und Chemotherapie sind wenig wirksam, und die Prognose ist sehr ernst.

X.3 Fasciitis nodularis

Klinik. Pseudotumoröse Proliferation, die sich aus dem Bindegewebe der Faszien und Septen entwickelt und vornehmlich bei Erwachsenen auftritt. Man findet sie im Lid- und Brauenbereich, unter der Conjunctiva im Bereich der Tenon-Kapsel oder in der Orbita in den Muskelscheiden.

Histopathologie. Es handelt sich um eine ziemlich gut abgegrenzte Fibroblastenvermehrung, die jedoch die benachbarten Gewebe infiltrieren kann. Die an der Peripherie dichtere Läsion ist lockerer in der Mitte, wo die durch eine hyaluronsäurereiche (Alcian-Blau positive) Grundsubstanz auseinandergedrängten Zellen ein sternartiges Aussehen annehmen. Auf Grund der unregelmäßigen, großen Kerne, der möglichen Mitosen, des raschen Wachstums wurde sie mitunter als pseudosarkomatös bezeichnet.

PLATE 29   PLANCHE 29   TAFEL 29

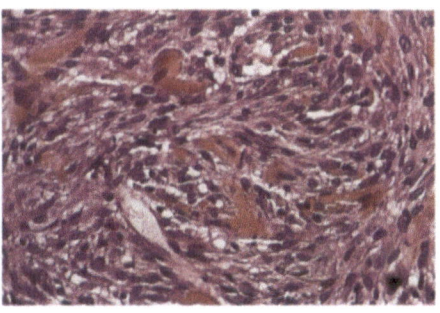

a

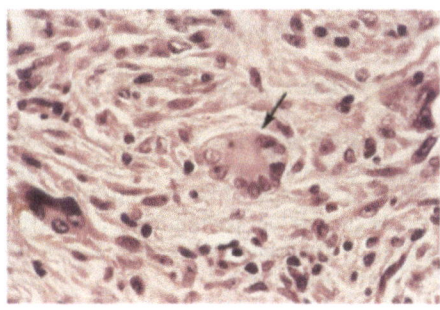

b

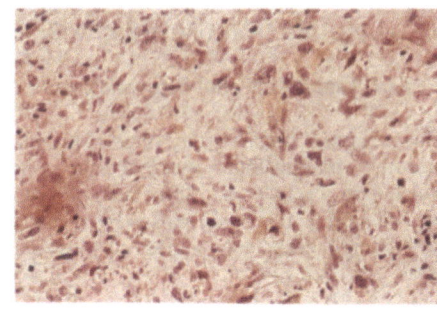

c

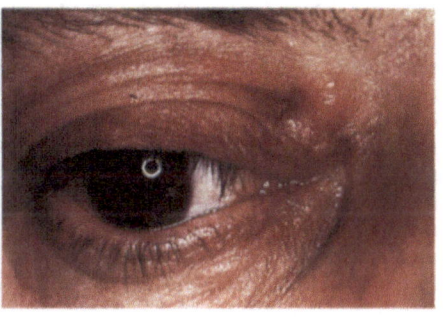

d

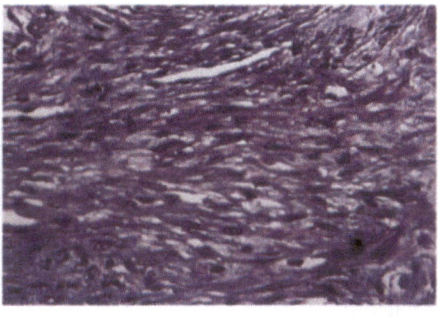

e

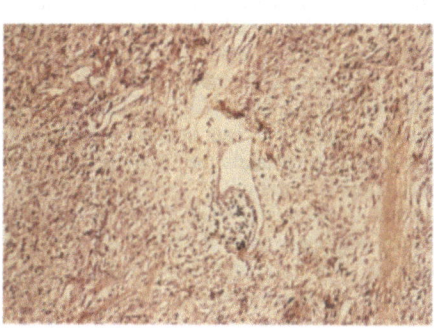

f

Fig. a. Benign fibrohistiocytoma.
The cells of the tumour are spindle-shaped fibroblasts and/or histiocyte-like, smaller, polyhedral cells with crescent or reniform nuclei. Some of these cells may contain lipidic vacuoles or deposits of haemosiderin. The cells are arranged in intertwined bundles; sometimes they are grouped around a connective or vascular core (storiform pattern).

Fig. b. Atypical fibrohistiocytoma.
This tumour shows a more pleomorphic cytological character; there are some dystrophic nuclei and some giant multinuclear cells which may look like Touton's cells (→), mitotic figures are not rare.

Fig. c. Malignant fibrohistiocytoma.
Absence of storiform character, nuclei are irregular in size and shape.

Fig. d. Nodular fasciitis of the eyelid and eyebrow region.
Nodular hyperhaemic lesion, hard, sometimes painful, deeply located although slightly adhering to the skin.

Fig. e. Nodular fasciitis (Masson's trichrome).
Periphery of the lesion. Spindle-shaped cells of a fibroblastic appearance, with elongated nuclei. A capillary is visible.

Fig. f. Nodular fasciitis.
Spindle-shaped cells mixed with inflammatory cells (suggestive of a reactive rather than a tumoral lesion).

Fig. a. Fibrohistiocytome bénin.
Tumeur constituée de cellules les unes fusiformes d'allure fibroblastique, les autres plus petites, polyédriques à noyau en virgule ou réniforme, d'aspect histiocytaire. Certaines d'entre-elles peuvent contenir des vacuoles lipidiques ou des dépôts d'hémosidérine. Elles se disposent en faisceaux entrecroisés ou enroulés autour d'un axe collagène ou vasculaire (disposition storiforme).

Fig. b. Fibrohistiocytome atypique.
Aspect cytologique nettement plus pléomorphe: certains noyaux sont dystrophiques; on rencontre des cellules géantes plurinucléées qui peuvent prendre l'allure de cellules de Touton (→), les mitoses ne sont pas rares.

Fig. c. Fibrohistiocytome malin.
Absence de disposition storiforme. Noyaux de taille et de forme irrégulières.

Fig. d. Fasciite nodulaire de la région palpébrosourcilière.
Lésion nodulaire, ferme, parfois douloureuse, profonde, mais parfois adhérente à la peau.

Fig. e. Fasciite nodulaire (Trichrome Masson).
Périphérie de la lésion. Cellules fusiformes à caractère fibroblastique, à noyaux allongés, entre lesquelles court un capillaire.

Fig. f. Fasciite nodulaire.
Aux cellules fusiformes se mêlent ici des cellules inflammatoires (argument en faveur d'une lésion réactionnelle plutôt que tumorale).

Abb. a. Gutartiges Fibrohistiozytom.
Der Tumor besteht aus spindelförmigen, fibroblastenähnlichen Zellen einerseits, aus kleineren, vieleckigen Zellen mit strich- oder nierenförmigem, eher histiozytärem Kern andererseits. Manche davon können Lipidvakuolen oder Hämosiderinablagerungen enthalten. Sie ordnen sich zu sich durchflechtenden Bündeln oder umgeben eine Kollagen- oder Gefäßachse (storiforme Anordnung).

Abb. b. Atypisches Fibrohistiozytom.
Der zytologische Befund ist eindeutig stärker polymorph: manche Kerne sind dystrophisch; es kommen plurinukleäre Riesenzellen vor, die das Aussehen von Touton-Zellen annehmen können (→), Mitosen sind nicht selten.

Abb. c. Bösartiges Fibrohistiozytom.
Keine storiforme Anordnung. Kerne von unregelmäßiger Form und Größe.

Abb. d. Fasciitis nodularis im Lid-Brauen-Bereich.
Knötchenförmige, feste, manchmal schmerzhafte Läsion, tief in die unteren Schichten eingelagert und gleichzeitig etwas an der Haut haftend.

Abb. e. Fasciitis nodularis (Trichromfärbung nach Masson).
Peripherie. Spindelförmige Zellen mit Fibroblastencharakter, länglichen Kernen, zwischen denen eine Kapillare verläuft.

Abb. f. Fasciitis nodularis.
Zu den Spindelzellen kommen hier entzündliche Zellen hinzu (was eher für eine reaktive als geschwulstartige Läsion spricht).

PLATE 30 PLANCHE 30 TAFEL 30

XI. TUMOURS OF MUSCULAR TISSUE

XI.1 Embryonal rhabdomyosarcoma

This malignant tumour seems to develop from primitive pluripotential mesenchymal cells which are capable of differentiating into striated muscle; this could explain the fact that they do not necessarily appear in muscular areas.

Clinical features. This tumour occurs selectively in children and in adolescents, 3/4 of the cases being diagnosed before the age of 10. Congenital cases exist. The presentation is of a rapidly developing proptosis (from several days to several weeks), which is often inflammatory in appearance. It is mostly localized in the nasal or supranasal region, invading the upper eyelid. Sometimes the tumour grows out towards the conjunctiva.

Histopathology. This diffuse tumour is made up of very dense cellular areas alternating with others which have a myxoid structure and with areas of necrosis. The cells which have a highly acidophilic cytoplasm can be spindle-shaped and can present a strap-like appearance. Alternately they may be thicker at their nuclear extremity ("comet-like"); in the myxoid areas they may have a star-like aspect; others can look globular with a central nucleus and a cytoplasm bearing huge vacuoles. There are 2 specific forms:

Alveolar rhabdomyosarcoma (Riopelle and Thériault). Fibrovascular septa divide the tumour into alveoli on the walls of which are inserted tumorous cells, very often of a cuboidal form. This pattern resembles the alveolar architecture of the lungs.

Botryoid rhadomyosarcoma. This is similar to other submucosal rhabdomyosarcomas of the body, and is made up of a dense superficial layer of mostly spindle shaped cells, under which the looser structure takes on a myxoid appearance.

Prognosis. The poor prognosis of these tumours which metastasize rapidly has improved noticeably during recent years, by the combined use of surgery, high voltage radiotherapy and chemotherapy.

XI. TUMEURS MUSCULAIRES

XI.1 Rhabdomyosarcome embryonnaire

Tumeur maligne paraissant dériver d'éléments mésenchymateux primitifs pluripotentiels possédant la capacité de se différencier en muscle strié, ce qui pourrait expliquer qu'elle n'apparaît pas obligatoirement dans des territoires musculaires.

Clinique. Elle se rencontre avant tout chez les enfants et les adolescents; les 3/4 des cas sont diagnostiqués avant l'âge de 10 ans et l'on connaît des formes congénitales. Le tableau est celui d'une exophtalmie d'évolution rapide (de quelques jours à quelques semaines) d'allure souvent inflammatoire, à localisation le plus souvent nasale ou supéro-nasale, envahissant la paupière supérieure. Parfois la tumeur s'extériorise vers la muqueuse conjonctivale.

Histopathologie. La tumeur, diffuse, est constituée de plages denses très cellulaires alternant avec des zones à structure myxoïde et des plages de nécrose. Les cellules à cytoplasme nettement acidophile peuvent être fusiformes, rubanées, épaissies parfois à leur extrémité nucléaire (aspect en "comète"); dans les zones myxoïdes, elles peuvent prendre une forme étoilée; d'autres enfin sont globuleuses avec un noyau central et un cytoplasme creusé de grosses vacuoles. Deux formes sont particulières:

Le rhabdomyosarcome alvéolaire (Riopelle et Thériault). Des septa fibrovasculaires cloisonnent la tumeur en alvéoles sur les parois desquelles s'insèrent des cellules tumorales souvent cubiques (disposition "en régime de dattes"). L'ensemble rappelle l'architecture des alvéoles pulmonaires.

Le rhabdomyosarcome botryoïde, semblable aux autres rhabdomyosarcomes sous-muqueux de l'organisme, est constitué d'une couche cellulaire dense superficielle comprenant en majorité des cellules fusiformes, sous laquelle l'agencement tumoral, plus lâche, prend une allure myxoïde.

Pronostic. Le pronostic redoutable de ces tumeurs, qui métastasent rapidement, s'est notablement amélioré ces dernières années par l'adjonction à la chirurgie, de la radiothérapie à haute énergie et de la chimiothérapie.

XI. MUSKELTUMOREN

XI.1 Embryonales Rhabdomyosarkom

Bösartiger Tumor, der von primitiven pluripotentiellen Mesenchymelementen auszugehen scheint und zur Differenzierung von quergestreiften Muskeln fähig ist, woraus man sich erklären könnte, warum er nicht nur in Muskelbereichen auftritt.

Klinik. Es ist vor allem bei Kindern und Jugendlichen anzutreffen, 3/4 aller Fälle werden vor dem Alter von 10 Jahren diagnostiziert; man kennt kongenitale Formen. Es kommt rasch zum Exophthalmus (wenige Tag bis zu wenigen Wochen) häufig mit Entzündungzeichen, meist nasal oder nasal oben und das ganze obere Lid mit einbeziehend. Manchmal durchbricht der Tumor die Bindehaut nach außen hin.

Histopathologie. Die diffuse Geschwulst besteht aus dichten, stark zellhaltigen Feldern, in denen Gebiete mit Schleimstruktur und Nekrose abwechseln. Die Zellen mit eindeutig acidophilem Zytoplasma können spindelförmig, bänderartig, manchmal am Kernende verdickt sein ("kometenhaftes" Aussehen); in den myxoiden Abschnitten können sie Sternform haben; andere sind wiederum rundlich mit zentralem Kern und mit von großen Vakuolen durchsetztem Zytoplasma. Es gibt zwei besondere Formen:

Das alveoläre Rhabdomyosarkom (Riopelle und Thériault). Fibrovaskuläre Septa teilen den Tumor in Alveolen ein, an deren Wänden sich Tumorzellen (häufig kubisch) einreihen (Anordnung in Form eines "Dattelbüschels"). Das Ganze erinnert and die Struktur der Lungenalveolen.

Das botryoide Rhabdomyosarkom, vergleichbar mit anderen submucösen Rhabdomyosarkomen des Organismus, besteht aus einer dichten oberflächlichen, mehrheitlich aus Spindelzellen bestehenden Zellschicht, unter der das lockerere Tumorgewebe einen myxoiden Aspekt annimmt.

Prognose. Die bedrohliche Prognose dieser Tumoren, die rasch Metastasen bilden, hat sich in den letzten Jahren, dank des kombinierten Einsatzes von Chirurgie, Radiotherapie mit hoher Energie und Chemotherapie, wesentlich verbessert.

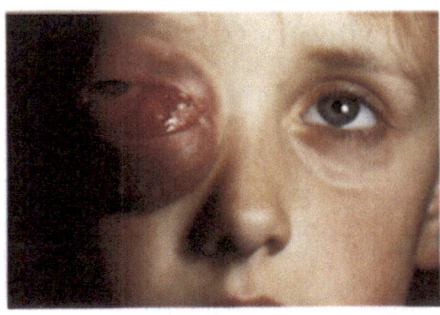

a

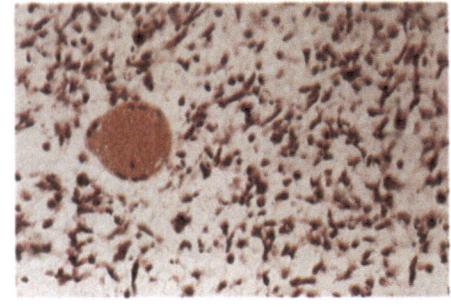

b

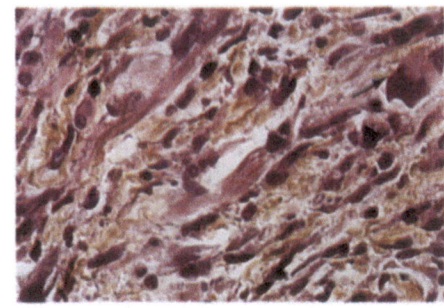

c

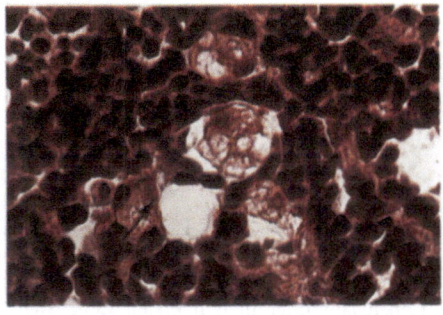

d

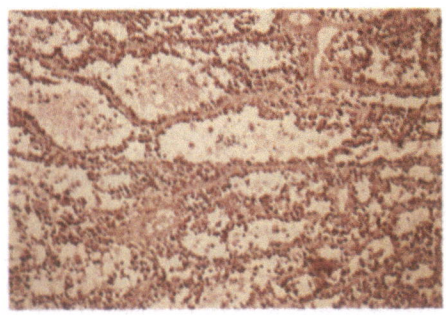

e

Fig. a. Embryonal rhabdomyosarcoma of the orbit. Inflammatory pseudo-phlegmonous looking proptosis. The tumour grows out under the conjunctiva as a reddish lobulate mass, resembling a "bunch of grapes" in appearance and is thus called "botryoid sarcoma".

Fig. b. Embryonal rhabdomyosarcoma.
Myxoid area crossed by a vessel. The cells, which are small, tend to have a star-like appearance.

Fig. c. Embryonal rhabdomyosarcoma.
Elongated, strap-like, rectangular cells, with a frequently monstrous looking nucleus (→) with characteristic striations in the cytoplasm. These striations visualised by the Masson's stain, and by Mallory's phosphotungstic hematoxylin stain, are often difficult to demonstrate, but are easily detected in ultra structural studies.

Fig. d. Embryonal rhabdomyocarcoma.
Large globular cell with a central nucleus surrounded by huge vacuoles containing glycogen ("spiderweb"-like cell) (→).

Fig. e. Alveolar rhabdomyosarcoma.
The tumour is divided into alveoli in which desquamating tumour cells take on a round shape.

Fig. a. Rhabdomyosarcome embryonnaire de l'orbite.
Exophtalmie d'allure inflammatoire pseudo-phlegmonneuse. La tumeur s'extériorise sous la conjonctive en une masse rougeâtre, lobulée "en grappe de raisin" d'où son nom de sarcome "botryoïde".

Fig. b. Rhabdomyosarcome embryonnaire.
Zone myxoïde traversée par un vaisseau. Les cellules, petites, ont tendance à prendre un aspect étoilé.

Fig. c. Rhabdomyosarcome embryonnaire.
Cellules allongées, rubanées, rectangulaires, à noyau souvent monstrueux (→) et dont le cytoplasme contient des striations caractéristiques. Ces striations, mises en évidence par les colorations de Masson, ou de Mallory à l'hématoxyline phosphotungstique, sont très inconstantes, mais se trouvent plus aisément en ultrastructure.

Fig. d. Rhabdomyosarcome embryonnaire.
Grosse cellule globuleuse à noyau central entouré de grandes vacuoles claires contenant du glycogène (cellule "en toile d'araignée") (→).

Fig. e. Rhabdomyosarcome alvéolaire.
La tumeur est divisée en alvéoles dans lesquelles desquament les cellules tumorales qui prennent une forme arrondie.

Abb. a. Embryonales Rhabdomyosarkom der Orbita.
Exophthalmus mit entzündlicher, pseudo-phlegmonöser Erscheinungsform. Der Tumor tritt unter der Bindehaut als rötliche Masse nach außen, die traubenförmig gelappt ist; daher der Name "botryoid".

Abb. b. Embryonales Rhabdomyosarkom.
Von einem Gefäß durchzogene Schleimzone. Die kleinen Zellen neigen zur Sternform.

Abb. c. Embryonales Rhabdomyosarkom.
Längliche, bandartige, rechteckige Zellen mit oft mißgebildetem Kern (→), deren Zytoplasma charakteristische Querstreifen aufweist. Diese Streifen, die mit Wolframphosphor-Hämatoxylin-Färbungen nach Masson, oder Mallory nachgewiesen werden, sind sehr unbeständig, aber finden sich leichter in Ultrastruktur.

Abb. d. Embryonales Rhabdomyosarkom.
Große perlenartige, rundliche Zelle mit einem zentralen Kern, der von großen, hellen, Glykogen enthaltenden Vakuolen umgeben ist ("Spinngeweb"-Zelle) (→).

Abb. e. Alveoläres Rhabdomyosarkom.
Die Geschwulst ist in Alveolen unterteilt, in die sich die Tumorzellen, eine rundliche Form annehmend, abstoßen.

PLATE 31　　　　　　　　　PLANCHE 31　　　　　　　　　TAFEL 31

XII. BENIGN PALPEBRO-ORBITAL VASCULAR TUMOURS

These tumours can appear as solitary lesions in the orbit or in the lid. They can also be present simultaneously in both localizations and communicate. Prudence is therefore essential in the surgical approach to palpebral angiomas. There is no absolute correlation between the clinical appearance and the histological type.

XII.1 Cavernous haemangioma

Clinical features. This is the most frequent tumour of the orbit in adults, inducing a progressive, painless, exophthalmos, giving way under pressure on the eyeball without bruit and without important functional impairment. In the eyelid, it has a variable, sometimes nodular appearance.

Histopathology. Generally encapsulated in the orbit, the tumour is made up of irregular vascular cavities, varying in size and containing red blood cells.

XII.2 Benign haemangio-endothelioma

Clinical features. Mostly encountered in nurslings and infants, it is relatively frequent in premature babies. It grows rapidly during the first year of life, remaining stationary for some time before spontaneously regressing and disappearing at puberty. General or even local corticosteroid therapy has been proposed to hasten this regression. In the eyelid, the lesion looks like a protruding nodule, sometimes lobulate, known as tuberous angioma or "strawberry angioma". As it grows in size it may impair vision either by palpebral occlusion or by direct compression on the eyeball. Surgery may become necessary as it is advisable to avoid radiotherapy. In the orbit, it provokes an early and rapidly growing exophthalmos.

Histopathology. The more or less lobulate tumour is made up of vascular tubes separated by thin walls of connective tissue.
Malignant types of haemangio-endothelioma exist (angiosarcoma), fortunately rarely in ophthalmology.

XII. TUMEURS VASCULAIRES BÉNIGNES PALPÉBRO-ORBITAIRES

Ces tumeurs sont soit isolées à localisation palpébrale ou orbitaire, soit à double localisation: elles sont alors communicantes. La prudence doit donc être de règle dans l'abord chirurgical des angiomes palpébraux. Il n'y a pas de corrélation absolue entre aspect clinique et type histologique.

XII.1 Angiome caverneux

Clinique. C'est, dans l'orbite la plus fréquente des tumeurs chez l'adulte, provoquant une exophtalmie progressive, indolore, réductible, sans souffle ni retentissement fonctionnel important. A la paupière son aspect est variable, parfois nodulaire.

Histopathologie. La tumeur, généralement encapsulée, est constituée de cavités vasculaires irrégulières de taille variable, contenant des hématies.

XII.2 Hémangio-endothéliome bénin

Clinique. Il se rencontre surtout chez le nourrisson et le jeune enfant avec une relative fréquence chez les prématurés. Il s'accroît rapidement dans la ou les premières années de la vie puis reste stationnaire avant de régresser spontanément pour s'effacer vers la puberté. On a proposé pour hâter cette régression une corticothérapie soit générale soit même locale. A la paupière il se présente comme un nodule saillant parfois lobulé et est connu alors sous le nom d'angiome tubéreux ou angiome "fraise". Lorsque sa taille devient trop importante il peut compromettre la vision soit par occlusion palpébrale soit par compression directe sur le globe; il peut devenir nécessaire alors d'intervenir chirurgicalement car il faut éviter la radiothérapie. Dans l'orbite il provoque une exophtalmie précoce et rapide.

Histopathologie. Tumeur plus ou moins lobulée constituée de tubes vasculaires séparés par de minces cloisons conjonctives.
Il existe des formes malignes d'hémangio-endothéliome (angiosarcomes) heureusement rares dans le domaine oculaire.

XII. GUTARTIGE GEFÄßTUMOREN DER LIDER UND ORBITA

Diese Geschwülste treten entweder einzeln am Lid oder in der Orbita auf, oder sie kommunizieren miteinander. Bei einem chirurgischen Eingriff an Lidangiomen ist deshalb Vorsicht geboten. Es besteht keine absolute Korrelation zwischen dem klinischen Aspekt und dem histologischen Typ.

XII.1 Kavernöses Hämangiom

Klinik. In der Orbita ist es die häufigste Geschwulst des Erwachsenen. Sie bewirkt einen progressiven, schmerzlosen, kompressiblen Exopthalmus, ohne Geräusch und ohne nennenswerte funktionelle Auswirkung. Am Lid ist das Aussehen unterschiedlich, manchmal knötchenartig.

Histopathologie. Die in der Orbita im allgemeinen abgekapselte Geschwulst besteht aus unregelmäßigen Gefäßhohlräumen unterschiedlicher Größe, die Erythrozyten enthalten.

XII.2 Gutartiges Hämangio-Endotheliom

Klinik. Es ist in erster Linie beim Säugling und Kleinkind und relativ häufig bei Frühgeborenen zu beobachten. Im ersten Lebensjahr oder in den ersten Lebensjahren wächst es rasch, bleibt dann stationär, um in der Pubertät spontan wieder zu verschwinden. Zur Beschleunigung dieser Rückbildung wurde eine allgemeine und auch lokale Kortikotherapie vorgeschlagen. Am Lid tritt es als vorstehendes Knötchen in Erscheinung und ist – wenn gelappt – als tuberöses Hämangiom bekannt. Wenn es zu große Ausmaße annimmt, kann es das Sehvermögen entweder durch Lidverschluß oder durch direkten Druck auf den Bulbus beeinträchtigen; ein chirurgischer Eingriff kann dann notwendig werden, da von einer Radiotherapie abzusehen ist. In der Orbita bewirkt es einen frühzeitigen, schnellen Exophthalmus.

Histopathologie. Mehr oder weniger gelappte Geschwulst, die aus Gefäßen besteht, die durch feinste Bindegwebswandungen voneinander getrennt sind.
Es gibt bösartige Formen des Hämangio-Endothelioms (Angiosarkome), die im Augenbereich glücklicherweise selten sind.

PLATE 31 PLANCHE 31 TAFEL 31

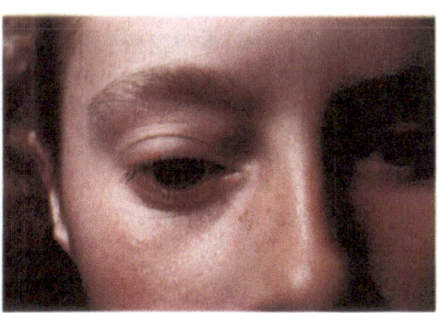

a

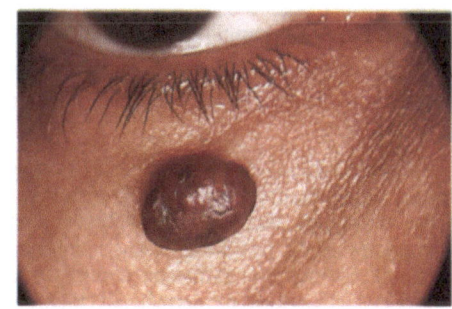

b

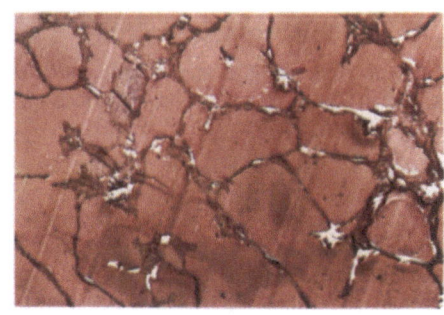

c

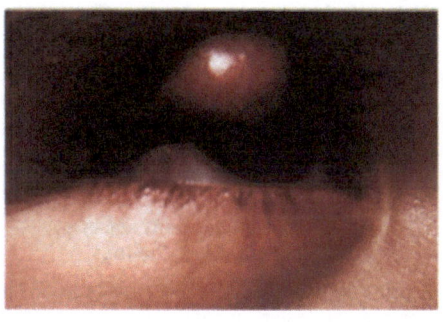

d

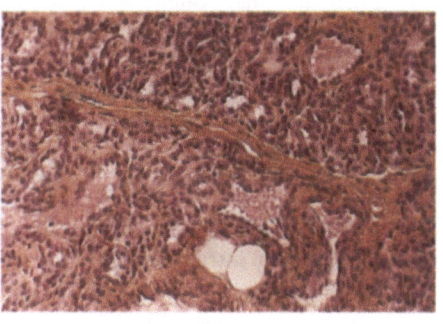

e

Fig. a. Cavernous haemangioma of the orbital supero-medial angle: inferolateral proptosis.

Fig. b. Cavernous haemangioma of the eyelid. Smooth renitent protruding nodule. Red to dark purple, it may in the latter case, be suggestive of a dome-shaped melanoma.

Fig. c. Cavernous haemangioma of the orbit. Tumour made up of irregularly shaped vascular cavities, variable in size, lined by a flattened endothelium, full of red blood cells which are separated by connective tissue partitions of differing thickness. Due to the stasis, thrombi may develop which may subsequently become calcified (phleboliths).

Fig. d. Benign haemangio-endothelioma of the eyelid in a nursling. Bright red protruding, painless and renitent nodule.

Fig. e. Benign haemangio-endothelioma. Dense gathering of vascular tubes in which high endothelial cells, sometimes presenting mitotic figures can even totally fill the vascular lumen. The staining of reticulin will confirm the intracavitary site of the cells.

Fig. a. Angiome caverneux de l'angle supéro-interne de l'orbite: exophtalmie inféro-temporale.

Fig. b. Angiome caverneux de la paupière. Nodule saillant lisse et rénitent. De teinte rouge à pourpre foncé il peut dans ce dernier cas faire discuter un mélanome en dôme.

Fig. c. Angiome caverneux de l'orbite. Tumeur constituée de cavités vasculaires de contour irrégulier, de taille inégale, bordées d'un endothélium aplati, remplies d'hématies et séparées par des cloisons conjonctives plus ou moins épaisses. Du fait de la stase des thrombis peuvent se former et même secondairement se calcifier (phlébolithes).

Fig. d. Hémangio-endothéliome bénin de la paupière chez un nourrisson. Nodule saillant rouge vif indolore et rénitent.

Fig. e. Hémangio-endothéliome bénin. Groupement dense de tubes vasculaires. A l'intérieur de ces tubes les cellules endothéliales, hautes, parfois en mitose, peuvent même oblitérer totalement la lumière vasculaire. La coloration de la réticuline authentifiera le siège intracavitaire des cellules.

Abb. a. Kavernöses Angiom im oberen inneren Winkel der Orbita: inferotemporaler Exophthalmus.

Abb. b. Kavernöses Hämangiom des Lids. Vorstehendes, glattes, nicht verschiebbares Knötchen. Mit seiner roten bis dunkelpurpurnen Färbung kann in diesem Fall ein kuppenförmig vorgewölbtes Melanom zur Diskussion stehen.

Abb. c. Kavernöses Hämangiom der Orbita. Geschwulst aus Gefäßen mit unregelmäßigen Umrissen, von ungleicher Größe, mit einem Plattenendothel ausgekleidet, mit Erythrozyten gefüllt und durch mehr oder weniger dichte Bindegewebswände voneinander getrennt. Auf Grund der Stase können sich Thromben bilden und sekundär sogar verkalken (Phlebolithen).

Abb. d. Gutartiges Hämangio-Endotheliom des Lids bei einem Säugling. Vorstehendes, hellrotes, schmerzloses und unverschiebbares Knötchen.

Abb. e. Gutartiges Hämangio-Endotheliom. Dichte Gruppierung von Gefäßen, die von hohen, manchmal in Mitose befindlichen Endothelzellen ausgekleidet sind. Die Retikulinfärbung bestätigt die intraluminäre Lage der Zellen. Letztere können die Lumina vollständig verschließen.

65

PLATE 32 PLANCHE 32 TAFEL 32

XII.3 Haemangio-pericytoma

Clinical features. It is more frequently observed in adults and mostly located in the superior sectors of the orbit.

Histopathology. It consists of fine capillaries encapsulated in cellular agglomerations of variable density. Recurrences are frequent and the possibility of malignant change renders the prognosis poor; the histological appearance is of little help for a long term prediction of the outcome. It is generally believed that the prognosis is better in children.

XII.4 Flat haemangioma

Clinical features. This angioma is generally observed at birth and better known clinically than histologically. It presents itself as a dark red to purple flat area, irregular in shape, showing no tendency to increase in size (Port-Wine stain). In the trigeminal nerve distribution area, it may be a part of the Sturge-Weber-Krabbe's Syndrome (encephalotrigeminal angiomatosis). (See Plate 53)

Histopathology. Dermal capillaries are more numerous than normal and are more dilated. It has, in fact, a more telangiectatic than angiomatous appearance.

XII.5 Intravascular vegetating haemangio-endothelioma

Clinical features. The lesion is a prominent tumour, painful at times, located in the dermis.

Histopathology. Papillary proliferation of endothelial cells within a venous or angiomatous cavity wherein local thrombosis may occur. The vascular structure is sometimes so much altered that the lesion may be misinterpreted as an angiosarcoma.

XIII. TUMOURS OF ADIPOSE ORBITAL TISSUE

XIII.1 Lipoma

Clinical features. True orbital lipomas are rare and are mostly observed in adults.

Histopathology. It is identical to that of palpebral or conjunctival lipoma (Plate 23, Chapter VI) but the existence of a capsule prevents its misinterpretation as a simple fatty hernia.

XIII.2 Liposarcoma

Clinical features. Although rarely observed in the orbit, it may be seen (unlike other localizations) in children or adolescents. Prognosis is poor (70% metastasize).

Histopathology. A large range of cells may be observed, from the most differentiated types, similar to those of a lipoma, to the polymorphous liposarcoma and the type with round pseudo-lymphoid cells.

PLATE 32   PLANCHE 32   TAFEL 32

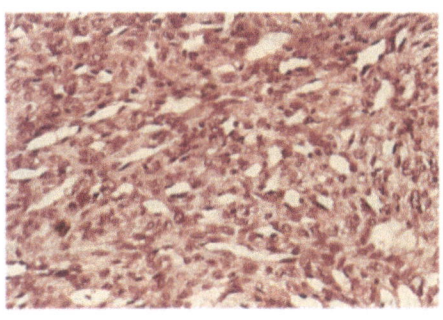

a

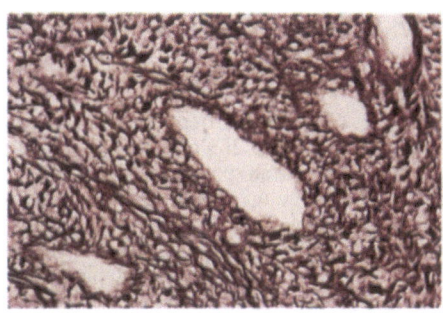

b

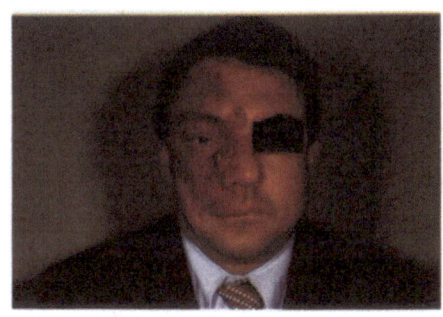

c

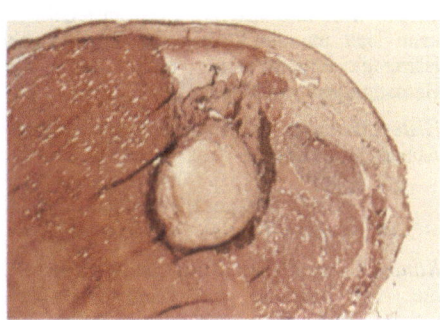

d

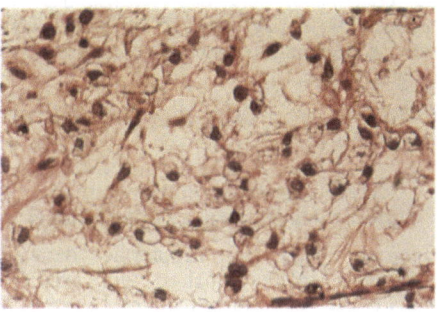

e

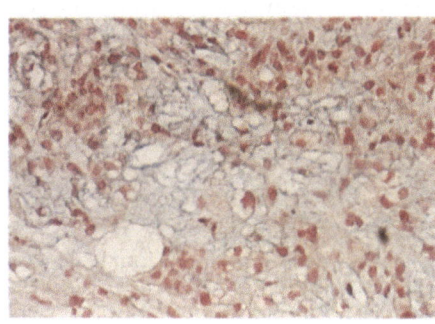

f

Fig. a. Haemangiopericytoma.
Tumour made up of capillaries separated by small spindle-shaped cells with the appearance of pericytes.

Fig. b. Haemangiopericytoma (Laidlaw).
The reticulin network surrounding the capillaries separates the tumour cells from one another. It shows that the latter proliferate outside the vascular wall.

Fig. c. Flat angioma of the face, in the trigeminal nerve area in a Sturge-Weber-Krabbe's disease.

Fig. d. Intravascular vegetating haemangio-endothelioma.
Venous cavity almost totally filled by a papillary proliferation of endothelial cells.

Fig. e. Orbital liposarcoma.
Tumour made up of lipoblasts, with their clear cytoplasm and a round central nucleus which looks swollen at times.

Fig. f. Myxoid liposarcoma (Alcian Blue).
Stroma with an exceptionally high content of acid mucopolysaccharides.

Fig. a. Hémangio-péricytome.
Tumeur constituée de capillaires séparés par de petites cellules fusiformes d'allure péricytaire.

Fig. b. Hémangio-péricytome (Laidlaw).
Le réseau de réticuline engainant les capillaires sépare les unes des autres les cellules tumorales. Celles-ci prolifèrent donc en dehors de la paroi vasculaire.

Fig. c. Angiome plan de la face couvrant le territoire du trijumeau dans une maladie de Sturge-Weber-Krabbe.

Fig. d. Hémangio-endothéliome végétant intravasculaire.
Cavité veineuse presque totalement occupée par une prolifération papilliforme de cellules endothéliales.

Fig. e. Liposarcome orbitaire.
Tumeur constituée de lipoblastes, cellules à cytoplasme clair, à noyau central arrondi parfois boursouflé.

Fig. f. Liposarcome myxoïde (Bleu Alcian).
Le stroma est particulièrement riche en mucopolysaccharides acides.

Abb. a. Hämangio-Perizytom.
Geschwulst bestehend aus Kapillaren, die durch kleine spindelförmige Zellen mit perizytären Eigenschaften voneinander getrennt sind.

Abb. b. Hämangio-Perizytom (Laidlaw).
Das die Kapillaren einhüllende Retikulinnetz zeigt, daß die proliferierenden Zellen außerhalb der Gefäßwand liegen.

Abb. c. Flaches Gesichtsangiom, das bei einer Sturge-Weber-Krabbe-Erkrankung den Trigeminusbereich bedeckt.

Abb. d. Wucherndes intravasales Hämangio-Endotheliom.
Venöser Hohlraum, der fast völlig von einer papillenartigen Wucherung der Endothelialzellen ausgefüllt ist.

Abb. e. Liposarkom der Orbita.
Der Tumor besteht aus Lipoblasten, Zellen mit hellem Zytoplasma, mit abgerundetem, zentralem, manchmal angeschwollenem Kern.

Abb. f. Myxoides Liposarkom (Alcian-Blau).
Das Stroma enthält besonders viel saure Mukopolysaccharide.

PLATE 33 PLANCHE 33 TAFEL 33

XIV. BONE TUMOURS

XIV.1 Osteoma

Clinical features. This is the most frequent bone tumour of the orbit. Mostly observed in young adults, it usually originates from the wall of a sinus, mainly from the frontal sinus. X rays show a dense, homogenous, well defined opacity. When of ethmoidal origin, the proptosis is more of an axial type. In the case of a sphenoidal osteoma, compression of the optic nerve may occur. The association of an osteoma with a polyposis of the colon and a soft tissue tumour is known as Gardner and Richards' syndrome, an autosomal dominant hereditary condition.

Histopathology. Histopathology is described with Fig. b.

XIV.2 Bone haemangioma

Clinical features. A rare tumour which, when observed, is mostly localized in the flat bones of the skull. It can be a cavernous angioma, haemangio-endothelioma or an haemangio-pericytoma.

Histopathology. Histopathology is described with Fig. d.

XIV.3 Giant cell tumour (osteoclastoma)

Clinical features. This neoplasm is derived from mesenchymal cells which develop into osteoclasts. Pain and palpebral oedema are the usual initial symptoms. The radiological image is that of an osteolysis with partitions. In fact, it occurs very rarely in the orbit, usually being found in the long bones. When it is suspected, a blood test for calcium and phosphorus is necessary in order to exclude hyperthyroidism and Recklinghausen's brown tumour.

Histopathology. Histopathology is described with Fig. e.

XIV.4 Osteosarcoma

Clinical features. This malignant tumour, seldom located in the orbit, is more often secondary to radiotherapy rather than primary. It may also aggravate the evolution of Paget's disease. It is sometimes observed in patients having had a retinoblastoma. Pain and swelling of the surrounding tissues are commonly associated with proptosis. From the radiological point of view, osteolytic and osteoformative areas are mixed.

Histopathology. Histopathology is described with Fig. f.

XIV.5 Mesenchymatous chondrosarcoma

Clinical features. It is an extremely rare tumour, but when observed it seems to be selectively located in the orbit.

Histopathology. This tumour consists of anaplastic mesenchymatous tissue, consisting of round or ovoid elements which, in places, undergo a rudimentary chondroid differentiation with imprecise delimitation. Its rich vascularization sometimes makes diagnosis difficult.

68

XIV. TUMEURS OSSEUSES

XIV.1 Ostéome

Clinique. C'est la plus fréquente des tumeurs osseuses de l'orbite. Il s'observe surtout chez l'adulte jeune. Son point de départ est en général la paroi d'un sinus, en particulier frontal. Aux rayons X, c'est une opacité dense, homogène, bien délimitée. Lorsque l'origine est ethmoïdale l'exophtalmie est plus axile. En cas d'ostéome sphénoïdal une compression du nerf optique est possible. L'association d'un ostéome à une polypose colique et à une tumeur des tissus mous réalise le syndrome de Gardner et Richards, d'hérédité autosomique dominante.

Histopathologie. L'histopathologie ne donne lieu à aucune difficulté de diagnostic (Fig. b).

XIV.2 Hémangiome de l'os

Clinique. Tumeur rare mais dont les os plats du crâne sont une des localisations de prédilection. Il peut s'agir d'angiome caverneux, d'hémangio-endothéliome ou d'hémangiopéricytome.

Histopathologie. L'histopathologie est décrite avec la Fig. d.

XIV.3 Tumeur à cellules géantes (tumeur à myéloplaxes, ostéoclastome)

Clinique. C'est un néoplasme dérivant d'éléments mésenchymateux qui évoluent vers l'ostéoclaste. Elle se manifeste en général par des douleurs et un oedème palpébral. Radiologiquement c'est une image ostéolytique avec des cloisonnements. Elle est, en fait, très rare dans l'orbite, son siège habituel étant les os longs. Il faut donc toujours réclamer un dosage de la calcémie et de la phosphorémie pour éliminer une hyperthyroïdie et une tumeur brune de Recklinghausen.

Histopathologie. L'histopathologie est décrite avec la Fig. e.

XIV.4 Ostéosarcome

Clinique. Très rare dans l'orbite cette tumeur maligne est plus souvent secondaire, succédant à des traitements par radiations, que primitive. Elle peut compliquer l'évolution de maladie de Paget. Elle s'observe tardivement, avec une certaine fréquence, chez les sujets ayant présenté un rétinoblastome. Elle se manifeste par des douleurs et un gonflement des tissus avoisinants. Radiologiquement, plages d'ostéolyse et d'ostéoformation sont mêlées.

Histopathologie. L'histopathologie est décrite avec la Fig. f.

XIX.5 Chondrosarcome mésenchymateux

Clinique. C'est une tumeur très rare mais dont l'orbite paraît être un des sièges d'élection.

Histopathologie. Elle est constituée d'un tissu mésenchymateux anaplasique comportant des éléments arrondis ou ovoïdes qui par places subissent une ébauche de différenciation chondroïde à limites floues. Son abondante vascularisation en rend parfois le diagnostic difficile.

XIV. KNOCHENTUMOREN

XIV.1 Osteom

Klinik. Es ist der am häufigsten vorkommende Knochentumor der Orbita. Er wird vor allem bei jungen Erwachsenen beobachtet. Sein Ausgangspunkt ist im allgemeinen die Wand eines Sinus, insbesondere der Stirnhöhle, und er bewirkt einen Exophthalmus. Im Röntgenbild erscheint er als dichter, gleichmäßiger, gut abgegrenzter Schatten. Wenn er vom Siebbein ausgeht, ist der Exophthalmus mehr axial. Geht er vom Keilbein aus, so ist Kompression des Sehnervs möglich. Das gemeinsame Auftreten eines Osteoms mit einer Polyposis des Kolons und eines Weichteiltumors ergibt das Gardner-Richards-Syndrom mit dominant autosomaler Heredität.

Histopathologie. Die histopathologie ist unter Abb. b beschrieben.

XIV.2 Knochenhämangiom

Klinik. Seltener Tumor, der sich vornehmlich an den flachen Schädelknochen ansiedelt. Es kann sich um ein kavernöses Angiom, ein Hämangio-Endotheliom oder um ein Hämangioperizytom handeln.

Histopathologie. Die Histopathologie ist unter Abb. d beschrieben.

XIV.3 Riesenzellentumor (Myeloplax-Tumor, Osteoklastom)

Klinik. Es handelt sich um eine Geschwulst, die von Mesenchymelementen ausgeht, welche sich zu einem Osteoklasten hin entwickeln. Es macht sich meist durch Schmerzen und ein Lidödem bemerkbar. Radiologisch typisch ist eine Osteolyse mit multiplen Septen. In der Orbita ist es sehr selten, da es sich gewöhnlich an langen Knochen ansiedelt. Mit Kalzämie- und Phosphorämieuntersuchung ist eine Überfunktion der Schilddrüse und ein brauner Recklinghausen Tumor auszuschließen.

Histopathologie. Die Histopathologie ist unter Abb. e beschrieben.

XIV.4 Osteosarkom

Klinik. Diese in der Orbita sehr seltene, bösartige Geschwulst tritt häufiger sekundär als Folge von Strahlenbehandlung und weniger als Primärtumor auf. Sie kann auch Komplikation einer Paget-Krankheit sein. Sie ist manchmal bei Personen, die vormals ein Retinoblastom aufwiesen, zu beobachten. Sie macht sich durch Schmerzen und Schwellung der umliegenden Gewebe bemerkbar. Radiologisch treten knochenauflösende und knochenbildende Bezirke gemischt auf.

Histopathologie. Die Histopathologie ist unter Abb. f beschrieben.

XIV.5 Mesenchymatöses Chondrosarkom

Klinik. Dies ist ein sehr seltener Tumor, der sich mit Vorliebe in der Orbita niederzulassen scheint.

Histopathologie. Er besteht aus mesenchymalem anaplastischem Gewebe mit abgerundeten oder ovoiden Elementen, mit stellenweisen Ansätzen zu unscharf abgegrenzter Knorpeldifferenzierung. Wegen der reichlichen Vaskularisierung ist die Diagnose mitunter schwierig.

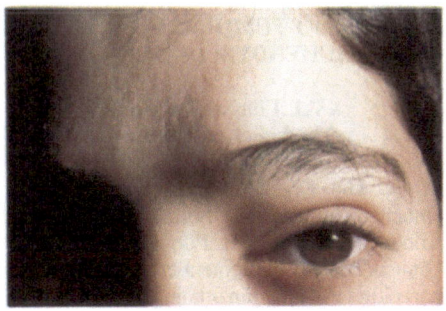

a

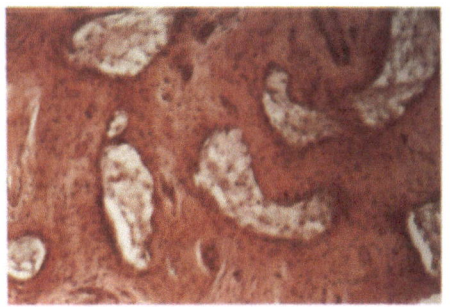

b

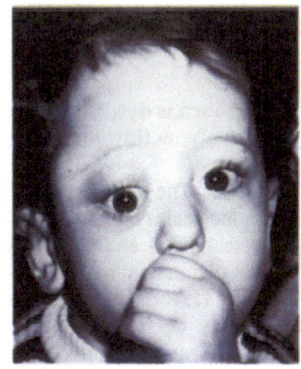

c

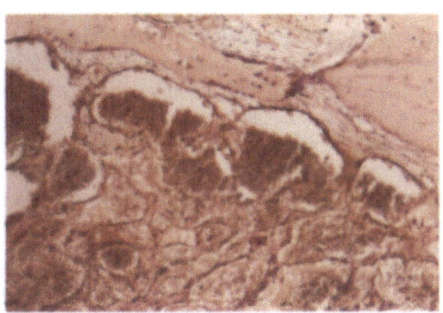

d

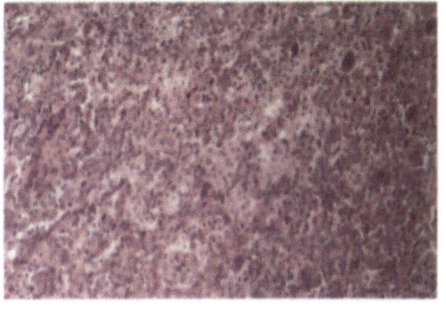

e

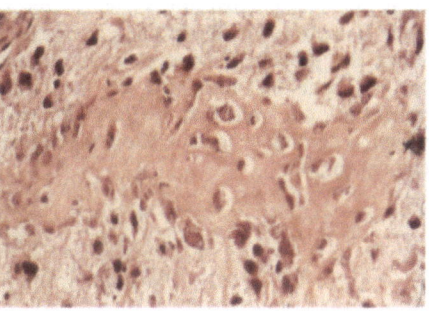

f

Fig. a. Orbital osteoma of frontal sinus origin in a child.
Lateral exophthalmos.

Fig. b. Orbital osteoma: structure of a mature lamellar bone.
Depending on the case, the condition is considered to be either a spongy osteoma or a compact eburnated osteoma.

Fig. c. Cavernous haemangioma of the bone, located in the orbit.
Progressive, lateralized exophthalmos, resisting pressure on the eyeball, often painful.

Fig. d. Cavernous haemangioma of the bone: thin walled irregular vascular cavities, growing between the bone strata.

Fig. e. Giant cell tumour.
Proliferation of ovoid or spindle shaped mononuclear cells. Multinucleated giant cells containing up to 50 or 100 nuclei and which are identical to osteoclasts can be observed. Some malignant cases have been described, with mitotic figures and atypical cells.

Fig. f. Orbital osteosarcoma.
Mesenchymatous proliferation, including spindle-shaped cells and osteoblastic looking cells surrounding the poorly defined bone framework. If distinct chondroid areas are also present the lesion is described as an osteo-chondro-sarcoma.

Fig. a. Ostéome orbitaire d'origine sinusienne frontale chez un enfant.
Exophtalmie latéralisée.

Fig. b. Ostéome orbitaire: structure d'un os mature, lamellaire.
Selon les cas on parle d'ostéome spongieux ou au contraire d'ostéome compact ou éburné.

Fig. c. Hémangiome caverneux osseux de l'orbite.
Exophtalmie latéralisée irréductible progressive, souvent douloureuse.

Fig. d. Hémangiome caverneux de l'os: cavités vasculaires irrégulières, se développant entre les travées osseuses.

Fig. e. Tumeur à cellules géantes.
Prolifération d'éléments ovoïdes ou fusiformes, mononucléés. On y rencontre des plasmodes géantes contenant jusqu'à 50 à 100 noyaux et identiques à des ostéoclastes. On a décrit des formes malignes avec mitoses et atypies cellulaires.

Fig. f. Ostéosarcome de l'orbite.
Prolifération mésenchymateuse faite de cellules fusiformes et d'éléments d'allure ostéoblastique entourant des travées osseuses mal limitées. Lorsqu'existent en outre des plages chondroïdes, il s'agit d'un ostéo-chondro-sarcome.

Abb. a. Osteom der Orbita, von der Stirnhöhle ausgehend, bei einem Kinde.
Seitlicher Exophthalmus.

Abb. b. Osteom der Orbita: Struktur eines reifen Lamellenknochens.
Man spricht je nachdem von einem schwammigen Osteom oder im Gegenteil von einem kompakten oder elfenbeinartig verdichteten Knochen.

Abb. c. Kavernöses Knochenhämangiom der Orbita.
Seitlicher Exophthalmus, progressiv, oft schmerzhaft, der sich nicht zurückdrängen läßt.

Abb. d. Kavernöses Knochen hämangiom: unregelmäßige Gefäßhöhlungen, die sich zwischen den Knochenbälkchen bilden.

Abb. e. Riesenzellentumor.
Proliferation von ovoiden oder spindelförmigen, mononukleären Elementen. Man findet Riesenzellen mit 50 bis 100 Kernen, die Osteoklasten gleich sind. Es wurden bösartige Formen mit Mitosen und Zellatypien beschrieben.

Abb. f. Osteosarkom der Orbita.
Mesenchymale Proliferation von spindelförmigen Zellen und osteoblastartigen Elementen, die schlecht abgegrenzte Knochenbalken umschließen. Sind außerdem knorpelartige Felder vorhanden, so handelt es sich um ein Osteo-Chondro-Sarkom.

PLATE 34 PLANCHE 34 TAFEL 34

XV. PSEUDO-TUMOROUS BONE DYSPLASIAS

XV.1 Fibrous dysplasia and ossifying fibroma

Clinical features. The disease may involve one bone (monosteal type) only or several bones (polyosteal type) and when associated with cutaneous pigmentation and a precocious puberty it is known as Albright-Fuller Syndrome. It may be found in children and adolescents. Its evolution stops in adulthood with bone growth. It manifests itself by a slow, painless, progressive proptosis, but if located in the posterior orbit, it may produce optic nerve atrophy. Radiologically, it is a sometimes heterogeneous hyperdensity, with a thickening of the bone, and passing through the synchondroses.

Histopathology. Under gross examination the tissue shows disseminated haemorrhagic areas; its characteristically granular consistency is explained by the histological features. When the growth of bone is important and brings about the formation of true bone trabeculae, one refers to *ossifying fibroma*, which, according to some authors, is a distinct clinical entity.

XV.2 Bone cyst aneurysm

Clinical features. This lesion may appear in young patients under the age of 20. Trauma may sometimes be considered the cause. It often manifests itself by pain and inflammatory signs which result in a congestive palpebral oedema. X rays show an invasive lesion destroying the inflated puffy looking osseous wall, the cavity of which is bound by a thin trabecular bone lamella.

Histopathology. Histological examination shows large vascular cavities, devoid of endothelium, in the connective tissue. The latter is characterized by haemorrhagic areas and haemosideric cells next to multinucleated giant cells recalling osteoclasts. At the periphery a bony lamella, called an osteoid band, surrounds the lesion.

XV. DYSPLASIES OSSEUSES PSEUDO-TUMORALES

XV.1 Dysplasie fibreuse et fibrome ossifiant

Clinique. La maladie peut intéresser un seul os (forme monostéale) ou plusieurs (forme polyostéale) et peut alors s'associer à des pigmentations cutanées et à une puberté précoce réalisant le syndrome d'Albright-Fuller. Elle se rencontre chez l'enfant et l'adolescent et son évolution cesse à l'âge adulte avec la croissance osseuse. Elle se révèle par une exophtalmie non douloureuse lente et progressive, mais dans ses localisations postérieures elle peut provoquer une atrophie optique. Radiologiquement c'est une hyperdensité parfois hétérogène avec épaississement de l'os et traversant les synchondroses.

Histopathologie. Macroscopiquement le tissu parfois parsemé de plages hémorragiques a une consistance sablonneuse caractéristique qu'explique l'image histologique. Quand la production osseuse est importante et aboutit à la formation de véritables travées osseuses on parle plutôt de *fibrome ossifiant* qui serait pour certains une entité distincte.

XV.2 Kyste anévrysmal de l'os

Clinique. C'est une lésion du sujet jeune apparaissant avant l'âge de 20 ans. Un traumatisme est parfois invoqué comme cause déclenchante. Elle se manifeste souvent par des douleurs et des signes inflammatoires que traduit un oedème congestif de la paupière. Radiologiquement c'est une lésion qui s'étend en détruisant la paroi osseuse qui apparaît soufflée, la cavité cernée d'une fine lamelle osseuse ayant un aspect trabéculé.

Histopathologie. L'examen histologique découvre de larges cavités vasculaires, sans limite endothéliale, dans un tissu conjonctif parsemé d'hémorragies et de cellules géantes multinucléées d'aspect ostéoclastique. A la périphérie une lamelle osseuse dite bande ostéoïde borde la lésion.

XV. PSEUDO-TUMORALE KNOCHENDYSPLASIEN

XV.1 Fibröse Dysplasie und verknöcherndes Fibrom

Klinik. Die Krankheit kann einen einzigen Knochen (monosteale Form) oder mehrere Knochen (polyosteale Form) betreffen; es können dann Hautpigmentierungen und eine vorzeitige Pubertät hinzukommen, so daß sich das Albright-Fuller Syndrom ergibt. Sie ist bei Kindern und Jugendlichen anzutreffen, und ihre Progredienz schließt im Erwachsenenalter mit dem Ende des Knochenwachstums. Sie zeigt sich als nicht schmerzhafter, langsamer und progredienter Exophthalmus, kann aber bei retrobulbärer Lage zu Sehnervenatrophie führen. Radiologisch findet man eine bisweilen heterogene Hyperdensität des Knochens, die die Synchondrosen durchdringt und mit einer Verdickung des Knochens einhergeht.

Histopathologie. Makroskopisch hat das manchmal von hämorrhagischen Feldern übersäte Gewebe eine charakteristische sandige Konsistenz, die durch das histologische Bild erklärt wird. Wenn die Knochenbildung ausgesprochen ist und zur Bildung richtiger Knochenbalken führt, spricht man eher von einem *verknöchernden Fibrom*, das laut einigen Autoren ein einheitliches Krankheitsbild sein soll.

XV.2 Aneurysmatische Knochenzyste

Klinik. Es handelt sich um eine Läsion junger Menschen, die vor 20 Jahren auftritt. Als auslösende Ursache wird manchmal ein Trauma genannt. Sie zeigt sich häufig durch Schmerzen und entzündliche Veränderungen im Lid (Ödem und Rötung). Das Röntgenbild zeigt eine invasive Läsion, welche die Knochenwand zerstört; diese erscheint wie aufgetrieben, und der von einer feinen Knochenlamelle umgebene Defekt hat eine trabekuläre Struktur.

Histopathologie. Die histologische Untersuchung ergibt weite Gefäßausschnitte ohne Endothelauskleidung, die in einem Bindegewebe liegen, das mit Blutungen, hämosiderinhaltigen Zellen neben vielkernigen Riesenzellen von osteoklastartigem Aspekt übersät ist. Peripher ist die Läsion von einer Knochenlamelle begrenzt, welche osteoider Saum genannt wird.

PLATE 34 PLANCHE 34 TAFEL 34

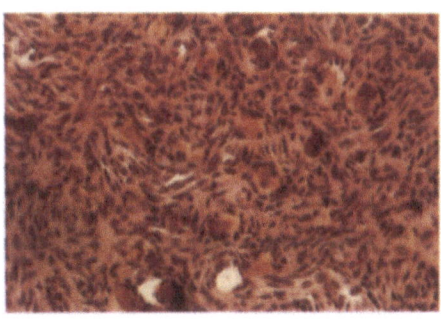

a

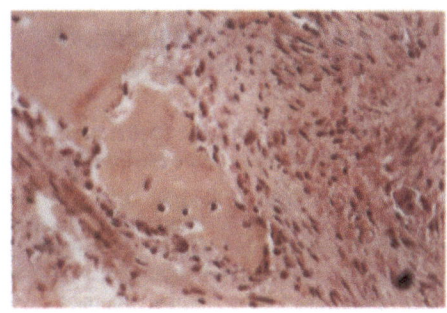

b

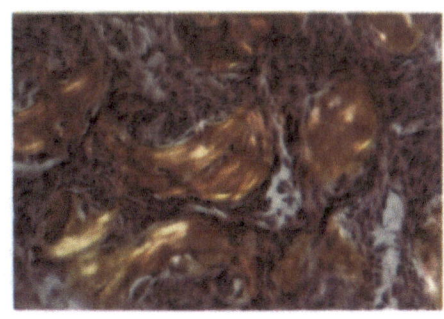

c

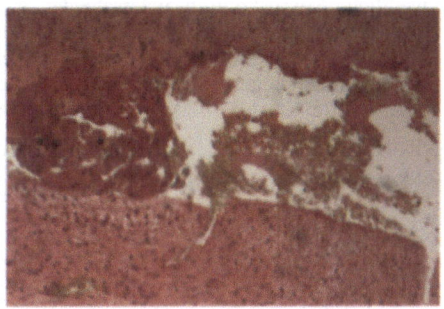

d

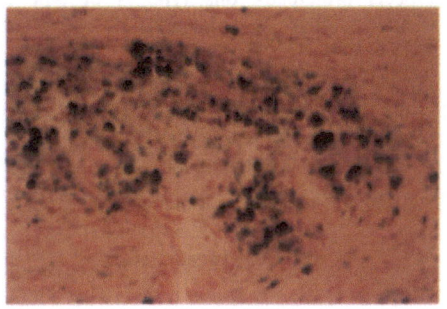

e

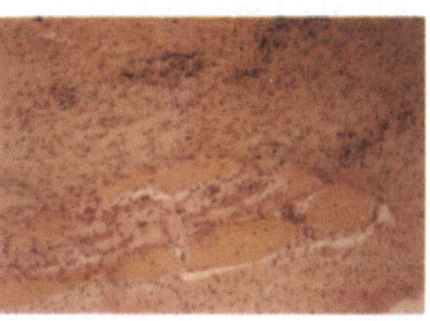

f

Fig. a. Fibrous dysplasia: histopathology.
Fibroblastic proliferation made up of small spindle-shaped cells arranged in a more or less spiral pattern around irregular, or fine osseous spicules without osteoblastic border.

Fig. b. Ossifying fibroma.
Within the fibroblastic proliferation bony lamellae with osteoblastic borders have developed.

Fig. c. Ossifying fibroma.
Examination in polarized light shows a lamellar pattern of the fibres denoting a maturation of the bones.

Fig. d. Bone cyst aneurysm.
Cavity filled with red blood cells, without endothelial lining but enclosed in a richly cellular connective tissue.

Fig. e. Bone cyst aneurysm (Perls stain).
Presence in the connective tissue of macrophages filled with haemosiderin which is stained with Prussian blue.

Fig. f. Bone cyst aneurysm.
At the periphery of the lesion, two elongated osseous lamellae forming the osteoid band can be seen in the connective tissue which also contains haemosiderin deposits.

Fig. a. Dysplasie fibreuse: histopathologie.
Prolifération fibroblastique faite de petites cellules fusiformes à disposition plus ou moins tourbillonnante autour d'une multitude de fines spicules osseuses irrégulières sans bordure ostéoblastique.

Fig. b. Fibrome ossifiant.
Au sein de la prolifération fibroblastique se sont développées des lamelles osseuses bordées d'ostéoblastes.

Fig. c. Fibrome ossifiant.
L'examen en lumière polarisée montre la disposition lamellaire des fibres témoignant d'une maturation osseuse.

Fig. d. Kyste anévrysmal de l'os.
Cavité remplie d'hématies, mais sans bordure endothéliale et creusée au sein d'un tissu conjonctif richement cellulaire.

Fig. e. Kyste anévrysmal de l'os (coloration de Perls).
Présence au sein du tissu conjonctif de macrophages chargés d'hémosidérine teintés en bleu par la méthode au Bleu de Prusse.

Fig. f. Kyste anévrysmal de l'os.
A la périphérie de la lésion on trouve au sein du tissu conjonctif qui contient des dépôts hémosidériniques deux lames osseuses allongées qui constituent la bande ostéoïde.

Abb. a. Fibröse Dysplasie: Histopathologie.
Fibroblastproliferation aus kleinen spindelförmigen Zellen mit mehr oder weniger wirbelartiger Anordnung um eine Vielzahl feiner, unregelmäßig geformter, Knochenbälkchen ohne Osteoblastensaum.

Abb. b. Verknöcherndes Fibrom.
Innerhalb der Fibroblastproliferation haben sich von Osteoblasten gesäumte Knochenlamellen gebildet.

Abb. c. Verknöcherndes Fibrom.
Die Untersuchung im polarisierten Licht zeigt die Lamellenanordnung der Fasern, Hinweis auf Knochenreifung.

Abb. d. Aneurysmatische Knochen-Zyste.
Mit Erythrozyten gefüllter Hohlraum ohne Endothel, inmitten eines zellreichen Bindegewebes.

Abb. e. Aneurysmatische Knochen-Zyste (Färbung nach Perls).
Im Bindegewebe befinden sich mit Hämosiderin beladene Makrophagen, in der Berliner Blaureaktion blaugefärbt.

Abb. f. Aneurysmatische Knochen-Zyste.
In der Peripherie der Läsion befinden sich in dem Hämosiderinablagerungen enthaltenden Bindegewebe zwei längliche Knochenlamellen, die den osteoiden Saum bilden.

PLATE 35   PLANCHE 35   TAFEL 35

XVI. TUMOURS OF THE NEURAL TISSUE OR NEURAL-LIKE TUMOURS

XVI.1 Schwannoma (neurinoma, neurilemmoma, peripheral glioma)

Clinical features. This tumour found in adults can be isolated or associated with other localizations (one should look for a neurofibromatosis in such cases). Growing from an orbital nerve, the tumour may be extraconical exerting lateral pressure on the eyeball, or intraconical, and cause diplopia. This evolves into an axial proptosis resisting pressure on the eyeball associated with a lowering of visual acuity. It is characterized by a painless, very gradual course.

Histopathology. Contrary to neurofibroma, schwannoma is limited to the proliferation of Schwann cells. The nerve fibres are pushed towards the periphery of the tumour which appears to be well encapsulated, is ovoid in shape and whitish on gross examination. On microscopical examination, it is possible to distinguish two main patterns called respectively Antoni A and B. In all cases, the intratumoral vessels present a thick hyalinized wall.

XVI.2 Orbital neurofibroma (see palpebral neurofibroma – Plate 24)

XVI.3 Granular cell tumour (formerly granular cell myoblastoma)

Clinical features. It is mainly observed in adults. It can involve the lid and the eyebrow and mimic a dermoid or intraorbital cyst, causing a painless and progressive exophthalmos resisting pressure on the eyeball.

Histopathology. The aspect of the cells with granular cytoplasm is characteristic. Recent work has suggested that they might be derived from Schwann cells.

XVI.4 Alveolar soft part sarcoma

Clinical features. This tumour is observed in adults, causing a progressive proptosis sometimes associated with a palpebro-conjunctival oedema.

Histopathology. The organoid structure of the tumour speaks for itself. The cells with a fine granular eosinophilic cytoplasm may contain pathognomonic PAS positive needle-like crystals. The histo-pathogenesis of this tumour remains unexplained. Some researchers have suggested that it might be a malignant form of a granular cell tumour.

XVI.5 Sympathoblastoma (neuroblastoma)

Clinical features. Although it is a metastasis from a mediastinal or retroperitoneal localization, the orbital site of this tumour is often revealing. Clinically it leads to proptosis which may be bilateral and associated with orbital ecchymosis and a possible increase of intracranial pressure (Hutchinson's syndrome). Such a clinical picture makes it necessary to test for catecholamines.

Histopathology. Characteristic are groups of cells arranged in a rosette-like pattern around a fibrillar centre (Homer-Wright rosettes).

XVI. TUMEURS DU TISSU NERVEUX OU ASSIMILÉES

XVI.1 Schwannome (neurinome, neurilemmome, gliome périphérique)

Clinique. Tumeur de l'adulte, elle peut être isolée ou associée à d'autres localisations (rechercher alors une neurofibromatose). Se développant sur un tronc nerveux orbitaire elle peut être extraconique, repoussant le globe latéralement, ou intraconique et se manifeste par une diplopie précédant une exophtalmie irréductible, axile, avec baisse de l'acuité visuelle. L'évolution est très progressive et indolore.

Histopathologie. A la différence du neurofibrome le schwannome est constitué d'une prolifération des seules cellules de Schwann. Les fibres nerveuses sont repoussées à la périphérie de la tumeur qui apparaît bien encapsulée, ovoïde, blanchâtre à la coupe. Microscopiquement on distingue deux aspects principaux dits type A et type B d'Antoni. Dans tous les cas les vaisseaux intra-tumoraux ont une paroi épaisse et hyalinisée.

XVI.2 Neurofibrome de l'orbite (voir Neurofibrome de la paupière – Planche 24)

XVI.3 Tumeur à cellules granuleuses (ancien myoblastome à cellules granuleuses)

Clinique. C'est plutôt une tumeur de l'adulte. Elle peut être palpébro-sourcilière et simuler un kyste dermoïde, ou intra-orbitaire et entraîner une exophtalmie progressive, irréductible et indolore.

Histopathologie. L'aspect des cellules à cytoplasme granuleux est caractéristique. A la lumière des études récentes, elles dériveraient des cellules de Schwann.

XVI.4 Sarcome alvéolaire des parties molles

Clinique. C'est une tumeur de l'adulte provoquant une exophtalmie progressive avec parfois un oedème palpébro-conjonctival.

Histopathologie. La structure organoïde de la tumeur est assez évocatrice. Les cellules à cytoplasme éosinophile finement granuleux, peuvent contenir des cristaux en aiguille, PAS positifs, pathognomoniques. L'histologie de cette tumeur n'est pas élucidée. Pour certains elle serait une forme maligne de la tumeur à cellules granuleuses.

XVI.5 Sympathoblastome (neuroblastome)

Clinique. Bien qu'il s'agisse d'une métastase d'une localisation médiastinale ou rétropéritonéale, la localisation orbitaire de cette tumeur est souvent révélatrice. Cliniquement elle réalise une exophtalmie qui peut être bilatérale accompagnée d'ecchymoses orbitaires et parfois d'hypertension intracrânienne (syndrome de Hutchinson). Un tel tableau doit faire pratiquer un dosage des catécholamines.

Histopathologie. En histopathologie il faut rechercher des groupements de cellules en rosettes autour d'un amas central fibrillaire (rosettes de Homer-Wright).

XVI. GESCHWÜLSTE DES NERVEN-GEWEBES UND VERWANDTER GEWEBSARTEN

XVI.1 Schwannom (Neurinom, Neurilemmom, peripheres Gliom)

Klinik. Tumor des Erwachsenen. Er kann einzeln oder gemeinsam mit anderen Lokalisationen (sodann auf eine Neurofibromatose hin zu untersuchen) auftreten. Er entwickelt sich in einem Orbitanerv und kann extrakonisch dann den Bulbus seitlich wegdrückend, oder intrakonisch sein, was sich durch Diplopie, gefolgt von einem axilen Exophthalmus, der sich nicht zurückdrängen läßt, sowie vermindertem Sehvermögen zeigt. Der Verlauf ist sehr progressiv und schmerzlos.

Histopathologie. Im Unterschied zum Neurofibrom besteht das Schwannom aus einer Wucherung, an der nur Schwannzellen beteiligt sind. Die Nervenfaser wird zur Peripherie des Tumors verdrängt, und dieser erscheint gut abgekapselt, ovoid, im Schnitt weißlich. Mikroskopisch unterscheidet man zwei Hauptaspekte vom sogenannten A-Typ und B-Typ nach Antoni. In allen Fällen haben die intratumoralen Gefäße ein dicke, hyalinisierte Wand.

XVI.2 Neurofibrom der Orbita (siehe Neurofibrom des Lids – Tafel 24)

XVI.3 Granulosazell-Tumor

Klinik. Dieser Tumor kommt eher beim Erwachsenen vor. Er kann im Lid-Brauenbereich auftreten und eine Dermoidzyste vortäuschen oder er kann intraorbital auftreten und einen progressiven, schmerzlosen Exophthalmus zur Folge haben, der nicht zurückgedrängt werden kann.

Histopathologie. Die Zellen mit ihrem granulären Zytoplasma haben ein charakteristisches Aussehen. Neueren Erkenntnissen zufolge sollen sie von den Schwannzellen ausgehen.

XVI.4 Alveoläres Weichteilsarkom

Klinik. Tumor des Erwachsenen mit progressivem Exophthalmus, manchmal mit Ödem an Lidern und Bindehaut.

Histopathologie. Die Struktur des Tumors ist bezeichnend. Die Zellen mit einem eosinophilen, fein granulären Zytoplasma können die pathognomonischen, PAS-positiven Nadelkristalle enthalten. Die Histologie dieses Tumors ist nicht geklärt. Nach Meinung Mancher handelt es sich um eine bösartige Form der Granulosazelltumors.

XVI.5 Sympathoblastom (Neuroblastom)

Klinik. Wenngleich es sich um eine Metastase bei mediastinalem oder retroperitonealem Befall handelt, ist das Auftreten dieses Tumors in der Orbita oft aufschlußreich. Klinisch bewirkt er einen Exophthalmus, der beidseitig sein kann, begleitet von orbitalen Ekchymosen und manchmal gleichzeitigem erhöhtem intracraniellem Liquordruck (Hutchinson-Syndrom). Ein solches klinisches Bild sollte zu einer Katecholaminbestimmung veranlassen.

Histopathologie. Histopathologisch ist nach rosettenartig um ein zentrales Fibrillenhäufchen angeordneten Zellgruppierungen zu suchen (Homer-Wrightsche Rosetten).

PLATE 35 PLANCHE 35 TAFEL 35

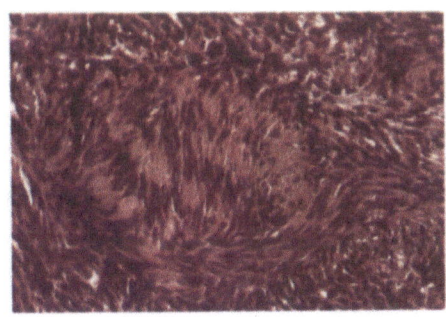

a

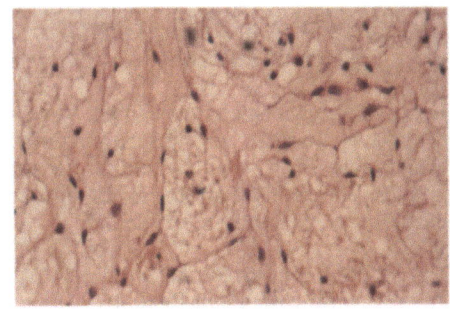

b

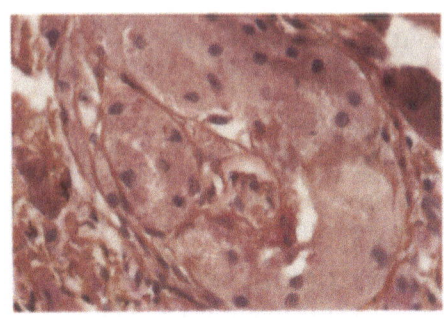

c

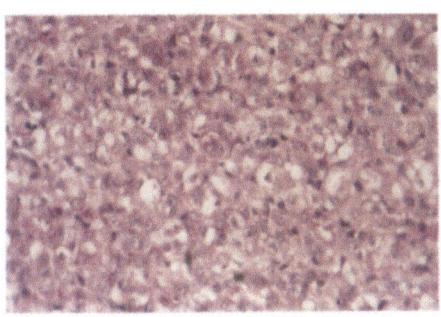

d

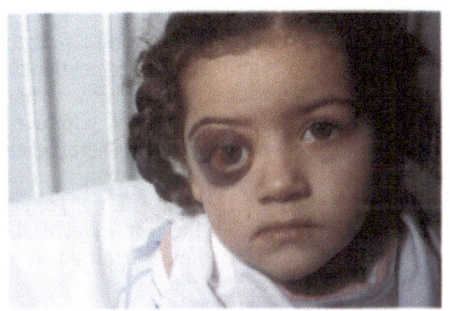

e

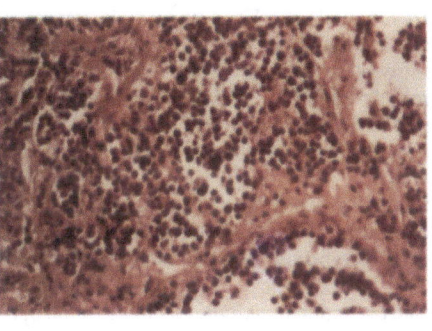

f

Fig. a. Orbital Schwannoma (Antoni A).
Spindle-shaped Schwann cells with elongated nuclei, are placed side by side to form a "palisade". The cells arranged in bundles resembling barrel-staves, form the characteristic Verocay's bodies.

Fig. b. Orbital Schwannoma (Antoni B).
The structure is less dense, the stroma oedematous, myxoid. According to Masson this aspect is degenerative due to a slow prolonged course.

Fig. c. Granular cell tumour.
Tumorous lobules consisting of large well defined oval cells, with a round nucleus. The cytoplasm is finely granular, discreetly eosinophilic and stains slightly with PAS.

Fig. d. Alveolar soft part sarcoma.
Pseudo-alveolar structure made of polygonal cells with a granular eosinophilic cytoplasm. Pseudo-endocrinic looking interlobular vascularization.

Fig. e. Sympathoblastoma.
Proptosis with characteristic palpebro-conjunctival ecchymosis.

Fig. f. Sympathoblastoma.
Undifferentiated cells with a poorly defined cytoplasm. The round nuclei have a high chromatin content. Cells are separated from one another by slightly fibrillar partitions.

Fig. a. Schwannome de l'orbite (Antoni A).
Cellules schwanniennes fusiformes à noyaux allongés disposées côte à côte en "palissade". Les faisceaux enroulés sur eux-mêmes en "douves de tonneau" forment les caractéristiques nodules de Verocay.

Fig. b. Schwannome de l'orbite (Antoni B).
Structure beaucoup plus lâche; stroma oedémateux, myxoïde. Il s'agirait pour Masson d'un aspect dégénératif dû à une évolution prolongée.

Fig. c. Tumeur à cellules granuleuses.
Lobules tumoraux constitués de grandes cellules ovalaires à limites nettes, à noyau arrondi, à cytoplasme finement granuleux discrètement éosinophile, prenant légèrement le PAS.

Fig. d. Sarcome alvéolaire des parties molles.
Structure pseudo-alvéolaire constituée de cellules polygonales à cytoplasme granuleux éosinophile. Vascularisation interlobulaire d'allure pseudo-endocrinienne.

Fig. e. Sympathoblastome.
Exophtalmie avec la caractéristique ecchymose palpébro-conjonctivale.

Fig. f. Sympathoblastome.
Cellules indifférenciées à cytoplasme mal défini, à noyau arrondi riche en chromatine, séparées par des cloisons délicatement fibrillaires.

Abb. a. Schwannom der Orbita (Antoni A).
Spindelförmige Schwannzellen mit länglichem Kern, "palissadenartig" nebeneinander angeordnet. Die in sich selbst fassdaubenartig eingerollten Bündel bilden die charakteristischen Verocay-Knötchen.

Abb. b. Schwannom der Orbita (Antoni B).
Viel lockerere Struktur: ödematöses, myxoides Stroma. Masson zufolge soll es sich um eine mit einem langen Krankheitsverlauf in Zusammenhang stehende Degenerationserscheinung handeln.

Abb. c. Granulosazelltumor.
Tumorläppchen, bestehend aus großen ovalen Zellen mit deutlichen Abgrenzungen, rundlichem Kern, fein granuliertem, diskret eosinophilem Zytoplasma, leicht PAS-positiv.

Abb. d. Alveoläres Weichteilsarkom.
Pseudoalveoläre Struktur, die aus polygonalen Zellen mit granulärem, eosinophilem Zytoplasma besteht. Vaskularisation zwischen den Läppchen mit pseudoendokrinem Aspekt.

Abb. e. Sympathoblastom.
Exophthalmus mit der charakteristischen Ekchymose an Lid und Bindehaut.

Abb. f. Sympathoblastom.
Undifferenzierte Zellen mit schlecht definiertem Zytoplasma, abgerundetem, chromatinreichem Kern, getrennt durch zarte fibrilläre Wände.

73

PLATE 36　　　　　PLANCHE 36　　　　　TAFEL 36

XVII. TUMOURS OF THE INTRA-ORBITAL OPTIC NERVE

The symptomatology of these tumours if that of an orbital tumour localized in the retrobulbar cone: axial proptosis with impairment of visual acuity. They may involve the optic nerve itself or its sheaths (meningioma).

XVII.1 Glioma (of the optic nerve and of chiasm of the child)

This glioma is a slowly developing benign tumour, often associated (12% to 37%) with a neurofibromatosis.

Clinical features. The proptosis resisting pressure on the eyeball is associated with a papilloedema followed by an optic atrophy. The widening of the optic canal shown by X rays and the thickening of the nerve observed by CAT confirm the diagnosis.

Histopathology. The tumour is made of spindle-shaped cells named pilocytic astrocytes, benign in appearance, without mitotic figures. These are sometimes associated with oligodendrocytes. Mucinous degenerative cavities may also be observed which can be stained with acid mucopolysaccharides. The sheaths may become thicker due to gliosis and reactive meningeal hyperplasia and/or vascular congestion.

The exceptional *malignant glioma* of the optic nerve and chiasm may occur *in adults* without signs of neurofibromatosis and rapidly cause bilateral blindness; it is fatal within a year. Histologically it is a malignant glioblastoma.

XVII.2 Meningiomas (of the intra-orbital optic nerve)

Clinical features. These tumours which may, at times, precede other localizations of neurofibromatosis occur mostly among the young. They produce axial proptosis, ocular motor paralysis, vision impairment. Chorioretinal striae and sometimes a papilledema may be observed. They may be either of intracranial origin and secondarily extend to the orbit, or else primitive, involving the meningeal sheaths of the intra-orbital optic nerve or of the optic foramen.

Histopathology. These meningiomas are, as a rule, tumours of a meningotheliomatous type. They may be scattered with calcium concretions (calcospherites); in case of proliferation of the latter they are called psammomas.

XVII. TUMEURS DU NERF OPTIQUE INTRA-ORBITAIRE

Leur symptomatologie est celle d'une tumeur de l'orbite localisée au cône rétrobulbaire: exophtalmie axile, avec baisse de l'acuité visuelle. Elles peuvent toucher le nerf optique lui-même ou ses gaines (méningiome).

XVII.1 Gliome (du nerf optique et du chiasma de l'enfant)

Ce gliome du nerf optique et du chiasma de *l'enfant* est une tumeur bénigne à évolution lente, associée souvent (12% à 37% selon les statistiques) à une neurofibromatose.

Clinique. Cliniquement l'exophtalmie, irréductible, s'accompagne d'un oedème papillaire, puis d'une atrophie optique. L'élargissement du canal optique aux RX et l'épaississement du nerf à la TDM affirment le diagnostic.

Histopathologie. La tumeur est formée d'astrocytes fusiformes, dits pilocytiques, d'aspect bénin, sans mitoses, parfois associés à des oligodendrocytes. On peut y trouver aussi des cavités de dégénérescence mucineuse prenant les colorants des mucopolysaccharides acides. Les gaines peuvent s'épaissir par gliose et hyperplasie méningée réactionnelles ou congestion vasculaire.

L'exceptionnel *gliome malin* du nerf optique et du chiasma se rencontre chez *l'adulte*, sans signes de neuro-fibromatose, conduisant rapidement à une cécité bilatérale et à la mort en moins d'un an. Histologiquement c'est un glioblastome malin.

XVII.2 Méningiomes (du nerf optique intra-orbitaire)

Clinique. Précédant parfois d'autres localisations de neurofibromatose, ces tumeurs apparaissent plutôt chez le sujet jeune. Elles provoquent exophtalmie axile, paralysies oculo-motrices, baisse de vision, stries choriorétiniennes et parfois oedème papillaire à l'ophtalmoscopie. Elles sont soit à point de départ intracrânien et atteignant l'orbite secondairement, soit primitives, touchant les méninges du nerf optique intra-orbitaire ou du canal optique.

Histopathologie. Ces méningiomes sont dans la règle des tumeurs de type méningothéliomateux. Ils peuvent être parsemés de concrétions calcaires (calcosphérites); lorsqu'elles sont nombreuses on parle de psammome.

XVII. GESCHWÜLSTE DES INTRAORBITALEN SEHNERVS

Die Symptomatologie ist die eines im retrobulbären Konus gelegenen Tumors der Orbita: axialer Exophthalmus mit Einbuße der Sehschärfe. Sie können den Sehnerven selbst oder seine Scheiden befallen (Meningiome).

XVII.1 Gliom (des Sehnervs und des Chiasmas des Kindes)

Das Gliom des Sehnervs und des Chiasmas des Kindes ist ein gutartiger, sich langsam entwickelnder Tumor, der oft (statistisch in 12% bis 37% der Fälle) mit einer Neurofibromatose einhergeht.

Klinik. Klinisch ist der nicht kompressible Exophthalmus mit einem Papillenödem, dann mit einer Optikusatrophie verbunden. Eine auf dem Röntgenbild sichtbare Erweiterung des Canalis opticus und die mit CT aufgezeigte Verdickung des Nervs bestätigen die Diagnose.

Histopathologie. Histopathologisch besteht der Tumor aus spindelförmigen, sogenannten pilozytären Astrozyten von gutartigem Aussehen, ohne Mitosen, die manchmal zusammen mit Oligodendrozyten auftreten. Es sind auch von Mukusdegeneration herrührende Hohlräume anzutreffen, die die Färbungen saurer Mukopolysaccharide annehmen. Die Scheiden können sich durch reaktive Gliose und Hyperplasie der Opticushüllen oder durch Gefäßkongestion verdicken.

Das außergewöhnlich seltene *bösartige Gliom* des Sehnervs und des Chiasmas tritt *beim Erwachsenen* auf ohne Anzeichen von Neurofibromatose, führt rasch zu bilateraler Erblindung und in weniger als einem Jahr zum Tod. Histologisch handelt es sich um ein bösartiges Glioblastom.

XVII.2 Meningiome (des intraorbitalen Sehnervs)

Klinik. Diese Geschwülste, die manchmal anderen Neurofibromatose-Lokalisierungen vorangehen, sind eher bei jungen Menschen anzutreffen. Sie haben einen axialen Exophthalmus, Augenmuskellähmungen, Einbuße des Sehvermögens, Aderhaut- und Netzhautstreifen, und manchmal ein ophtalmoskopisch festzustellendes Papillenödem zur Folge. Sie haben entweder einen intrakraniellen Ausgangspunkt und erreichen sekundär die Orbita oder sind Primärgeschwulste in den Hüllen des intraorbitalen Sehnervs oder des Canalis opticus.

Histopathologie. Histopathologisch sind diese Meningiome in der Regel Tumoren vom meningotheliomatösen Typ. Sie können mit sandkornartigen Ablagerungen (Kalkospheriten) durchsetzt sein; sind diese zahlreich, spricht man von einem Psammon.

PLATE 36 PLANCHE 36 TAFEL 36

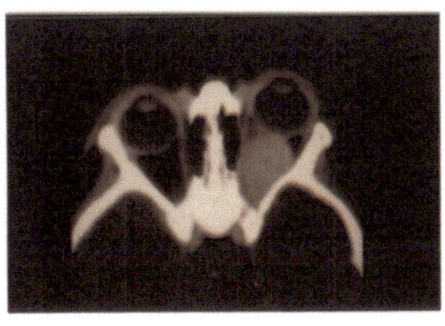

a

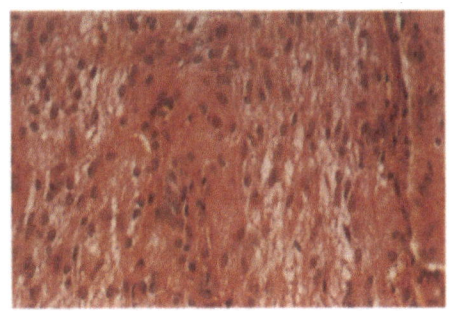

b

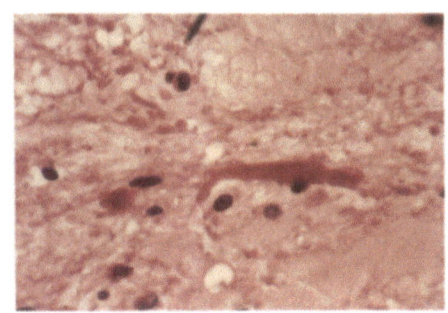

c

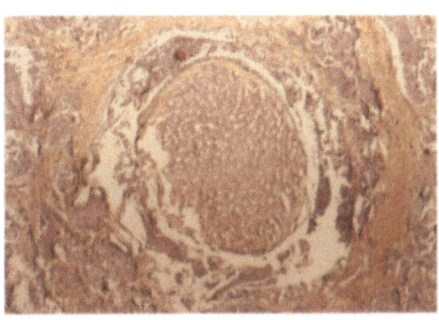

d

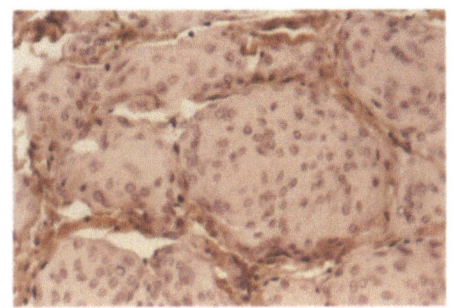

e

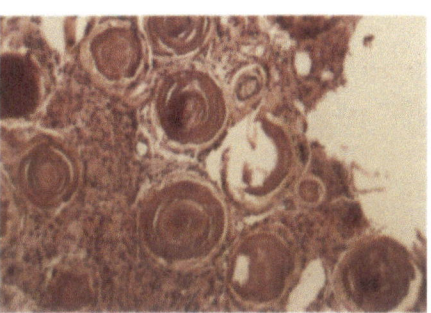

f

Fig. a. CAT image of a glioma of the right optic nerve showing thickening of the nerve and proptosis.

Fig. b. Glioma of the optic nerve.
Bundles of spindle-shaped astrocytes with fibrillary expansions (pilocytic astrocytes).

Fig. c. Glioma of the optic nerve.
Rosenthal's fibres, anhistic, eosinophilic, globular or ovoid thickening of degenerative glial cells.

Fig. d. Meningioma of the optic nerve sheaths.
Thickening of the sheath due to a meningotheliomatous tumour proliferation surrounding the atrophic optic nerve.

Fig. e. Meningotheliomatous meningioma.
"Epitheliomatous"-looking areas, made of small cells with imprecise limits, a clear small nucleus, arranged in lobuli, isolated by connective tissue partitions.

Fig. f. Psammoma.
Numerous laminated, calcified structures scattered in the meningotheliomatous lobuli and which give an "arenaceous" appearance to the lesion.

Fig. a. Image TDM d'un gliome du nerf optique droit montrant l'épaississement du nerf et l'exophtalmie.

Fig. b. Gliome du nerf optique.
Faisceaux d'astrocytes fusiformes à expansions fibrillaires (astrocytes pilocytiques).

Fig. c. Gliome du nerf optique.
Fibres de Rosenthal, épaississement anhiste, éosinophile, globuleux ou ovoïde de cellules gliales dégénérées.

Fig. d. Méningiome de la gaine du nerf optique.
Epaississement de la gaine par une prolifération tumorale méningothéliomateuse entourant un nerf optique atrophique.

Fig. e. Méningiome méningothéliomateux.
Plages d'aspect "épithéliomateux" de petites cellules à limites indécises, à petit noyau clair, disposées en lobules séparés par des cloisons conjonctives.

Fig. f. Psammome.
Nombreuses concrétions calcaires parsemant les lobules méningothéliomateux et donnant à la lésion un caractère "arénacé".

Abb. a. CT-Bild eines rechtseitigen Sehnervenglioms, das die Verdickung des Sehnervs und den Exophthalmus zeigt.

Abb. b. Gliom des Sehnervs.
Stränge spindelförmiger Astrozyten mit fibrillären Auswüchsen (pilozytische Astrozyten).

Abb. c. Gliom des Sehnervs.
Rosenthal-Fasern, amorphe, eosinophile, kugelförmige oder ovoide Verdickung von degenerierten Gliazellen.

Abb. d. Meningiom der Sehnervenscheide.
Verdickung der Scheide durch eine meningotheliomatöse Tumorproliferation, die einen atrophischen Sehnerv umgibt.

Abb. e. Meningotheliomatöses Meningiom.
"Epitheliomatös" wirkende Felder mit kleinen, unscharf abgegrenzten Zellen mit kleinem, hellem Kern, die lappenartig angeordnet und durch Bindegewebssepten getrennt sind.

Abb. f. Psammom.
Zahlreiche Kalkablagerungen in den meningotheliomatösen Läppchen liegen dem Namen "sandkornartig" zugrunde.

XVIII. HAEMATO-SARCOMAS

XVIII.1 Lymphomas
(non-Hodgkinian lymphomas)

Clinical features. First appearing after the age of 30, reaching a maximum around 60, these tumours practically never occur in children, with the exception of Burkitt's lymphoma. In the orbit (Plate 37, Fig. a) they produce an exophthalmos, without ocular motor paralysis or lowering of visual acuity. These tumours occur mainly in the upper part of the orbit as "a plate" deeply sunken towards the back. When accessible, they feel firm to the touch. They may also grow further beneath the conjunctiva, or even be solely subconjunctival (Plate 37, Fig. b).

Histopathology. The present classifications of lymphomas are based rather on pathophysiological than on morphological criteria, on the principle that tumorous cells are derived from the same clone, the maturation of which has been stopped at a given stage. No universal nomenclature has been adopted as yet. We will therefore use the Kiel classification and within brackets, its equivalent in the international formulation for clinical use (Working formulation). As a rule, in the ocular adnexa, lymphomas develop from B lymphocyte proliferation.

See Plate 37 on page 79.

XVIII. HÉMATOSARCOMES

XVIII.1 Lymphomes
(non Hodgkiniens)

Clinique. Apparaissant après le 30e année avec un maximum aux alentours de 60 ans, ces tumeurs ne se rencontrent pratiquement pas chez l'enfant, à l'exception du lymphome de Burkitt. Dans l'orbite (Planche 37, Fig. a) elles provoquent une exophtalmie sans paralysie oculomotrice ni baisse d'acuité visuelle. Elles siègent plus souvent à la partie supérieure de l'orbite, s'enfonçant vers l'arrière "en semelle". Lorsqu'elles sont palpables on note leur consistance ferme. Elles peuvent également se prolonger sous la conjonctive ou même être uniquement sous-conjonctivales (Planche 37, Fig. b).

Histopathologie. Les classifications actuelles des lymphomes se réfèrent plutôt à des critères physiopathologiques que morphologiques, partant du principe que les cellules tumorales dérivent d'un même clone bloqué à un stade de maturation donné. Il n'y a pas encore néanmoins de nomenclature universellement adoptée. En conséquence nous utiliserons la classification de Kiel tout en donnant entre parenthèses son équivalent dans la formulation internationale à usage clinique (Working formulation). En règle dans les annexes oculaires les lymphomes sont issus de la prolifération de lymphocytes B.

Voir Planché 37 à la page 79.

XVIII. HÄMATOSARKOME

XVIII.1 Lymphome
(Non Hodgkin-Lymphome)

Klinik. Diese nach dem 30. Lebensjahr, mit einem Maximum bei 60 Jahren auftauchenden Tumoren sind, mit Ausnahme des Burkitt-Lymphoms, beim Kind praktisch nicht anzutreffen. In der Orbita (Tafel 37, Abb. a) bewirken sie einen Exophthalmus ohne Augenmuskellähmung und ohne Einbuße des Sehvermögens. Sie sind häufig im oberen Teil der Orbita lokalisiert und schieben sich "sohlenartig" nach hinten. Sind sie palpabel, so fällt ihre derbe Konsistenz auf.
Sie können sich ebenfalls unter der Bindehaut fortsetzen oder auch nur subkonjunktival auftreten (Tafel 37, Abb. b).

Histopathologie. Die derzeitigen Lymphomklassifizierungen stützen sich eher auf physiopathologische als auf morphologische Kriterien, wobei sie von dem Prinzip ausgehen, daß die Tumorzellen von ein und demselben, in einem bestimmten Reifestadium blockierten Klon abstammen. Es gibt aber noch keine universell eingeführte Nomenklatur. Wir verwenden deshalb die Kielsche Klassifizierung und geben in Klammern die entsprechende internationale Formulierung für den klinischen Gebrauch (Working formulation). Im allgemeinen gehen die Lymphome der Augenadnexe aus B-Lymphozytenwucherungen hervor.

Siehe Tafel 37 auf Seite 79.

PLATE 37 PLANCHE 37 TAFEL 37

Lymphocytic lymphomas (Fig. c.)
(diffuse lymphomas with small lymphocytes)

They appear usually as a complication during the evolution of a chronic lymphoid leukosis and often take the form of a pericorneal ring.

Lymphoplasmacytoid-lymphomas Lennert's lymphomas (Fig. d.)
(diffuse lymphomas with small lymphocytes with plasmacytic differentiation, or mixed diffuse lymphomas with small and large cells)

This is perhaps the commonest type found present in the ocular area. These lymphomas reflect the evolution of the lymphocyte towards an immunosecreting cell. They may be preceded by the lacrimal localization of a Sjögren's syndrome or by a pseudolymphoma. They may remain isolated without systemic manifestation or be part of the picture of Waldenström's disease. The prognosis is generally good.

Centrocyto-centroblastic lymphomas
(follicular lymphomas with small cells, mixed or with large cells; mixed diffuse lymphomas or large cell lymphomas)

Their structure is follicular in most cases (Fig. e) similar to the germinating centres of the lymph nodes: indeed, for maturing forms, such as cleft nucleate centrocytes and centroblasts, are associated with lymphocytes and plasma cells (Fig. f.) The diffuse non-follicular forms are the least frequently observed.

Centrocytic lymphomas
(diffuse lymphomas with small or large cleaved cells)

Consisting of diffuse and regular infiltration of centrocytes, these lymphomas occur very rarely in the ocular area.

Centroblastic lymphomas
(diffuse lymphomas with large cells)

They are principally made up of centroblasts mainly associated with some immunoblasts. These cells may secrete monoclonal immunoglobulin.

B lymphoblastic lymphomas
(lymphomas with small noncleaved cells)

These are Burkitt's lymphomas affecting precisely the orbito-palpebral region, sometimes originating in the maxillary bone. These lymphomas occur in children aged 2 to 12, particularly in regions with a high incidence of malaria, above all in equatorial Africa. Contrary to other forms of lymphoma, exophthalmos develops abruptly, grows rapidly and is sometimes associated with visceral implications; fortunately its drastic progression may be arrested by cyclophosphamide.

Histopathology. See Plate 38, Fig. a.

78

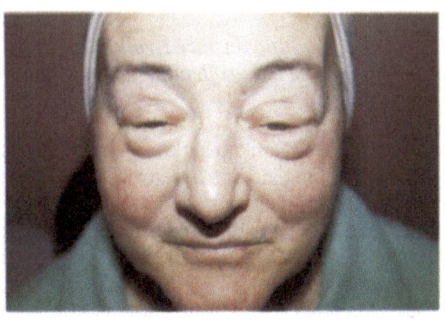

a

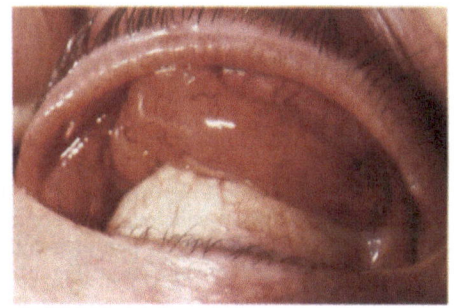

b

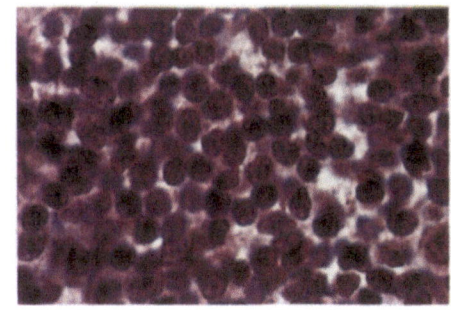

c

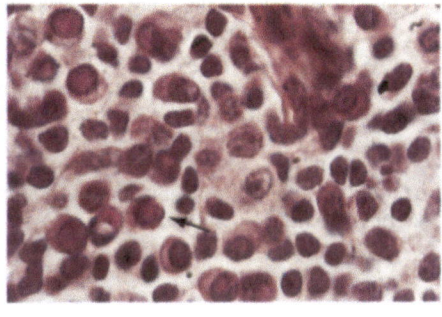

d

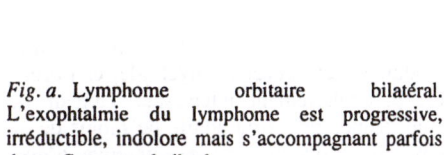

e

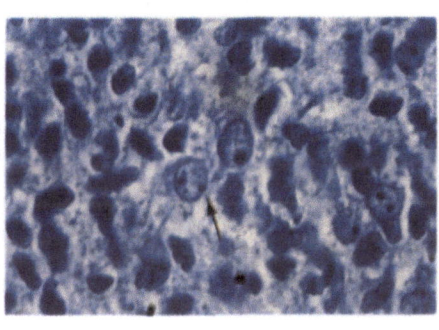

f

Fig. a. Bilateral orbital lymphoma. Progressive, irreducible, painless proptosis, often accompanied by swelling of the eyelids.

Fig. b. Subconjunctival lymphoma. A salmon pink, smooth, soft, elongated mass which fills up the fornix.

Fig. c. Lymphocytic lymphoma. A diffuse homogeneous layer of small mature lymphocytes with round nucleus and barely visible cytoplasm.

Fig. d. Lymphoplasmacytoid lymphoma (PAS). Lymphocytes, plasma cells and intermediary lympho-plasmacytic cells with an eccentric nucleus and widespread cytoplasm. This cytoplasm and the intranuclear round vacuoles (→) are strongly stained by PAS. The inclusions are made up of monoclonal IgM, which means that they present one and the same light chain. These light chains can make intratumorous amyloid deposits possible.

Fig. e. Centrocytic-centroblastic follicular lymphoma (low power). This tumour is made up of giant lymphoid follicules, in a regular pattern. It is the classical Brill-Symmers giant follicular lymphoma.

Fig. f. Centrocytic-centroblastic lymphoma (Giemsa's staining). On one hand, mainly centrocytes with small irregular nuclei can be observed, on the other hand, mainly centroblasts with larger nuclei containing less chromatin and with 2 to 3 nucleoles adhering to the nuclear membrane (→).

Fig. a. Lymphome orbitaire bilatéral. L'exophtalmie du lymphome est progressive, irréductible, indolore mais s'accompagnant parfois de gonflement palpébral.

Fig. b. Lymphome sous-conjonctival. Masse oblongue, lisse, d'un rose saumon, molle, remplissant le cul-de-sac.

Fig. c. Lymphome lymphocytique. Nappe diffuse homogène de petits lymphocytes matures à noyau arrondi, à cytoplasme peu visible.

Fig. d. Lymphome lymphoplasmocytaire (PAS). Lymphocytes, plasmocytes, et éléments intermédiaires lympho-plasmocytoïdes à noyau excentré et à cytoplasme étendu. Ce cytoplasme se teinte fortement par le PAS, ainsi que des vacuoles arrondies intra-nucléaires (→). Les inclusions sont constituées d'IgM monoclonale c'est-à-dire ne comportant qu'un seul et même type de chaîne légère. Ces chaînes légères peuvent être à l'origine de dépôts amyloïdes intra-tumoraux.

Fig. e. Lymphome centrocyto-centroblastique folliculaire (faible grossissement). La structure de cette tumeur est faite de follicules lymphoïdes géants régulièrement disposés. C'est le classique lymphome giganto-folliculaire de Brill-Symmers.

Fig. f. Lymphome centrocyto-centroblastique (coloration Giemsa). On trouve d'une part des centrocytes à petit noyau irrégulier, d'autre part des centroblastes à noyau plus grand moins riche en chromatine et possédant 2 à 3 nucléoles plaqués contre la membrane nucléaire (→).

Abb. a. Beidseitiges Lymphom der Orbita. Der durch das Lymphom verursachte Exophthalmus ist progressiv, nicht kompressibel, schmerzlos, manchmal aber von einer Schwellung der Lider begleitet.

Abb. b. Subkonjunktivales Lymphom. Längliche, glatte, lachsfarbene, weiche Masse, welche die Umschlagsfalte ausfüllt.

Abb. c. Lymphozytäres Lymphom. Diffuses, homogenes Feld kleiner, voll entwickelter Lymphozyten mit rundlichem Kern, wenig sichtbarem Zytoplasma.

Abb. d. Lymphoplasmozytäres Lymphom (PAS-Färbung). Lymphozyten, Plasmozyten und Lympho-plamozytoide Zwischenformen mit exzentrisch gelagertem Kern und ausgedehntem Zytoplasma. Dieses Zytoplasma färbt sich ebenso wie die rundlichen Vakuolen im Kerninneren stark mit PAS (→). Die Einschlüsse bestehen aus monoklonalem IgM, d.h. sie bestehen immunchemisch aus ein und derselben leichten Kette. Weil leichte Ketten vorhanden sind, werden Amyloidablagerungen im Inneren des Tumors möglich.

Abb. e. Zentrozyto-zentroblastisches Lymphom (schwache Vergrößerung). Dieser Tumor besitzt eine Struktur aus lymphoiden Riesenfollikeln in regelmäßiger Anordnung. Dies ist das klassische Großfollikellymphom nach Brill-Symmers.

Abb. f. Zentrozyto-zentroblastisches Lymphom (Giemsa-Färbung). Man findet einerseits Zentrozyten mit kleinem, unregelmäßigem Kern, andererseits Zentroblasten mit größerem, weniger chromatinreichem Kern und 2 bis 3 gegen die Kernwand gepreßten Nukleolen (→).

PLATE 38 PLANCHE 38 TAFEL 38

B immunoblastic lymphomas
(lymphomas with large immunoblastic cells)

These are the reticulosarcomas of former classifications. They appear after the age of sixty but are preceded sometimes by signs of disimmunity. Their prognosis is poor. They are almost totally made up of immunoblasts (Fig. b).

XVIII.2 Plasmacytomas

Clinical features (Fig. c).They are made of neoplastic plasma cells and, in the orbit, may be:
- either a localization of a myeloma (Kahler's disease) with its sharply circumscribed defects throughout the bone with no reactive marginal sclerosis on Xrays, its medullar plasmacytosis above 10% and its myelomatous proteins in urine and serum;
- or develop without any bone involvement. This is the extramedullar plasmacytoma, which may be primary, or secondary to another localization (mostly bronchial). It is often "non-secreting" i.e. without paraproteinemia.

Histopathology. It is characterized by a homogeneous proliferation of abnormal plasma cells (Fig. d).

XVIII.3 Granulocytic sarcoma
(chloroma, myeloid sarcoma)

Clinical features. It is an extramedullary localization of myeloid leukemia, affecting the orbit particularly. This tumour occurs in young patients, children or adults under 30 years of age. It provokes a rapidly evolving proptosis, often accompanied by changes in the orbital bony frame but which may precede the haematic manifestations of the disease by months, or even by years, making diagnosis especially difficult. Uveal localizations are equally possible (Plate 54, Chapter XXIV.4, Fig. a, b).

Histopathology. Classically the tumour takes on a greenish colour (chloroma) due to the presence of an enzyme, myeloperoxydase, but this is an unstable, labile coloration. Histopathologically, it is a diffuse infiltrating proliferation of immature granulocytes (Fig. e) the identification of which can be made easier by Leder's histoenzymological staining (Fig. f).

B immunoblastiques B
(lymphomes à grandes cellules immunoblastiques)

Ce sont les réticulosarcomes des anciennes classifications. Survenant après 60 ans ils sont cliniquement primitifs, parfois précédés de manifestations dysimmunitaires. Leur pronostic est redoutable. Ils sont à peu près entièrement constitués d'immunoblastes (Fig. b).

XVIII.2 Plasmocytomes

Clinique (Fig. c). Composés de plasmocytes néoplasiques ils peuvent dans l'orbite:
- soit représenter une localisation d'un myélome (maladie de Kahler) avec ses images radiologiques ostéolytiques en géodes, sa plasmocytose médullaire supérieure à 10% et ses protéines myélomateuses sériques et urinaires;
- soit se développer en-dehors de toute atteinte osseuse, c'est le plasmocytome extra-médullaire primitif ou secondaire à une autre localisation (bronchique notamment). Il est souvent "non excrétant" c'est-à-dire sans paraprotéine circulante.

Histopathologie. L'image est celle d'une prolifération régulière de plasmocytes anormaux (Fig. d).

XVIII.3 Sarcome granulocytaire
(chlorome, sarcome myéloïde)

Clinique. C'est une localisation extra-médullaire de leucémie myéloïde, et l'orbite est particulièrement intéressée. Tumeur du sujet jeune, enfant ou adulte de moins de 30 ans, elle provoque une exophtalmie d'évolution rapide s'accompagnant souvent d'altérations du cadre osseux. Mais elle peut précéder de plusieurs mois voire années les manifestations sanguines de la maladie, ce qui rend le diagnostic particulièrement délicat. Des localisations uvéales sont également possibles (Planche 54, Chapitre XXIV.4, Fig. a,b).

Histopathologie. Classiquement la tumeur a une coloration verdâtre (chlorome) due à la présence d'une enzyme la myéloperoxydase mais cette teinte est inconstante et labile. Histopathologiquement c'est une prolifération diffuse et infiltrante de granulocytes immatures (Fig. e) dont l'identification peut être facilitée par la coloration histo-enzymologique de Leder (Fig. f).

B-immunoblastäre Lymphome
(Lymphome mit großen Immunoblasten)

Es sind die Retikulosarkome der früheren Klassifizierungen. Sie treten nach 60 Jahren auf und benehmen sich wie Primärgeschwülste; manchmal gehen ihnen dysimmunologische Manifestationen voran. Ihre Prognose ist schlecht. Sie bestehen fast ausschließlich aus Immunoblasten (Abb. b).

XVIII.2 Plasmozytome

Klinik (Abb. c). Sie enthalten neoplastische Plasmozyten und können in der Orbita:
- entweder beim Myelom (Kahler-Krankheit) mit den "ausgestanzten" Osteolysen auf den Röntgenbildern, einer medullären Plasmozytose von über 10% und den myelomatösen Proteinen in Serum und Urin auftreten;
- oder sich außerhalb jeder Knochenerkrankung entwickeln; dies ist das extramedulläre primäre oder sekundäre Plasmozytom mit anderer (hauptsächlich bronchialer) Lokalisation. Es ist häufig "nicht exkretierend", das heißt es tritt im Blut kein Paraprotein auf.

Histopathologie. Regelmäßige Proliferation anormaler Plasmozyten (Abb. d).

XVIII.3 Granulozytäres Sarkom
(chlorom, myeloides Sarkom)

Klinik. Dies ist eine extramedulläre Lokalisation der myeloischen Leukämie, wobei insbesondere die Orbita betroffen ist, ein Tumor des jungen Menschen, des Kindes oder Erwachsenen unter 30. Er bewirkt einen sich rasch entwickelnden Exophthalmus, häufig Alterationen der Knochenwand. Er kann aber mehrere Monate oder sogar Jahre den Manifestationen der Krankheit im Blut vorangehen, was die Diagnose besonders schwierig macht. Uvea-Lokalisationen sind ebenfalls möglich. (Tafel 54, Kapitel XXIV.4, Abb. a, b).

Histopathologie. Die Geschwulst hat klassischerweise eine grünliche Farbe (daher Chlorom), die auf das Vorhandensein der Myeloperoxydase zurückzuführen ist; diese Färbung ist jedoch nicht konstant, und labil. Histologisch ist es eine diffus infiltrierende Proliferation von unreifen Granulozyten (Abb. e), die mit der histo-enzymologischen Lederschen Färbung leichter zu identifizieren sind (Abb. f).

PLATE 38   PLANCHE 38   TAFEL 38

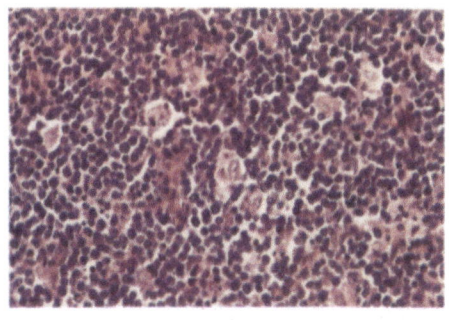

a

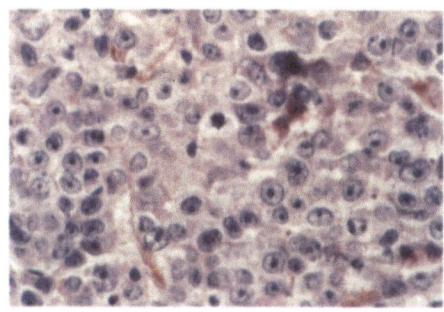

b

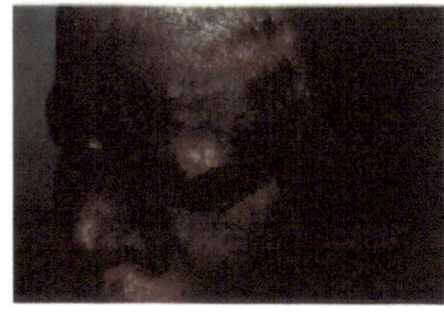

c

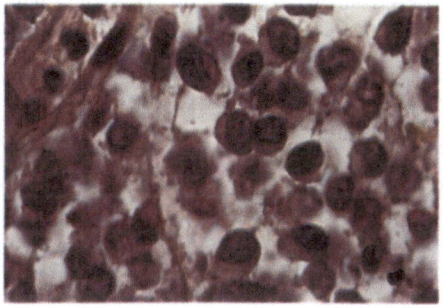

d

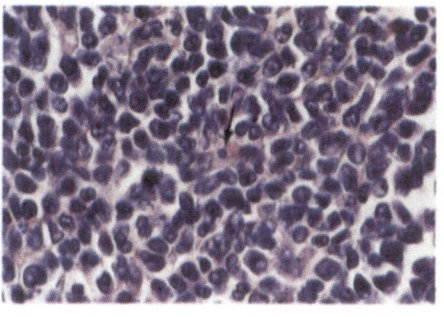

e

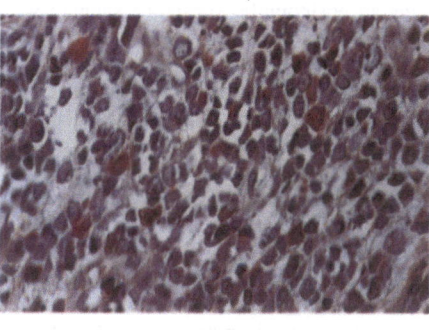

f

Fig. a. Burkitt's lymphoma.
Proliferation of cells with a round noncleaved nucleus, often mitotic: they could be intermediaries between lymphocytes and centroblasts (Lennert). Large macrophages containing so-called tingible bodies are disseminated in this proliferation, giving the characteristic appearance of a "starry sky". The genome of the Eptein-Barr virus is present in the nucleus of the tumorous cells and 90 per cent of patients show a chromosomic abnormality (translocation 8–14). (See text p. 78.)

Fig. b. B-Immunoblastic lymphoma.
The tumour is entirely made up of large cells with a widespread basophilic cytoplasm, a round or oval nucleus with a large central nucleolus.

Fig. c. Orbital plasmacytoma having invaded the lid of a man of African origin.

Fig. d. Orbital plasmacytoma.
Large sized, abnormal plasma cells often binucleate. The nuclei present a high content of chromatin. They produce a monoclonal protein, in general IgA, and may therefore be accompanied by a local amyloid deposit.

Fig. e. Orbital granulocytic sarcoma.
Proliferation of non-differentiated cells with a round, oval or kidney-shaped nucleus with disseminated chromatin. The presence of eosinophilic granulations in some cells of myelocytic appearance (→) contributes to the diagnosis.

Fig. f. Granulocytic sarcoma. Leder's staining shows the esterase activity of the cells (stained in red). This staining can only be used for tissue previously fixed in formaldehyde.

Fig. a. Lymphome de Burkitt.
Prolifération de cellules à noyau arrondi non clivé souvent en mitose qui seraient des éléments intermédiaires entre lymphocytes et centroblastes (Lennert). Cette prolifération est parsemée de grands macrophages à corps tingibles qui donnent un aspect caractéristique "en ciel étoilé". Le génome du virus Epstein-Barr est présent dans le noyau des cellules tumorales et 90% des sujets atteints présentent une anomalie chromosomique (translocation 8–14). (Voir texte p. 78.)

Fig. b. Lymphome immunoblastique B.
Tumeur presque entièrement constituée de grandes cellules à cytoplasme étendu, basophile, à noyau arrondi ou ovalaire avec un gros nucléole central.

Fig. c. Plasmocytome de l'orbite propagé à la paupière chez un Africain.

Fig. d. Plasmocytome de l'orbite.
Plasmocytes anormaux de grande taille souvent binucléés, à noyau riche en chromatine. Ils élaborent une protéine monoclonale en général IgA et peuvent donc s'accompagner de dépôt local de substance amyloïde.

Fig. e. Sarcome granulocytaire de l'orbite.
Prolifération de cellules indifférenciées à noyau arrondi, ovalaire ou réniforme, à chromatine dispersée. La présence de granulations éosinophiles dans certains éléments d'allure myélocytaire (→) aide beaucoup au diagnostic.

Fig. f. Sarcome granulocytaire, coloration de Leder montrant l'activité estérasique des cellules (colorées en rouge). Cette coloration ne peut être utilisée que sur pièces fixées au formol.

Abb. a. Burkitt-Lymphom.
Proliferation von Zellen mit rundlichem, nicht gespaltenem, oft in Mitose befindlichem Kern, die eine Zwischenform zwischen Lymphozyten und Zentroblasten sein sollen (Lennert). Diese Proliferation ist mit Kerntrümmermakrophagen übersät, die ein charakteristisches Bild ergeben ("Sternenhimmel" – "starry sky"). Das Genom des Epstein-Barr-Virus ist im Kern der Tumorzellen vorhanden, und 90% der Erkrankten weisen eine Chromosomenaberration auf (8–14-Translokation). (Siehe text p. 78.)

Abb. b. B-Immunoblastäres Lymphom.
Der Tumor besteht fast gänzlich aus großen Zellen mit ausgedehntem, basophilem Zytoplasma, mit rundlichem oder ovalem Kern mit einem großen Nukleolus in der Mitte.

Abb. c. In das Lid sich ausbreitendes Plasmozytom der Orbita bei einem Afrikaner.

Abb. d. Plasmozytom der Orbita.
Anormale, große, oft zweikernige Plasmozyten mit chromatinreichen Kernen. Sie produzieren ein monoklonales Protein (im allgemeinen IgA) und können also mit lokaler Amyloidablagerung einhergehen.

Abb. e. Granulozytäres Sarkom der Orbita.
Proliferation undifferenzierter Zellen mit rundlichem, ovalem oder nierenförmigem Kern mit versprengtem Chromatin. Das Vorhandensein eosinophiler Granulationen in manchen myelozytär wirkenden Elementen (→) erleichtert die Diagnose.

Abb. f. Granulozytäres Sarkom, Ledersche Färbung, welche die Esterase-Aktivität der (rot gefärbten) Zellen anzeigt. Diese Färbung kann nur auf formolfixierten Schnitten verwendet werden.

PLATE 39 PLANCHE 39 TAFEL 39

XIX. TUMOURS OF THE LACRIMAL GLAND

XIX.1 Benign mixed tumour (pleomorphic adenoma)

Clinical features. A typically adult condition, this is the most common tumour of the lacrimal gland. It results in an inferonasal exophthalmos. On palpation it is a firm, uneven painless mass, mobile under the skin, separated from the eyeball and the bone structures. It may cause diplopia. Slow in its evolution, it may sometimes recur a few years after excision. Moreover, these late relapses may contain foci tending to malignant change.

Histopathology. These tumours present both epithelial and connective components (formerly "mixed tumours"). The epithelial component is made up of tubular, canalicular formations, lined by one or two layers of cubical cells, surrounding a lumen which contains an eosinophilic substance staining with PAS. At the periphery of these tubes, the myoepithelial cells stretch themselves out, becoming spindle shaped or stellate in appearance and become isolated in the connective tissue, resulting in an adamantinoid appearance.

Apart from these glandular formations, areas of variable density or strands of epithelial cells can be observed which may undergo an epidermoid metaplasia with horny cysts. The more or less abundant stroma is of variable composition and is more or less "modified" (Leroux), hyaline and myxoid with a high content of acid mucopolysaccharides, or even chondroid. This tumour seems to be well limited, surrounded by a pseudocapsule which, in part, is merely a condensation of the surrounding supporting tissue. It is necessary to check that tumour nodules are not included in this capsule or even stuck to its external face. If this is the case one should fear recurrences which, in turn, would not be encapsulated.

XIX. TUMEURS DE LA GLANDE LACRYMALE

XIX.1 Tumeur bénigne mixte (adénome pléomorphe)

Clinique. Apanage de l'adulte c'est la plus fréquente des tumeurs de la glande lacrymale. Elle se manifeste par une exopthalmie inféronasale. A la palpation c'est une masse ferme bosselée, indolore, mobile sous la peau, indépendante du globe et du plan osseux. Elle peut entraîner une diplopie. D'évolution lente elle est susceptible de récidiver parfois des années après l'exérèse; ces récidives tardives peuvent d'ailleurs présenter des foyers de transformation maligne.

Histopathologie. Ce sont des tumeurs à double composante épithéliale et conjonctive ("tumeur mixte"). La composante épithéliale est faite de formations tubulaires, canaliculaires, bordées de une ou deux couches de cellules cubiques, entourant une lumière contenant une substance éosinophile prenant le PAS. A la périphérie de ces tubes les cellules myoépithéliales s'allongent, prennent un aspect fusiforme ou étoilé et s'isolent dans le tissu conjonctif environnant lui donnant une allure adamantoïde.

En-dehors de ces formations glandulaires on trouve des plages et des travées plus ou moins denses de cellules épithéliales qui peuvent subir une métaphasie épidermoïde avec kystes cornés. Le stroma plus ou moins abondant est de structure variable plus ou moins "remaniée" (Leroux), hyaline, myxoïde, riche en muco-polysaccharides acides, voire chondroïde. Cette tumeur paraît bien circonscrite, entourée d'une pseudocapsule qui n'est, en partie, qu'une condensation du tissu de soutien environnant. Il faut s'assurer que des nodules tumoraux ne sont pas inclus dans cette capsule, voire même accolés à sa face externe car une telle constatation doit faire craindre des récidives qui, elles, ne sont pas encapsulées.

XIX. TUMOREN DER TRÄNENDRÜSE

XIX.1 Gutartiger Tumor (Pleomorphes Adenom)

Klinik. Diese dem Erwachsenen vorbehaltene Geschwulst ist die häufigste unter den Tumoren der Tränendrüse. Sie ist durch einen Exophthalmus nach nasal unten gekennzeichnet. Beim Betasten spürt man eine derbe, höckrige, indolente Masse, beweglich unter der Haut, unabhängig von Bulbus und Knochenwand. Sie kann eine Diplopie zur Folge haben. Die sich langsam entwickelnde Geschwulst kann manchmal Jahre nach der Exstirpation rezidivieren; von diesen späten Rezidiven können übrigens bösartige Umwandlungen ausgehen.

Histopathologie. Es sind Tumoren mit doppelter, vom Epithel und vom Bindegewebe abstammender Komponente, daher die frühere Bezeichnung "Mischtumor". Der vom Epithel herrührende Teil besteht aus röhren- und schlauchartigen Gebilden, die von einer oder zwei Schichten kubischer Zellen ausgekleidet sind und in deren Innerem eine eosinophile, PAS-positive Substanz liegt. An der Peripherie dieser Schläuche werden die Myoepithelzellen länglicher, erhalten ein spindel- oder sternförmiges Aussehen und heben sich von dem umgebenden Bindegewebe ab, das einen adamantoiden Aspekt bekommt.

Neben diesen Drüsengebilden sind mehr oder weniger dichte Felder oder Stränge aus Epithelzellen anzutreffen, die eine epidermoide Metaplasie mit Hornzysten erfahren können. Das mehr oder weniger reichlich vorhandene Stroma ist wechselnd, mehr oder weniger "umgebildet" (Leroux), von hyaliner, myxoider Struktur, reich an sauren Mukopolysacchariden; es kann sogar knorpelartig sein. Dieser Tumor scheint klar abgegrenzt zu sein, er ist von einer Pseudokapsel umgeben, die zum Teil nur eine Kondensierung des umliegenden Stützgewebes ist. Es ist darauf zu achten, daß keine Tumorknötchen in dieser Kapsel eingeschlossen sind oder gar an deren Außenseite anhängen, denn eine solche Feststellung läßt Rezidiven befürchten, die ihrerseits nicht eingekapselt sind.

PLATE 39 PLANCHE 39 TAFEL 39

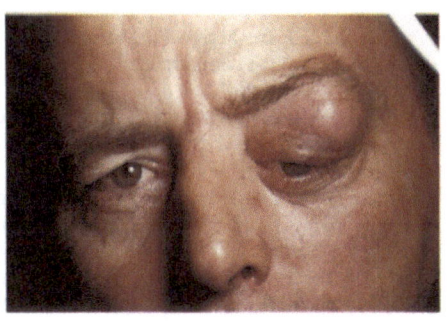

a

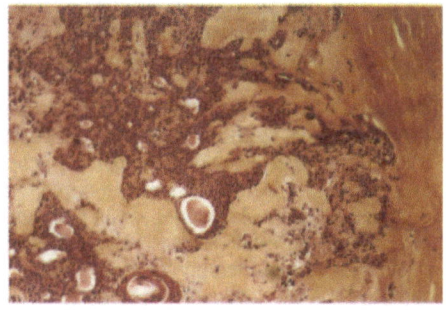

b

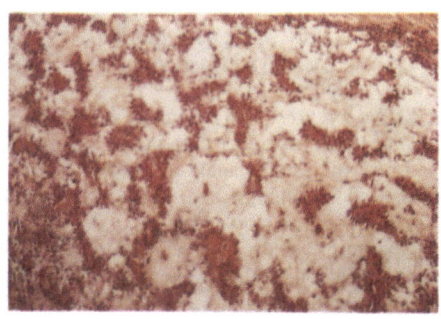

c

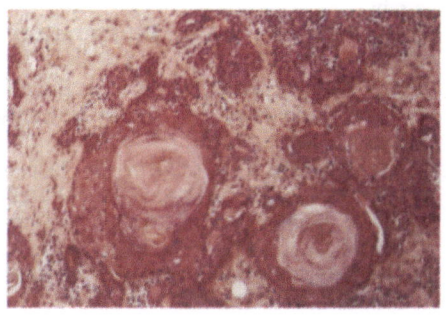

d

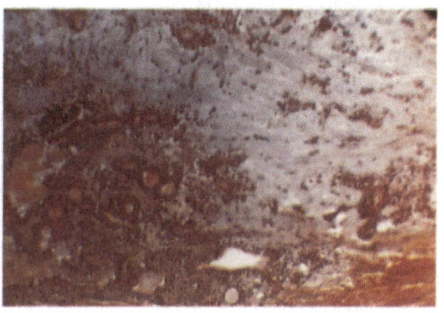

e

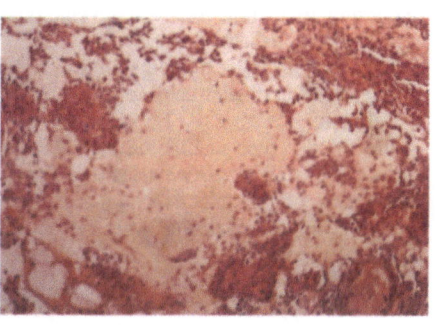

f

Fig. a. Pleomorphic adenoma of the lacrimal gland. This tumour is located in the superotemporal orbital region (fossa lacrimalis) and pushes the eyeball downwards and inwards.

Fig. b. Pleomorphic adenoma of the lacrimal gland. Frameworks made up of glandular epithelial cells amongst which exist individual canalicular formations with eosinophilic contents. The connective stroma is dense.

Fig. c. Pleomorphic adenoma of the lacrimal gland. Adamantinoid structure: myoepithelial cells surrounding epithelial islands are isolated in a myxoid stroma and take on a star-like form.

Fig. d. Pleomorphic adenoma of the lacrimal gland. Epidermoid metaplasia within the strands of epithelial cells, with formation of horn pearls.

Fig. e. Pleomorphic adenoma of the lacrimal gland. Mucoid stroma stained pale blue by Alcian blue.

Fig. f. Pleomorphic adenoma of the lacrimal gland. Chondroid metaplasia of the stroma.

Fig. a. Adénome pléomorphe de la glande lacrymale.
La tumeur siège dans l'angle supéro-externe de l'orbite (loge lacrymale) et refoule le globe en bas et en-dedans.

Fig. b. Adénome pléomorphe de la glande lacrymale.
Travées de cellules épithéliales glandulaires au sein desquelles s'individualisent des formations caniculaires à contenu éosinophile. Le stroma conjonctif est dense.

Fig. c. Adénome pléomorphe de la glande lacrymale.
Structure adamantoïde: les cellules myoépithéliales qui bordent les îlots épithéliaux, s'isolent au sein d'un stroma myxoïde et prennent une forme étoilée.

Fig. d. Adénome pléomorphe de la glande lacrymale.
Métaplasie épidermoïde au sein des travées épithéliales avec formation de globes cornés.

Fig. e. Adénome pléomorphe de la glande lacrymale.
Stroma mucoïde coloré en bleu pâle par le Bleu Alcian.

Fig. f. Adénome pléomorphe de la glande lacrymale.
Métaplasie chondroïde du stroma.

Abb. a. Pleomorphes Adenom der Tränendrüse.
Die Geschwulst sitzt im oberen äußeren Winkel der Orbita (Tränendrüsenloge) und drückt den Bulbus nach unten und innen.

Abb. b. Pleomorphes Adenom der Tränendrüse.
Stränge mit Drüsenepithelzellen, in denen sich röhrchenartige Formationen mit eosinophilen Inhalt gebildet haben. Dichtes Bindegewebsstroma.

Abb. c. Pleomorphes Adenom der Tränendrüse.
Adamantoide Struktur: die Myoepithelzellen, die die Epithelinseln umgeben, heben sich innerhalb eines myxoiden Stromas ab und nehmen Sternform an.

Abb. d. Pleomorphes Adenom der Tränendrüse.
Epidermoide Metaplasie innerhalb der Epithelstränge mit Bildung von Hornperlen.

Abb. e. Pleomorphes Adenom der Tränendrüse.
Schleimähnliches Stroma, mit Alcian Blau hellblau gefärbt.

Abb. f. Pleomorphes Adenom der Tränendrüse.
Knorpelige Metaplasie des Stromas.

PLATE 40 PLANCHE 40 TAFEL 40

XIX.2 Malignant tumours of the lacrimal gland

Clinical features. The proptosis is identical to that of pleomorphic adenoma but its evolution is rapid and accompanied by palpebral ptosis and oedema, diplopia and, above all, pain. X ray examination may reveal bone destruction in the temporal fossa. Where there is a pre-existing pleomorphic adenoma, it develops abruptly and rapidly in size.

Histopathology. Several histological varieties exist.

XIX.2.1 Adenoid cystic carcinoma

This is the most commonly occurring carcinoma of the lacrimal gland. It is classically known, due to its architecture, by the name of "cylindroma", but it could be mistaken for a certain variety of cutaneous carcinoma which has a totally different prognosis.
According to cellular density, several types may be distinguished:
- the "cribriform" carcinoma in which the strands of epithelial cells form a lace-like network;
- the tubular type carcinoma in which the formations are smaller and take on the appearance of glandular canals bounded by 2 to 3 layers of cells, sometimes surrounded by a basement membrane and drowned in a hyaline stroma;
- the solid type, also called basaloid type, is more dense and may be difficult to diagnose.

Tumour strands may penetrate the surrounding nerve sheaths, which is an aggravating factor in this infiltrative, destructive and metastasizing tumour.

XIX.2.2 Carcinoma within a pleomorphic adenoma (malignant mixed tumour)

The malignant change occurs only after a very long evolution and often after several recurrences. Besides some areas which maintain the appearance of a pleomorphic adenoma, clearly carcinogenic areas can be seen, some of them anaplastic, poorly differentiated, others adenoid cystic.

XIX.2.3 Other carcinomas

Much less frequent are:
- mucus-secreting adenocarcinoma: identical to that of the salivary gland;
- non differentiated anaplastic adenocarcinoma: made up of cellular tubes consisting of cells of poorly differentiated glandular type;
- mucoepidermoid tumour: in this proliferation originating in the canalicular epithelium, epidermoid structures and areas exhibiting secretion of mucin are associated.

XIX.2 Tumeurs malignes de la glande lacrymale

Clinique. L'exophtalmie est identique à celle de l'adénome pléomorphe mais elle est d'évolution rapide s'accompagnant de ptosis avec oedème palpébral, de diplopie, de douleurs surtout. L'examen radiographique peut mettre en évidence une destruction osseuse dans la fosse temporale. Lorsqu'existait auparavant un adénome pléomorphe, il augmente brusquement et rapidement de taille.

Histopathologie. Il en existe plusieurs variétés histologiques.

XIX.2.1 Carcinome adénoïde kystique

C'est le plus fréquent. Il est connu classiquement du fait de son architecture sous le nom de "cylindrome" mais il risque alors d'être confondu avec certains carcinomes cutanés de pronostic tout-à-fait différent.
Selon la densité cellulaire on distingue plusieurs types:
- le type "cribriforme" dans lequel des cordons de cellules myoépithéliales dessinent un réseau en dentelle;
- le type tubulaire où les formations sont plus petites et prennent l'allure de canaux glandulaires bordés de 2 à 3 couches cellulaires, parfois entourés d'une basale et noyés dans un stroma hyalin;
- le type solide, dit aussi basaloïde, plus dense et pouvant poser de difficiles problèmes diagnostiques.

Des cordons tumoraux peuvent infiltrer les gaines des nerfs avoisinants ce qui est un élément péjoratif dans ces tumeurs très infiltrantes, destructrices et métastasiantes.

XIX.2.2 Carcinome dans un adénome pléomorphe (tumeur mixte maligne)

Cette transformation maligne n'apparait qu'après un très long temps d'évolution et souvent après plusieurs récidives. A côté de plages conservant la physionomie d'un adénome pléomorphe on trouve des secteurs franchement carcinomateux, soit peu différenciés anaplasiques, soit adénoïdes kystiques.

XIX.2.3 Autres carcinomes

Ils sont beaucoup plus rares. Ce sont:
- l'adénocarcinome muco-sécrétant: identique à celui des glandes salivaires;
- l'adénocarcinome anaplasique ou indifférencié: constitué de boyaux cellulaires faits de cellules de type glandulaire peu différenciées;
- la tumeur muco-épidermoïde: où la prolifération née de l'épithélium canaliculaire associe des structures épidermoïdes à des structures mucipares sécrétantes.

XIX.2 Bösartige Tumoren der Tränendrüse

Klinik. Der Exophthalmus ist derselbe wie beim pleomorphen Adenom, er entwickelt sich aber schnell und geht mit Ptosis, Lidödem, Diplopie und vor allem Schmerzen einher. Die Radiographie kann eine Knochenzerstörung in der Fossa temporalis sichtbar machen. Sofern zuvor ein pleomorphes Adenom bestanden hat, vergrößert es sich plötzlich und schnell.

Histopathologie. Es gibt mehrere histologische Arten.

XIX.2.1 Adenoidzystisches Karzinom

Es ist das häufigste. Auf Grund seines Aufbaus ist es unter der Bezeichnung "Zylindrom" bekannt, wobei allerdings das Risiko einer Verwechslung mit bestimmten Hautkarzinomen mit völlig anderer Prognose besteht.
Entsprechend der Zelldichte unterscheidet man mehrere Typen:
- den "siebähnlichen" Typ, in dem Stränge von Myoepithelzellen ein spitzenartigs Netz bilden;
- den tubulären Typ, in dem die Tumorverbände kleiner sind und wie Drüsenkanäle aussehen, die von 2 bis 3 Zellschichten ausgekleidet und manchmal von einer Basalschicht umgeben und in ein hyalines Stroma eingetaucht sind;
- der solide, auch basaloid genannte, dichtere Typ, der schwierige diagnostische Probleme stellen kann.

Tumorstränge können die benachbarten Nervenscheiden infiltrieren, was bei diesen stark infiltrierenden, destruktiven und metastasebildenden Tumoren ein nachteiliges Element ist.

XIX.2.2 Karzinom in einem pleomorphen Adenom (bösartiger Mischtumor)

Diese bösartige Umwandlung tritt erst nach einer sehr langen Entwicklungszeit und oft nach mehreren Rezidiven in Erscheinung. Neben Abschnitten, die dem Bild eines pleomorphen Adenoms entsprechen, finden sich ausgesprochen karzinomatöse, entweder wenig differenziert anaplastische oder adenoid zystische Bereiche.

XIX.2.3 Andere Karzinome

Sie sind viel seltener. Dazu gehören:
- das schleimbildende Adenokarzinom: identisch mit dem entsprechenden der Speicheldrüsen;
- das anaplastische oder undifferenzierte Adenokarzinom: es setzt sich aus Zellschläuchen zusammen, die aus wenig differenzierten drüsenartigen Zellen bestehen;
- der muco-epidermoide Tumor: bei dem die Proliferation, welche vom Kanälchenepithel ausgeht, epidermoide neben schleimgebenden Strukturen aufweist.

PLATE 40 PLANCHE 40 TAFEL 40

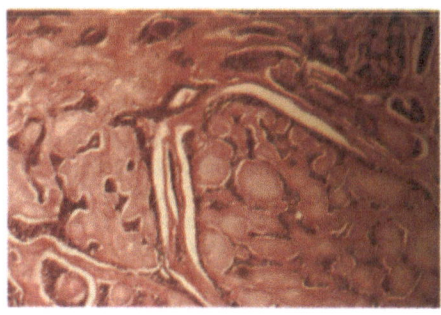

a

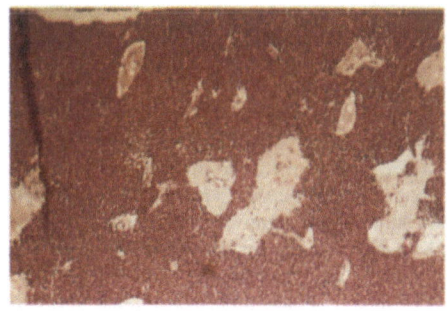

b

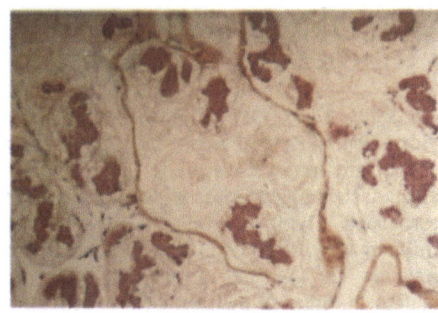

c

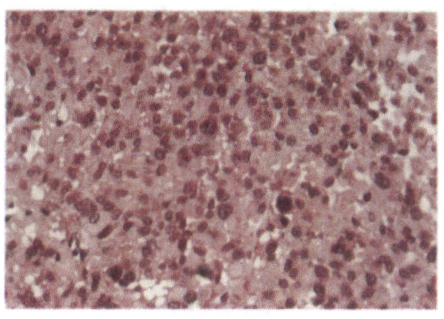

d

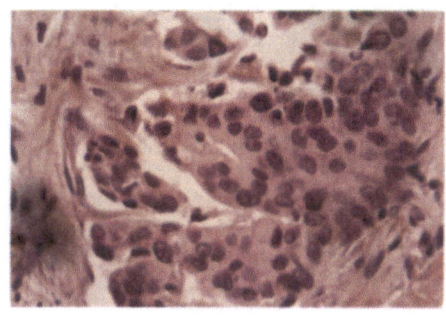

e

Fig. a. Cylindroma of the lacrimal gland.
"Cribriform" appearance: the cellular strands bind the round or oval cavities which contain an amorphous PAS positive substance. This substance secreted by the tumorous cells may become so abundant that it severs the cellular strands, which are reduced to thin threads and lost in a hyaline stroma.

Fig. b. Cylindroma of the lacrimal gland.
A solid form in which massive cellular areas (more or less lobulated) appear scattered with basophilic small round cavities, canalicular in appearance. This structure is seldom isolated and is, in general, situated next to more characteristic areas.

Fig. c. Mucus secreting adenocarcinoma.
The tumour cells secrete an abundant mucoid substance which floods the stroma and isolates the epithelial formations.

Fig. d. Anaplastic adenocarcinoma.
The cells are of glandular type, non differentiated, round or polygonal in shape with nuclei which are frequently seen to be monstrous.

Fig. e. Anaplastic adenocarcinoma.
Under high power, the outline of a glandular canalicule can be seen among the proliferating cells.

Fig. a. Cylindrome de la glande lacrymale.
Aspect "cribriforme": les cordons cellulaires limitent des cavités arrondies ou ovalaires contenant un matériel amorphe PAS positif. Cette substance sécrétée par les cellules tumorales peut devenir si abondante qu'elle dissocie les cordons cellulaires, qui se trouvent réduits à des minces lames au sein d'un stroma hyalin.

Fig. b. Cylindrome de la glande lacrymale.
Forme solide où les plages cellulaires sont massives, basophiles, parsemées de petites cavités arrondies. Cette structure est rarement isolée et voisine en général avec des zones plus caractéristiques.

Fig. c. Adénocarcinome muco-sécrétant.
Les cellules tumorales sécrètent une substance mucoïde abondante qui envahit le stroma isolant les formations épithéliales.

Fig. d. Adénocarcinome anaplasique.
Les cellules, de type glandulaire, sont indifférenciées, arrondies ou polygonales avec des noyaux souvent monstrueux.

Fig. e. Adénocarcinome anaplasique.
A un plus fort grossissement on distingue cependant une ébauche canaliculaire au sein de la prolifération cellulaire.

Abb. a. Zylindrom der Tränendrüse.
"Siebartiges" Aussehen: Zellstränge begrenzen die rundlichen oder ovalen, amorphes, PAS-positives Material enthaltenden Hohlräume. Diese von den Tumorzellen sezernierte Substanz kann in so großer Menge anfallen, daß sie die Zellstränge aufreißt und dissoziiert, so daß diese nur noch als feine Lamellen innerhalb eines hyalinen Stromas erkennbar sind.

Abb. b. Zylindrom der Tränendrüse.
Solide Form, in der die mehr oder weniger lappenartig angeordneten Zellfelder dicht, basophil, von kleinen abgerundeten, kanalförmigen Hohlräumen übersät sind. Diese Struktur tritt selten vereinzelt auf und ist meist in der Nähe charakteristischerer Zonen anzutreffen.

Abb. c. Schleimbildendes Adenokarzinom.
Die Tumorzellen sezernieren eine reichliche schleimartige Substanz, die in das Stroma eindringt, wobei die epithelialen Formationen isoliert werden.

Abb. d. Anaplastisches Karzinom.
Die den Tumor bildenden Zellen sind drüsenartig, undifferenziert, rundlich oder polygonal mit häufig vergrößerten Kernen.

Abb. e. Anaplastisches Adenokarzinom.
Bei stärkerer Vergrößerung ist in der Zellproliferation die Andeutung eines Kanälchens zu erkennen.

PLATE 41 PLANCHE 41 TAFEL 41

XX. TUMOURS OF THE LACRIMAL SAC

Clinical features. Tumours of the lacrimal sac, either benign or malignant, primary in most cases, are rarely observed and clinically appear as a palpable mass with epiphora often associated with chronic dacryocystitis. Inflammatory or mycotic pseudo-tumours are frequent (25%). 75% of true tumours are malignant. Signs of malignancy are: patients's age, the return flow of blood-mixed fluid when pressure is exerted, epistaxis, fistulization, bone destruction, proptosis.

Histopathology. These tumours derive from the epithelium of the sac, sometimes of the canaliculus.

Papillomas

According to the way they develop, papillomas may be classified as intra-canalicular exophytic tumours, inverted (in the chorion) or mixed. From the cytological point of view, three varieties may be differentiated: a malpighian form with occasional foci of dyskeratosis, a so-called transitional form with cylindrical cells recalling those of the nasolacrimal canal, and a mixed form.

Carcinoma

The carcinoma may occur de novo or within a papilloma. Cytologically three categories may also be observed: a malpighian form, a transitional variety and adenocarcinoma. The worst prognosis applies to the transitional form. Death may occur by local invasion or lymphatic metastases.

Oncocytoma

Oncocytoma is often discovered accidentally during the histological examination of a dacryocystitis. Its structure is identical to that of its homonym affecting the caruncle (Plate 9, Chapter I.1.6).

XX. TUMEURS DU SAC LACRYMAL

Clinique. Les tumeurs du sac lacrymal, bénignes ou malignes, primaires pour la plupart, sont rares et se manifestent cliniquement par une masse palpable, accompagnée d'épiphora et souvent de dacryocystite chronique. Les pseudo-tumeurs, inflammatoires ou mycosiques sont fréquentes (25%). Sur l'ensemble des vraies tumeurs 75% sont malignes. En faveur de la malignité parlent: l'âge, le reflux de liquide sanglant à la pression, l'épistaxis, la fistulisation, la destruction osseuse, l'exophtalmie.

Histopathologie. Ces tumeurs dérivent de l'épithélium du sac, parfois du canalicule.

Papillomes

Les papillomes, selon leur mode de croissance, peuvent être divisés en exophytiques intrasacculaires, inversés dans le chorion ou mixtes. Selon leur type cytologique on distingue également trois variétés: une forme malpighienne, montrant occasionnellement des foyers de dyskératose, une forme dite transitionnelle, à cellules cylindriques rappelant celles du canal lacrymo-nasal, et une forme mixte.

Carcinome

Le carcinome peut apparaître de novo ou au sein d'un papillome. Cytologiquement on distingue ici aussi trois catégories: une forme malpighienne, une variété "transitionnelle" et l'adénocarcinome. Ce sont les formes transitionnelles qui ont le pronostic le pire. La mort peut survenir par invasion locale ou par métastases lymphatiques.

Oncocytome

L'oncocytome est souvent une découverte fortuite lors de l'examen histologique d'une dacryocystite. Sa structure est identique à celle de son homonyme à la caroncule (Planche 9, Chapitre I.1.6).

XX. TUMOREN DES TRÄNENSACKS

Klinik. Geschwülste des Tränensacks, ob gutartig oder bösartig, zumeist primär, kommen selten vor und sind *klinisch* durch eine tastbare Masse erkennbar, einhergehend mit Epiphora und oft mit chronischer Dakryozystitis. Entzündliche oder durch Mykose hervorgerufene Pseudo-Tumoren treten häufig auf (25%). 75% aller echten Tumoren sind bösartig. Für Bösartigkeit sprechen: das Alter, Reflux einer blutigen Flüssigkeit bei Druck, Epistaxis, Fistelbildung, Knochenzerstörung, Exophthalmus.

Histopathologie. Histopathologisch gehen sie vom Epithel des Tränensackes, manchmal der Tränenkanälchen aus.

Papillome

Papillome können je nach ihrer Wachstumsart in exophytische (im Innern des Tränensacks), umgekehrte (in der Wand wachsende) oder gemischte unterteilt werden. Ihrem zytologischen Typ zufolge unterscheidet man ebenfalls drei Arten: eine epidermoide Form, bei der gelegentlich Dyskeratoseherde auftreten, eine sogenannte transitorische Form, (Übergangsform) mit Zylinderzellen die an die Zellen im Tränennasenkanal erinnern und eine gemischte Form.

Karzinom

Das Karzinom kann entweder de novo oder im Zusammenhang mit einem Papillom auftreten. Man unterscheidet hier ebenfalls drei Kategorien: eine epidermoide Form, eine "Übergangsform" und das Adenokarzinom. Für die Übergangsform ist die Prognose am schlechtesten. Der Tod kann durch lokale Ausbreitung oder durch lymphatische Metastasen verursacht werden.

Onkozytom

Das Onkozytom wird oft zufällig bei der histologischen Untersuchung einer Dakryozystitis entdeckt. Es hat dieselbe Struktur wie die gleichnamige Geschwulst der Karunkel (Tafel 9, Kapitel I.1.6).

PLATE 41   PLANCHE 41   TAFEL 41

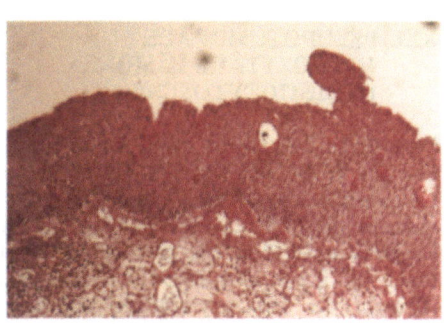

a

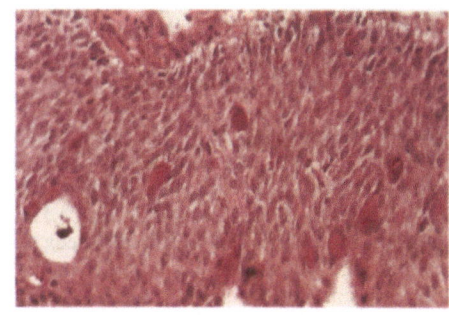

b

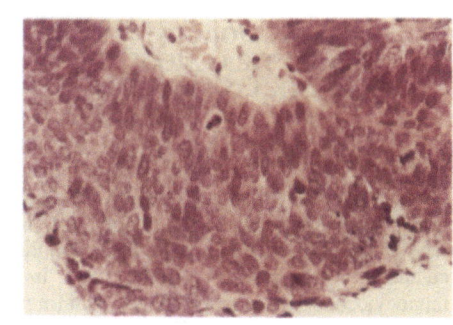

c

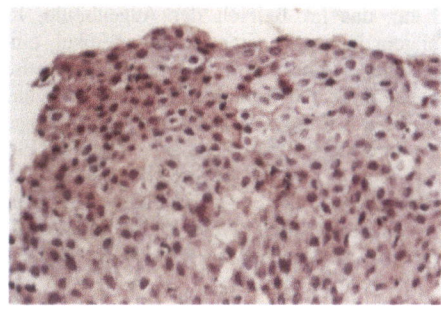

d

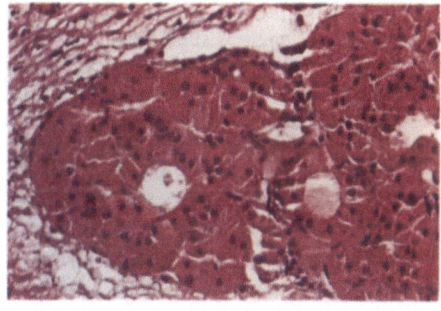

e

Fig. a. Transitional papilloma of the lacrimal sac. Uniform thickening of the epithelium, the cells of which have kept their usual characteristics. The mucous cells are easily identified by PAS.

Fig. b. Same as above, under higher power (PAS). Presence of a superadded inflammatory infiltrate with polymorphonuclear cells.

Fig. c. Transitional carcinoma of the lacrimal sac, discovered during the surgical operation of a fistulized dacryocystitis in a 7-year old child.

Fig. d. Transitional carcinoma of the lacrimal sac. Recurrent tumour showing a superficial epidermoid metaplasia.

Fig. e. Oncocytoma of the lacrimal sac.

Fig. a. Papillome transitionnel du sac lacrymal. Epaississement uniforme de l'épithélium dont les cellules ont gardé leurs caractéristiques habituelles. Les cellules à mucus sont bien reconnaissables grâce au PAS.

Fig. b. Le même à un plus fort grossissement (PAS).
Présence d'un infiltrat inflammatoire à polynucléaires surajouté.

Fig. c. Carcinome transitionnel du sac lacrymal, découvert au cours d'une intervention pour dacryocystite fistulisée chez une enfant de 7 ans.

Fig. d. Carcinome transitionnel du sac lacrymal. Tumeur récidivée présentant une métaplasie épidermoïde en surface.

Fig. e. Oncocytome du sac lacrymal.

Abb. a. Übergangsform des Tränensackpapilloms. Gleichmäßige Verdickung des Epithels, dessen Zellen ihre gewohnten Merkmale beibehalten haben. Die Schleimzellen sind dank PAS-Färbung leicht zu erkennen.

Abb. b. Dasselbe bei stärkerer Vergrößerung (PAS).
Ein zusätzliches, polynukleäres, entzündliches Infiltrat.

Abb. c. Übergangsform des Tränensackkarzinoms, das bei einem Eingriff wegen Dakryozystitis mit Fistelbildung bei einem siebenjährigen Kind vorgefunden wurde.

Abb. d. Übergangsform des Tränensackkarzinoms. Rezidivierende Geschwulst, die eine oberflächliche epidermoide Metaplasie aufweist.

Abb. e. Onkozytom des Tränensacks.

PLATE 42 PLANCHE 42 TAFEL 42

XXI. PSEUDO-TUMOROUS HISTIOCYTIC LESIONS (X HISTIOCYTOSES)

These diseases are characterized by the proliferation of histiocytes presenting typical intracytoplasmic structures on E.M.: Birbeck granules or Langerhans' rods. They are, in fact, identical to those which are present in the cutaneous Langerhans' cells, as immunocytochemical studies have confirmed ("Langerhans' histiocytoses").
In progressive order of seriousness, they are:
– eosinophilic granuloma of bone;
– Hand-Schüller-Christian disease;
– Letterer-Siwe disease.
Only the first two occur in the orbit with any frequency.

XXI.1 Eosinophilic granuloma of bone

Clinical features. In most cases, the condition occurs in a young child who presents with a soft, painful tumefaction (generally in the supero-lateral sector, at the rim of the orbit) causing occasional headaches, accompanied by a more or less erythematous palpebral oedema with, at times, skin fistulization. Radiologically, the irregular, serrated lytic lesion is characteristic. Other localizations, especially in the ribs, must be looked-for.

Histopathology. From the histological point of view, the tissue is vascularized and fragile, consisting of globular histiocytes sometimes associated with multinuclear giant cells, polymorphonuclear eosinophils and inflammatory cells.

XXI.2 Hand-Schüller-Christian disease

Clinical features. This is the chronic disseminated form of the histiocytosis X, which also appears mostly in children and is marked by the characteristic triad: proptosis (often bilateral), diabetes insipidus and bony lacunae of the dome of the skull.

Histopathology. Apart from mono- and multinuclear histiocytes and eosinophils, large xanthomatous cells with a lipid rich foamy cytoplasm can be observed. Birbeck granules are found on E.M.

XXI.3 Sinus histiocytosis (Rosai and Dorfman); histiocytose macrophagique lymphocytaire (Destombes)

Clinical features. This lymph node disease which is mainly observed in young Africans may also involve the orbit and produce a unilateral or bilateral proptosis.

Histopathology. Hyperchromatic cells (lymphocytes) and pale-staining structures (large macrophages of characteristic appearance) justify, especially in the orbit, the French term "histiocytose macrophagique lymphocytaire".

XXI. LÉSIONS HISTIOCYTAIRES PSEUDO-TUMORALES (HISTIOCYTOSES X)

Maladies caractérisées par la prolifération d'histiocytes qui contiennent, à l'échelle ultrastructurale, des organelles particulières: les granules de Birbeck ou bâtonnets de Langerhans. Ils sont en effet identiques à ceux des cellules de Langerhans de la peau comme l'ont confirmé les études immunocytochimiques ("Histiocytoses langerhansiennes").
Ce sont par ordre de gravité croissante:
– le granulome éosinophile de l'os;
– la maladie de Hand-Schüller-Christian;
– la maladie de Letterer-Siwe.
Seules les deux premières se rencontrent dans l'orbite avec une certaine fréquence.

XXI.1 Granulome éosinophile de l'os

Clinique. Il s'agit le plus souvent d'un jeune enfant présentant sur le pourtour orbitaire en général à l'angle supéro-externe une tuméfaction mollasse, douloureuse, pouvant occasionner des céphalées, accompagnée d'un oedème palpébral plus ou moins érythémateux avec parfois fistulisation à la peau. L'image radiologique lacunaire irrégulière est caractéristique. D'autres localisations, particulièrement costales, sont à rechercher.

Histopathologie. Le tissu prélevé, vascularisé et friable est constitué d'histiocytes globuleux avec parfois des plasmodes plurinucléées, des polynucléaires éosinophiles et des cellules inflammatoires.

XXI.2 Maladie de Hand-Schüller-Christian

Clinique. C'est la forme disséminée chronique de l 'histiocytose X. Elle apparaît également surtout chez l'enfant et se révèle par la triade caractéristique: exophtalmie souvent bilatérale, diabète insipide et lacunes osseuses de la voûte crânienne.

Histopathologie. Outre des histiocytes mono et plurinucléés et des éosinophiles, on trouve de grandes cellules xanthomateuses à cytoplasme spumeux riche en lipides, ainsi que des granules de Birbeck en microscopie électronique.

XXI.3 Histiocytose sinusale (Rosai et Dorfman); histiocytose macrophagique lymphocytaire (Destombes)

Clinique. Cette maladie ganglionnaire, apanage des sujets jeunes souvent mélanodermes peut également se localiser dans l'orbite.

Histopathologie. L'histopathologie montre des plages cellulaires les unes sombres (cellules lymphocytaires), les autres claires (grandes cellules macrophagiques d'aspect caractéristique). Elles justifient la dénomination "d'histiocytose macrophagique lymphocytaire", plus exacte dans l'orbite.

XXI. PSEUDOTUMORALE HISTIOZYTÄRE LÄSIONEN (X-HISTIOZYTOSEN)

Diese Krankheiten sind durch die Proliferation von Histiozyten geprägt, welche in der Ultrastruktur besondere Organellen aufweisen: die Birbeckschen Granula oder Langerhans-Stäbchen. Sie sind identisch mit denen der Langerhans-Zellen der Haut, wie Arbeiten der Immunzytochemie bestätigen ("Langerhanssche Histiozytosen"). Es sind dies mit zunehmendem Schweregrad der Erkrankung:
– das eosinophile Granulom des Knochens;
– die Hand-Schüller-Christian Krankheit;
– die Letterer-Siwe Krankheit.
Nur die beiden ersteren sind mit einiger Häufigkeit in der Orbita anzutreffen.

XXI.1 Eosinophilisches Granulom des Knochens

Klinik. Betroffen ist zumeist ein kleineres Kind, das im Bereich der Augenhöhle, im allgemeinen im oberen äußeren Winkel, eine weiche, schmerzhafte Schwellung aufweist. Diese kann Kopfschmerzen verursachen und mit einem Lidödem, das mehr oder weniger erythematös ist (manchmal sogar mit einer Fistel durch die Haut) einhergehen. Das Röntgenbild mit den scharfrandigen Defekten ist charakteristisch. Nach anderen Lokalisationen, insbesondere im Bereich der Rippen, sollte gesucht werden.

Histopathologie. Die weiche, vaskularisierte und zerbrechliche Gewebeprobe besteht aus kugeligen Histiozyten, manchmal mit mehrkernigen Plasmodien, eosinophilen polynukleären und entzündlichen Zellen.

XXI.2 Hand-Schüller-Christian Krankheit

Klinik. Es ist die disseminierte chronische Form der X-Histiozytose. Sie tritt ebenfalls vor allem beim kleinen Kind auf und hat drei charakteristische Merkmale: Exophthalmus, oft beidseitig, Diabetes insipidus und Knochendefekte im Scheitel des Schädels.

Histopathologie. Neben den ein- und mehrkernigen Histiozyten und den Eosinophilen findet man große xanthomatöse Zellen mit schaumigem, lipidreichem Zytoplasma, sowie, im Elektronomikroskop, Birbeck-Granula.

XXI.3 Sinus Histiozytose (Rosai und Dorfman); Histiocytose macrophagique lymphocytaire (Destombes)

Klinik. Diese vorwiegend bei jungen, oft dunkelhäutigen Menschen anzutreffende Lymphknotenkrankheit ist auch in der Orbita zu finden.

Histopathologie. Die Histopathologie zeigt teils dunkle (lymphozytäre Zellen), teils helle Zellfelder (große charakteristische Makrophagen). Sie rechtfertigen die für die Orbita zutreffendere Bezeichnung "lymphozytäre Makrophagen-Histiozytose".

PLATE 42 PLANCHE 42 TAFEL 42

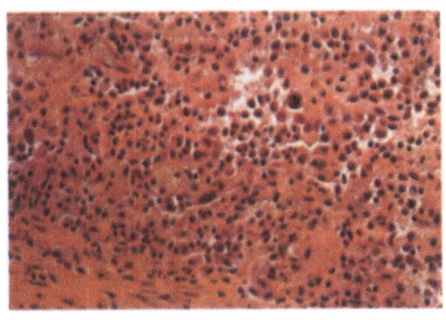

a

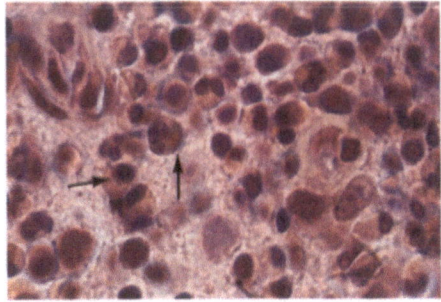

b

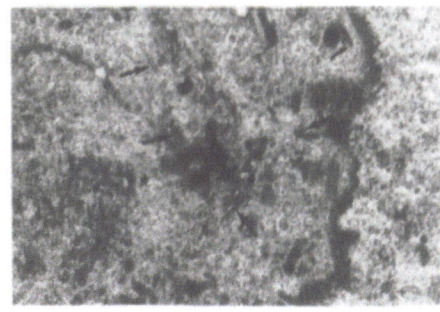

c

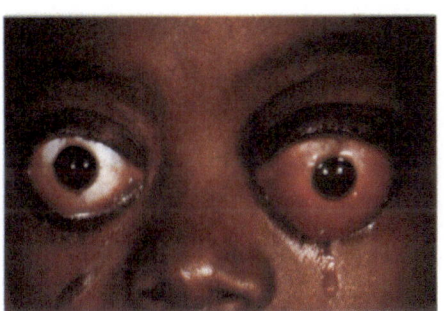

d

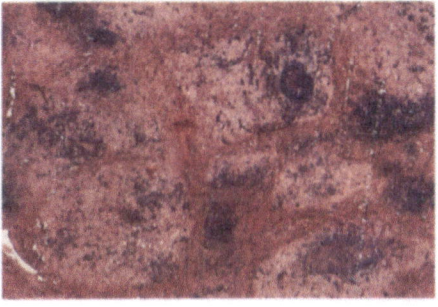

e

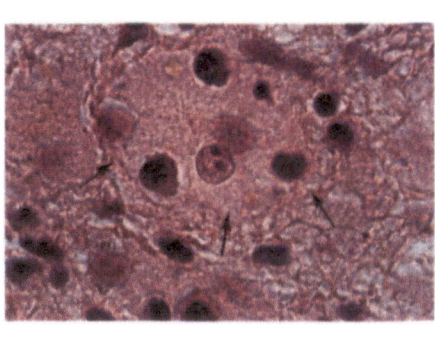

f

Fig. a. Eosinophilic granuloma of bone.
Non-homogeneous histiocytic proliferation, bearing scattered prenecrotic areas.

Fig. b. Eosinophilic granuloma of bone.
Globular histiocytic cells with a round or reniform nucleus; sometimes binuclear. Presence of many cells with eosinophilic granules (→)

Fig. c. Eosinophilic granuloma of bone (electron microscopy).
Presence of Langerhans' rods (→), 1µ long organelles having a central striated line which gives them a "zip fastener" appearance. These rods are located either within the cytoplasm or in contact with the plasmic membrane.

Fig. d. Sinus histiocytosis.
Bilateral proptosis developing rapidly in a 7-year old child, without pain or diplopia. The general state of health was good.

Fig. e. Sinus histiocytosis.
Mottled appearance of the tissue: light areas (histiocytes) alternating with dark areas (lymphocytes and plasma cells).

Fig. f. Sinus histiocytosis.
Large macrophage with a round nucleus (→) and a pale staining cytoplasm, showing vacuoles filled with intact-looking lymphocytic cells (emperopolesis).

Fig. a. Granulome éosinophile de l'os.
Prolifération histiocytaire inhomogène parsemée de plages prénécrotiques.

Fig. b. Granulome éosinophile de l'os.
Cellules histiocytaires, globuleuses à noyau arrondi ou réniforme; certaines sont binucléées. Présence de nombreuses cellules à granulations éosinophiles (→).

Fig. c. Granulome éosinophile de l'os (microscopie électronique).
Présence de bâtonnets de Langerhans (→), organelles de 1 µ de longueur parcourues par une densification linéaire centrale qui leur donne un aspect en "fermeture éclair". Ces bâtonnets sont situés soit en plein cytoplasme, soit au contact de la membrane plasmique.

Fig. d. Histiocytose macrophagique lymphocytaire.
Exophtalmie bilatérale d'évolution rapide chez un enfant de 7 ans. Il n'existait cependant ni douleurs, ni diplopie et l'état général était satisfaisant.

Fig. e. Histiocytose macrophagique lymphocytaire.
Aspect bariolé du prélèvement: plages claires (histiocytes) alternant avec les plages sombres (lymphocytes et plasmocytes).

Fig. f. Histiocytose macrophagique lymphocytaire.
Grande cellule macrophagique à noyau arrondi (→), à cytoplasme clair, creusé de vacuoles contenant des cellules lymphocytaires apparemment intactes (emperopolesis).

Abb. a. Eosinophiles Granulom des Knochens.
Nekrose- und Hämorrhagiefelder im Bereich der histiozytären Wucherung erklären die Konsistenz der Läsion.

Abb. b. Eosinophiles Granulom.
Histiozytäre, kugelige Zellen mit rundlichem oder nierenförmigem Kern; manche haben zwei Kerne. Es sind zahlreiche Zellen mit eosinophilen Granula vorhanden (→).

Abb. c. Histiozytäre Zelle eines eosinophilen Granuloms des Knochens (Elektronenmikroskopie). Langerhans-Stäbchen (→), Organellen von 1µ Länge, die eine lineare zentrale Verdichtung durchläuft und ihnen ein "reißverschlußartiges" Aussehen gibt. Diese Stäbchen liegen entweder mitten im Zytoplasma oder stehen mit der Plasmamembran in Berührung.

Abb. d. Sinus-Histiozytose.
Beidseitiger, sich schnell entwickelnder Exophthalmus bei einem 7 jährigen Kind. Es bestanden weder Schmerzen noch Diplopie, und der Allgemeinzustand war zufriedenstellend.

Abb. e. Sinus-Histiozytose.
Buntscheckiges Erscheinungsbild der Biopsie: helle Felder (Histiozyten), die sich mit dunklen Feldern (Lymphozyten und Plasmozyten) abwechseln.

Abb. f. Sinus-Histiozytose.
Großer Makrophage (→) mit rundlichem, gut mit Nukleolen besetztem Kern, hellem, granulösem Zytoplasma mit Vakuolen, die scheinbar intakte lymphozytäre Zellen enthalten (Emperopolesis).

C

Tumours of the uvea

*

Tumeurs de l'uvée

*

Geschwülste der Uvea

PLATE 43　　　　　　　　PLANCHE 43　　　　　　　　TAFEL 43

XXII. IRIS TUMOURS

XXII.1 Iris cysts

Clinical features. They are recognized on slit lamp examination with retro-illumination.

XXII.1.1 Primary cysts of the iris pigment epithelium

Originating from a separation of the anterior and posterior layers, they may bulge into the posterior chamber or prolapse through the pupil. Some cystic proliferations may break free and settle in the inferior sinus. Their differentiation from a peripheral iris tumour is usually made possible by inducing iris movements and by gonioscopy.

XXII.1.2 Secondary cystic proliferation

Except for cysts induced by miotic therapy, secondary cystic proliferatons result from post-traumatic epithelial downgrowth. These lesions grow, close to the corneal wound.

Histopathology. Cysts are lined by a stratified squamous epithelium, and are filled with a clear, mucinous or, rarely, keratinized material.

XXII.2 Iris pigmented tumours

XXII.2.1 Adenomas of the iris pigment epithelium

These exceptional tumours are difficult to differentiate clinically from melanomas and histologically from hyperplasia.

XXII.2.2 Melanocytic tumours of the iris stroma

Clinical features. They represent the commonest primary iris tumours. They occur mainly in lightly pigmented individuals and are detected earlier in life than ciliary or posterior uveal melanocytic tumours. The patients are frequently aware of a dark spot on the iris or of heterochromia.

XXII. TUMEURS IRIENNES

XXII.1 Kystes iriens

Clinique. Cliniquement ils sont identifiables à l'examen biomicroscopique en rétro-illumination.

XXII.1.1 Kystes spontanés de l'épithélium pigmentaire irien

Résultant de la séparation des couches antérieure et postérieure, ils bombent dans la chambre postérieure ou dans l'aire pupillaire. Certains peuvent se détacher vers le sinus inférieur et doivent être distingués d'une tumeur irienne par la mobilisation et à la gonioscopie.

XXII.1.2 Proliférations secondaires kystiques

La cause principale, mis à part les myotiques forts, est l'invasion épithéliale post-traumatique.

Histopathologie. Ces lésions situées, en regard de la plaie cornéenne, sont revêtues d'un épithélium malpighien stratifié. Le contenu peut être clair, mucineux, exceptionnellement kératinisé.

XXII.2 Tumeurs pigmentées de l'iris

XXII.2.1 Adénomes de l'épithélium pigmentaire irien

Ces tumeurs, exceptionnelles, sont difficiles à distinguer des mélanomes cliniquement et des hyperplasies, histologiquement.

XXII.2.2 Tumeurs mélaniques du stroma irien

Clinique. Ce sont les plus fréquentes des tumeurs iriennes. Elles surviennent surtout chez les sujets à teint clair et sont décelées plus tôt dans la vie que les tumeurs ciliochoroïdiennes. Les patients signalent une tache sombre sur l'iris ou une hétérochromie.

XXII. TUMOREN DER REGENBOGENHAUT

XXII.1 Iriszysten

Klinik. Klinisch sind sie mit der Spaltlampe bei retrograder Beleuchtung zu erkennen.

XXII.1.1 Spontane Zysten des Pigmentepithels der Iris

Sie entstehen durch die Trennung der vorderen von der hinteren Schicht und wölben sich bauchig in die Hinterkammer oder im Pupillarbereich vor. Manche können sich zum unteren Kammerwinkel hin ablösen und müssen von einem eigentlichen Iristumor durch ihre Beweglichkeit sowie gonioskopisch unterschieden werden.

XXII.1.2 Sekundäre Zysten

Die Hauptursache, von einer Behandlung mit starken Miotika abgesehen, ist die Epitheleinwachsung nach einer Verletzung. Sie liegen, gegenüber der Hornhautwunde.

Histopathologie. Histopathologisch sind sie mit einem mehrschichtigen Plattenepithel ausgekleidet. Der Inhalt kann hell, schleimig sein, in Ausnahmefällen aus Hornmassen bestehen.

XXII.2 Pigmentierte Tumoren der Iris

XXII.2.1 Adenom des Pigmentepithels der Iris

Diese äußerst seltenen Tumoren sind klinisch schwer von Melanomen, histologisch schwer von Hyperplasien zu unterscheiden.

XXII.2.2 Melanotische Tumoren des Irisstromas

Klinik. Es sind die häufigsten Geschwülste der Regenbogenhaut. Sie treten vor allem bei hellhäutigen Menschen auf und werden frühzeitiger als die cilio-choroidalen Tumoren erkannt. Die Patienten weisen einen dunklen Fleck auf der Iris oder eine Heterochromie auf.

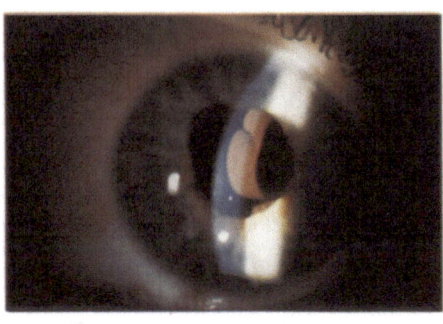

a

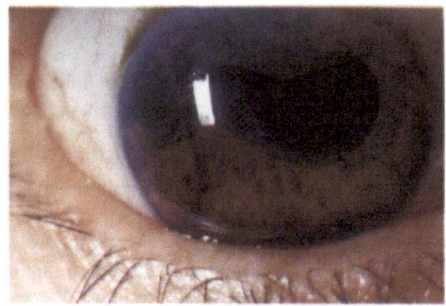

b

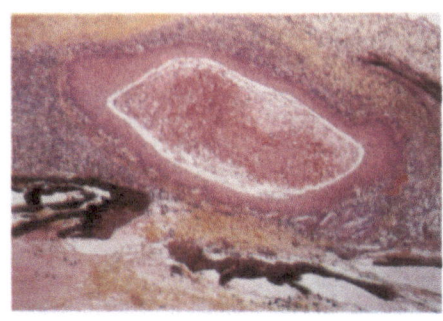

c

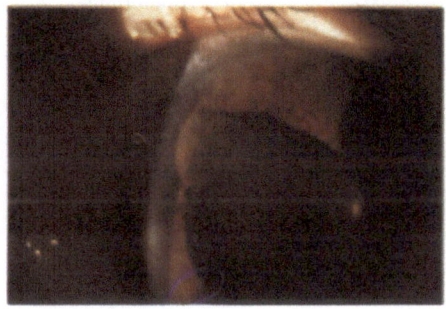

d

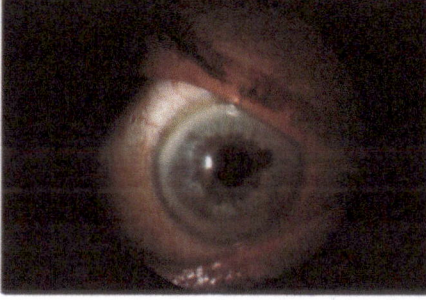

e

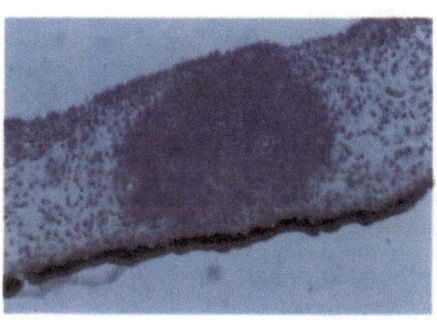

f

Fig. a. Large cyst of iris pigment epithelium occurring at the pupillary margin.

Fig. b. Anterior segment photograph of cystic epithelial downgrowth in an aphakic eye.

Fig. c. Micrography: epithelial downgrowth following trauma.
The cyst is lined by stratified squamous epithelium. The lumen is filled with desquamated epithelial cells.

Fig. d. Anterior segment photograph.
Adenoma of the iris pigment epithelium: mottled appearance of the tumour near the sphincter.

Fig. e. Anterior segment photograph.
Pigmented iris naevus near pupillary margin with ectropion iridis.

Fig. f. Micrographic section of spindle cell iris naevus extending to the anterior surface of the iris. The cells are spindle-shaped, compact and cohesive.

Fig. a. Volumineux kyste de l'épithélium pigmentaire irien au niveau du rebord pupillaire.

Fig. b. Photographie du segment antérieur montrant une invasion épithéliale kystique survenant dans un oeil aphaque.

Fig. c. Micrographie: invasion épithéliale posttraumatique.
Le kyste est bordé d'un épithélium malpighien stratifié. La lumière contient des cellules épithéliales desquamées.

Fig. d. Photographie du segment antérieur.
Adénome de l'épithélium pigmentaire irien: aspect en mottes de la tumeur près du sphincter.

Fig. e. Photographie du segment antérieur.
Naevus irien pigmenté près du bord pupillaire avec ectropion uvéal.

Fig. f. Micrographie d'un naevus irien à cellules fusiformes s'étendant jusqu'à la surface antérieure de l'iris. Les cellules sont fusiformes, compactes et cohésives.

Abb. a. Umfangreiche Zyste des Iris-Pigmentepithels am Pupillenrand.

Abb. b. Photographie des vorderen Segments, die eine zystische Epithelinvasion in einem aphaken Auge zeigt.

Abb. c. Mikrophotographie: Posttraumatische Epithelinvasion.
Die Zyste ist von einem mehrschichtigen Plattenepithel eingefaßt. Das Lumen enthält abgeschilferte Epithelzellen.

Abb. d. Photographie des vorderen Segments.
Adenom des Pigmentepithels der Iris: feinscholliger Aspekt des Tumors in der Nähe des Sphinkters.

Abb. e. Photographie des vorderen Segments.
Pigmentierter Irisnaevus in Pupillenrandnähe mit Ectropium uvae.

Abb. f. Mikrophotographie eines Irisnaevus mit Spindelzellen, der sich bis zur Irisvorderfläche ausdehnt. Die Zellen sind spindelförmig, kompakt und liegen eng beieinander.

93

PLATE 44   PLANCHE 44   TAFEL 44

Clinical features (continued)

In *neurofibromatosis*, Lisch nodules, composed of a proliferation of melanocytic cells, are very common (94%) and sometimes helpful in establishing the diagnosis. They do not differ clinically and pathologically from naevi.

The favourable prognosis of iris melanocytic tumours has long been noted. Recent clinicopathologic reappraisal of these lesions has shown that:
- 90% of tumours previously diagnosed as melanomas are actually *naevi*;
- very few clinical features indicate the malignant nature of the lesion. Ectropion iridis, sector cataract, hyphema, necrosis are no longer considered as suggesting a malignant transformation. The only significant features, which should be looked for, are unilateral elevated intraocular pressure, rapid growth, high vascularity, ring involvement, ciliary body involvement;
- some cytologically benign lesions may tend to local invasiveness and secondary glaucoma, leading to the anatomical or functional loss of the eye;
- metastases from iris melanomas are exceptional and long delayed.

Current histopathologic classification includes:
- melanocytosis
  (Plate 49, Chapter XXIV.1.3);
- melanocytomas
  (Plate 47, Chapter XXIII.2.1 and Plate 63, Chapter XXX);
- naevi (5 types) composed of either or all of the following: epithelioïd cells, spindle cells, arranged into nests or fascicles, with or without surface plaque proliferation;
- melanomas; spindle, epithelioid or mixed types.

A conservative approach is now advocated for these tumours.

Clinique (suite)

Dans la *neurofibromatose*, les nodules de Lisch, composés d'une prolifération de cellules mélanocytiques, sont très fréquents (94%) et parfois utiles au diagnostic. Ils ne diffèrent pas cliniquement et histologiquement des naevi.

Le bon pronostic des tumeurs pigmentées iriennes est une notion classique. Récemment, la réévaluation clinico-pathologique de ces tumeurs a montré que:
- 90% des tumeurs autrefois appelées mélanomes sont des *naevi*;
- très peu de critères cliniques peuvent indiquer la malignité d'une lésion. Ectropion uvéal, cataracte en secteur, hyphéma, nécrose, ne sont plus considérés comme suggestifs de malignité. Seules une élévation unilatérale de pression intra-oculaire, une croissance rapide, une vascularisation abondante, une atteinte annulaire et/ou du corps ciliaire sont des éléments de suspicion et doivent être recherchés;
- certaines lésions cytologiquement bénignes peuvent pourtant entraîner un envahissement local, un glaucome secondaire et entraîner la perte anatomo-fonctionnelle d'un oeil;
- les métastases de mélanomes iriens sont exceptionnelles et très tardives.

La classification histologique actuelle comprend:
- mélanocytose
  (Planche 49, Chapitre XXIV.1.3);
- mélanocytomes
  (Planche 47, Chapitre XXIII.2.1 et Planche 63, Chapitre XXX);
- naevi (5 types) composés de cellules "épithélioïdes" et/ou fusiformes, arrangées en thèques ou faisceaux, avec ou sans prolifération en plaque à la face antérieure;
- mélanomes, fusiformes, épithélioïdes ou mixtes.

Une attitude conservatrice prolongée est aujourd'hui la règle face à ces tumeurs.

Klinik (Fortsetzung)

Bei der *Neurofibromatose* treten sehr häufig Lisch-Knötchen auf (94%), die durch eine Proliferation von Melanozyten zustande kommen und manchmal diagnostisch von Nutzen sein können. Sie unterscheiden sich weder klinisch noch histologisch von melanocytären Naevi.

Die günstige Prognose der pigmentierten Iristumoren ist allgemein bekannt. Eine klinisch-pathologische Neubewertung dieser Tumoren hat kürzlich ergeben, daß:
- 90% der früher Melanome benannten Tumoren *Naevi* sind;
- sehr wenige klinische Kriterien als Hinweis für die Bösartigkeit einer Läsion gelten können. Ectropium uveae, sektorenförmiger Katarakt, Hyphäma, Nekrose werden nicht mehr als Hinweise für Bösartigkeit betrachtet. Nur ein einseitiges Ansteigen des inneren Augendrucks, ein schnelles Wachstum, eine starke Vaskularisierung, eine ringförmige Ausbreitung im Kammerwinkel und/oder in den Ciliarkörper hinein sind malignitätsverdächtige Zeichen, nach denen speziell zu forschen ist;
- gewisse zytologisch gutartige Läsionen können jedoch eine lokale Ausbreitung, ein Sekundärglaukom und den anatomisch-funktionellen Verlust eines Auges zur Folge haben;
- Metastasen von Irismelanomen treten nur ausnahmsweise und dann sehr spät auf.

Die gegenwärtige histologische Klassifizierung beinhaltet:
- Melanozytose
  (Tafel 49, Kapitel XXIV.1.3);
- Melanozytome
  (Tafel 47, Kapitel XXIII.2.1 und Tafel 63, Kapitel XXX);
- Naevi (5 Typen), bestehend aus "Epitheloid-" und/oder Spindelzellen (eventuell gemischt), die nest- oder bündelförmig angeordnet sind, mit oder ohne oberflächlichem Überzug;
- Melanome: spindelförmig, epitheloid oder gemischt.

Eine langfristige konservative Haltung ist heute angesichts solcher Geschwülste die Regel.

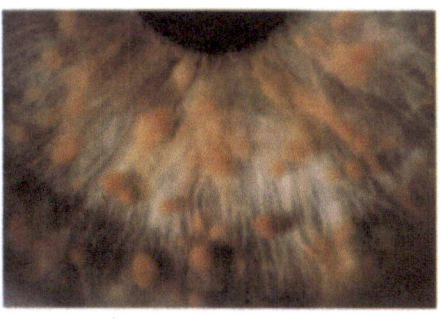

a

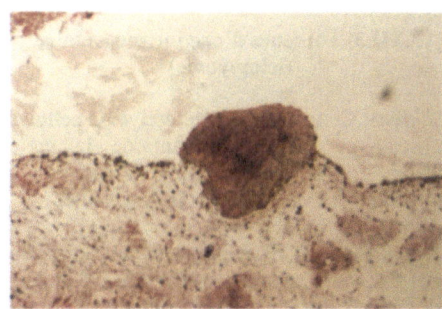

b

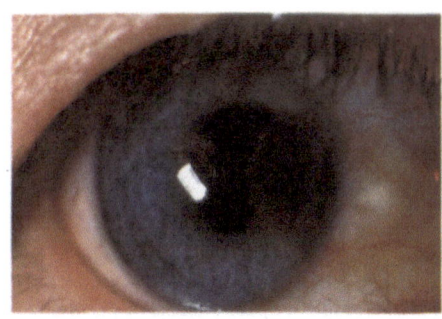

c

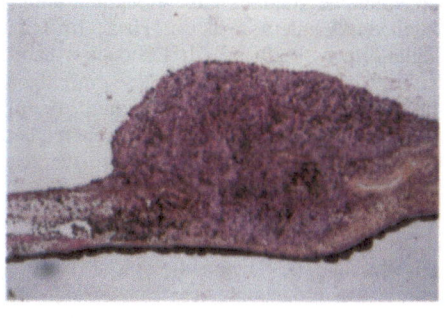

d

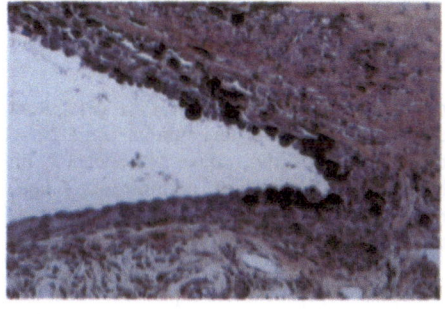

e

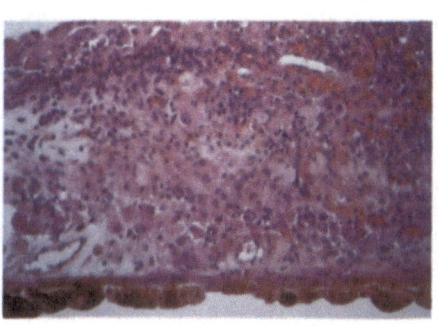

f

Fig. a. Lisch iris nodules in patient with neurofibromatosis.

Fig. b. Lisch nodule of neurofibromatosis.
Iris nodule composed of spindle-shaped naevus cells.

Fig. c. Clinical appearance of a large pigmented iris melanoma.

Fig. d. Histopathological section of pigmented iris melanoma.
The tumour involves all the iris stroma and extends along iris anterior surface, where cell cohesion is reduced.

Fig. e. Continued.
The tumour invades the anterior chamber angle and the ciliary body. Pigment-laden macrophages are present.

Fig. f. Continued.
The tumour is composed of large and smaller epithelioid cells with prominent nucleoli.

Fig. a. Nodules iriens de Lisch chez un patient atteint de neurofibromatose.

Fig. b. Nodules iriens de Lisch dans la neurofibromatose.
Les nodules iriens sont composés de cellules naeviques fusiformes.

Fig. c. Aspect clinique d'un volumineux mélanome irien pigmenté.

Fig. d. Aspect histopathologique d'un mélanome irien pigmenté.
La tumeur envahit toute l'épaisseur du stroma irien et s'étend jusqu'à la surface antérieure où la cohésion des cellules diminue.

Fig. e. Même cas.
La tumeur envahit l'angle camérulaire et le corps ciliaire. On note la présence de mélanophages.

Fig. f. Même cas.
La tumeur est composée de cellules épithélioïdes de taille variable avec des nucléoles bien visibles.

Abb. a. Lisch-Knötchen der Iris bei einem an Neurofibromatose erkrankten Patienten.

Abb. b. Lisch-Knötchen der Iris bei Neurofibromatose.
Die Irisknötchen setzen sich aus spindelförmigen Naevuszellen zusammen.

Abb. c. Klinischer Aspekt eines voluminösen pigmentierten Irismelanoms.

Abb. d. Histopathologischer Aspekt eines pigmentierten Irismelanoms.
Die Geschwulst dringt in die gesamte Dicke des Irisstromas ein und dehnt sich bis zur vorderen Oberfläche aus, wo der Zusammenhalt der Zellen abnimmt.

Abb. e. Derselbe Fall.
Der Tumor dringt in die Kammerbucht und in den Ziliarkörper ein. Auffällig ist das Vorhandensein von Melanophagen.

Abb. f. Derselbe Fall.
Der Tumor besteht aus epitheloiden Zellen unterschiedlicher Größe mit deutlich sichtbaren Nukleolen.

PLATE 45 PLANCHE 45 TAFEL 45

XXII.3 Iris myogenic tumours (leiomyoma)

Clinical features. This rare tumour arises from neural-crest-derived smooth muscle cells. It appears clinically as a slow-growing, slightly prominent, grayish-white nodule.

Histopathology. Classical histopathologic features are the abundance of fibrillary cell processes and the spindle-shape of the interlacing cells. Electron microscopic demonstration of cytoplasmic myofibrils, basement membrane production and plasmalemmal vesicles is sometimes necessary to rule out an amelanotic spindle-cell melanoma or a neurogenic tumour.

XXII.4 Juvenile xanthogranuloma

This lesion is a chronic granulomatous inflammatory reaction affecting young children. The most frequently involved sites are the skin, the iris and the ciliary body.

Clinical features. Iris lesions usually appear as unilateral, nodular or diffuse tumours, often associated with spontaneous hyphema. They may induce severe ocular complications such as repeated haemorrhage and secondary glaucoma.

Histopathology. The lesion is characterized by a chronic granulomatous inflammation with multinucleated giant cells of the Touton variety. Abundant vascularity with thin-walled, dilated, blood vessels may be confusing. Extensive bleeding may result from biopsy. Yet, diagnosis must be established clinically or through biopsy of an extra-ocular lesion, to allow the introduction of corticosteroids with, often, good results.

XXII.5 Metastases to the iris

Metastases to the iris, although rare, may reveal a carcinoma, usually from the lung or breast. Iris involvement may present clinically as a solitary nodule, iridocyclitis, hyphaema, or secondary glaucoma. Paracentesis is sometimes useful to allow a cytological diagnosis.

XXII.3 Tumeurs d'origine musculaire (leiomyome)

Clinique. Cette tumeur rare, dérive de cellules musculaires lisses provenant de la crête neurale. Elle se présente cliniquement comme un nodule peu saillant, à croissance lente.

Histopathologie. Histologiquement les critères sont l'abondance de prolongements cellulaires fibrillaires et la forme fusiforme des cellules entrelacées. Cependant la démonstration ultrastructurale de myofibrilles cytoplasmiques, de formation de membrane basale, de vésicules plasmalemmales est parfois nécessaire pour éliminer une tumeur mélanocytique non pigmentée, une tumeur neurogénique.

XXII.4 Xanthogranulome juvénile

Cette lésion est une réaction inflammatoire chronique granulomateuse touchant les jeunes enfants, le plus souvent au niveau cutané, irien, ou ciliaire.

Clinique. Les lésions iriennes se présentent cliniquement comme une tumeur unilatérale, nodulaire ou diffuse, souvent associée à un hyphéma spontané. Des complications oculaires sévères sont possibles: hémorragies récidivantes, glaucome secondaire...

Histopathologie. Histologiquement une inflammation chronique granulomateuse avec cellules géantes de type Touton est typique. L'abondance des vaisseaux dilatés, à paroi fine, peut être trompeuse. Les biopsies iriennes peuvent se compliquer d'hémorragies. Cependant le diagnostic doit être établi cliniquement ou par biopsie d'une lésion extra-oculaire pour permettre une corticothérapie souvent efficace.

XXII.5 Métastases iriennes

Quoique rares, elles peuvent être révélatrices d'un carcinome, généralement mammaire ou pulmonaire, sous l'aspect clinique d'un nodule irien, d'une irido-cyclite, d'un hyphéma, d'un glaucome secondaire. La paracentèse peut parfois permettre un diagnostic cytologique.

XXII.3 Myogene Tumoren (Leiomyom)

Klinik. Dieser seltene Tumor stammt von den glatten Muskelzellen ab, die sich von der Neuralleiste ableiten. Klinisch hat er die Form eines wenig vorstehenden, langsam wachsenden Knötchens.

Histopathologie. Die histopathologischen Kriterien sind ein Reichtum an Fibrillärzellprozessen und die Spindelform der umschlungenen Zellen. Manchmal ist jedoch der ultrastrukturelle Nachweis von cytoplasmatischen Myofibrillen, einer Basalmembran, von plasmolemmalen Bläschen notwendig, um eine nicht pigmentierte Melanozytengeschwulst oder eine neurogene Geschwulst auszuschließen.

XXII.4 Juveniles Xanthogranulom

Klinik. Diese Läsion ist eine chronische entzündliche granulomatöse Reaktion, die bei kleineren Kindern meist in Haut, Iris oder Ziliarkörper auftritt. Irisläsionen haben *klinisch* die Form eines einseitigen, knötchenartigen oder diffusen Tumors, der oft mit einem spontanen Hyphäma einhergeht. Schwerwiegende Komplikationen für das Auge sind möglich: wiederholte Blutungen, Sekundärglaukom...

Histopathologie. Histopathologisch ist eine chronische granulomatöse Entzündung mit Riesenzellen vom Typ Touton charakteristisch. Die Vielzahl erweiterter, feinwändiger Gefäße kann irreführen. Irisbiopsien können Komplikationen durch Blutungen hervorrufen. Die Diagnose ist jedoch klinisch oder durch Hautbiopsie zu stellen, damit die oft wirksame Kortikotherapie eingeleitet werden kann.

XXII.5 Iris Metastasen

Sie sind zwar selten, können aber in Form eines Irisknötchens, einer Iridozyklitis, eines Hyphämas, eines Sekundärglaukoms ein metastasierendes Carcinom, der Mamma oder der Lunge, entdecken lassen. Die Vorderkammerpunktion ermöglicht manchmal eine zytologische Diagnose.

PLATE 45   PLANCHE 45   TAFEL 45

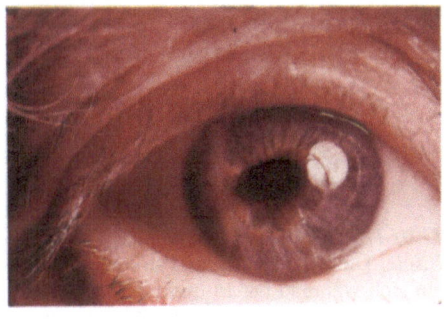

a

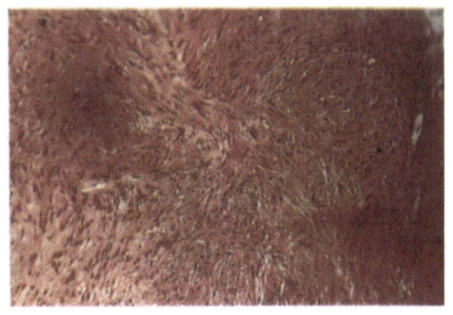

b

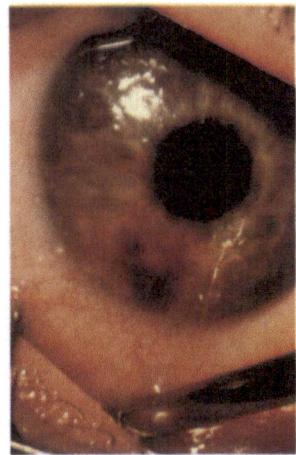

c

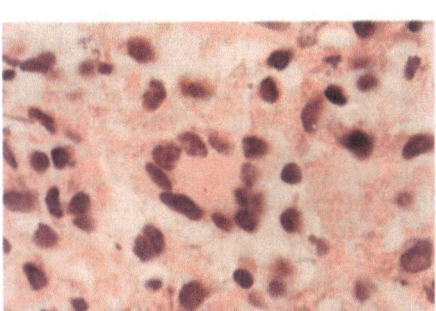

d

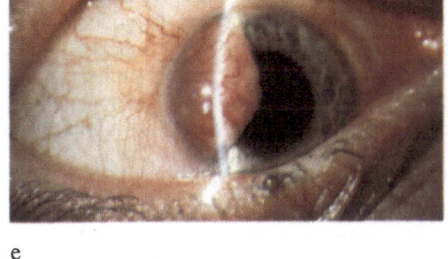

e

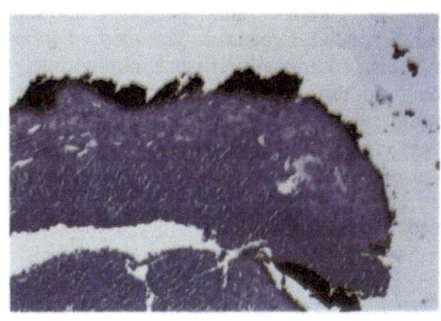

f

Fig. a. Iris Leiomyoma: clinical appearance.
Note pupillary irregularity and ectropion iridis.

Fig. b. Iris Leiomyoma: histopathology.
Histopathologic features include interlacing bundles of uniform, non-pigmented spindle-shaped cells with abundant fibrillary processes.

Fig. c. Anterior segment photograph: showing juvenile xanthogranuloma of iris presenting as a large localized iris nodule.

Fig. d. Histopathological features of juvenile xanthogranuloma of iris.
Chronic granulomatous inflammation with multinucleated giant cell of the Touton variety.

Fig. e. Metastasis to the iris.
Anterior segment photograph showing a large, non-pigmented iris tumour with prominent vascularity.

Fig. f. Histopathology (same patient).
The iris stroma is invaded by metastatic undifferentiated carcinoma. The primary was not found.

Fig. a. Leiomyome irien: aspect clinique.
Noter la déformation pupillaire et l'ectropion uvéal.

Fig. b. Leiomyome irien: histopathologie.
Aspect histopathologique montrant des faisceaux entrecroisés composés de cellules fusiformes non pigmentées de type uniforme avec d'abondants prolongements cellulaires fibrillaires.

Fig. c. Photographie de segment antérieur: xanthogranulome juvénile irien se présentant comme un volumineux nodule irien localisé.

Fig. d. Aspect histopathologique d'un xanthogranulome juvénile de l'iris.
Inflammation chronique granulomateuse avec cellule géante multinucléée de type Touton.

Fig. e. Métastase irienne.
Photographie du segment antérieur montrant une importante tumeur irienne très vascularisée.

Fig. f. Histopathologie (de la même tumeur).
Le stroma irien est envahi par un carcinome métastatique indifférencié. La tumeur primitive n'a pas été retrouvée.

Abb. a. Leiomyom der Iris: Klinischer Aspekt.
Zu beachten ist die verformte Pupille und das Ectropium uveae.

Abb. b. Leiomyom der Iris: Histopathologie.
Histopathologischer Aspekt: verschlungene Bündel nicht pigmentierter Spindelzellen von einheitlichem Typ mit einer Fülle von Fibrillarzellverlängerungen.

Abb. c. Photographie des vorderen Segments: Juveniles Xanthogranulom der Iris, das wie ein voluminös lokalisiertes Irisknötchen in Erscheinung tritt.

Abb. d. Histopathologischer Aspekt eines juvenilen Xanthogranuloms der Iris.
Chronische granulomatöse Entzündung mit multinukleärer Touton-Riesenzelle.

Abb. e. Iris-Metastase.
Photographie des vorderen Segments, die einen stark vaskularisierten, umfangreichen Iristumor aufzeigt.

Abb. f. Histopathologie (desselben Tumors).
Das Irisstroma ist von einem undifferenzierten, metastatischen Karzinom durchdrungen. Der Primärtumor wurde nicht aufgefunden.

97

PLATE 46   PLANCHE 46   TAFEL 46

XXIII. TUMOURS OF CILIARY BODY

XXIII.1 Epithelial tumours

XXIII.1.1 Tumours of non-pigmented epithelium

XXIII.1.1a Medullo-epitheliomas (diktyomas)
Clinical features. These congenital tumours arise during embryonic development from the immature medullary epithelium. They usually present, around 4 to 7 years, as a small mass or as multiple cysts in the iris or ciliary body. Unilateral poor vision, pain or leukocoria are the most common symptoms. Glaucoma is often associated.

Histopathology. The *non-teratoid form* is characteristically composed of sheets of poorly differentiated neuro-epithelial cells forming uni or multilayered tubules or papillae. These sheets are polarized, i.e. producing primary vitreous and external limiting membrane-like structures. The *teratoid form* contains, additionally, tissues not normally found in this location e.g.: cerebral tissue, hyaline cartilage, skeletal muscle. In both types criteria for malignancy include: production of poorly differentiated cells resembling retinoblasts, numerous mitotic figures, pleomorphism, invasion of the uvea, extraocular extension. The mortality rate is 10%.

XXIII.1.1b Adult-type tumours
Except for Fuchs' "adenoma", i.e. the hyperplastic lesion commonly seen in the elderly, these tumours comprise adenomas and adenocarcinomas, composed of a variably pigmented proliferation of cuboidal and columnar cells forming a papillary or tubular pattern. The last four criteria for malignancy described above are relevant here.

XXIII.1.2 Tumours of the ciliary pigment epithelium

Except for the presence of pigment granules, these tumours do not differ from the previous ones. Cytoplasmic vacuoles containing neuraminidase-sensitive sialomucin may be present, helping to differentiate these tumours from metastatic adenocarcinomas. In none of these tumours, even the cytologically malignant varieties, was there evidence of extra-ocular extension.

XXIII. TUMEURS DU CORPS CILIAIRE

XXIII.1 Tumeurs épithéliales

XXIII.1.1 Tumeurs de l'épithélium non pigmenté

XXIII.1.1a Médullo-épithéliomes (diktyomes)
Aspects cliniques. Ces tumeurs congénitales se développent pendant la vie embryonnaire à partir de l'épithélium médullaire immature. Elles apparaissent vers 4 à 7 ans, comme une petite masse ou des kystes multiples de l'iris ou du corps ciliaire. Amblyopie unilatérale, douleur ou leucocorie sont les signes les plus fréquents. Un glaucome est souvent associé.

Histopathologie. Dans la *forme non tératoïde* des travées de cellules neuro-épithéliales peu différenciées forment des tubules ou des papilles, uni- ou multistratifiées. L'élaboration de vitré primitif et de membrane limitante externe traduit la polarisation. Dans la *forme tératoïde* d'autres tissus, anormaux dans le corps ciliaire, sont associés: cérébral, cartilagineux, musculaire. Dans les deux formes les critères de malignité sont: la production de cellules indifférenciées, proches de rétinoblastes, l'abondance de mitoses, le pléomorphisme, l'invasion du stroma uvéal, l'extériorisation. 10% des cas sont mortels.

XXIII.1.1b Tumeurs de type adulte
Mis à part le banal "adénome" de Fuchs, traduisant une hyperplasie chez le sujet âgé, il s'agit d'adénomes et d'adénocarcinomes, composés de cellules cuboïdes ou cylindriques agencées en papilles ou tubules, de pigmentation variable. Les quatre derniers critères de malignité décrits ci-dessus sont applicables ici.

XXIII.1.2 Tumeurs de l'épithélium pigmenté ciliaire

Ces tumeurs, mise à part l'abondance de granules pigmentaires, sont analogues aux précédentes. Des vacuoles cytoplasmiques contiennent une sialomucine sensible à la neuraminidase, ce qui facilite la distinction entre adénocarcinomes primitifs et métastatiques. Aucune extension extra-oculaire n'a été observée, même dans les formes cytologiquement malignes.

XXIII. TUMOREN DES ZILIARKÖRPERS

XXIII.1 Epitheliale Geschwülste

XXIII.1.1 Tumoren des nichtpigmentierten Ziliarepithels

XXIII.1.1a Medullo-Epitheliome (Diktyome)
Klinik. Diese kongenitalen Tumoren entwickeln sich während der Embryonalzeit aus dem unreifen Epithel. Sie treten im Alter von etwa 4 bis 7 Jahren als kleine Neubildung oder multiple Zysten der Iris oder des Ziliarkörpers in Erscheinung. Einseitige Amblyopie, Schmerz oder Leukokorie sind die häufigsten Symptome, oft mit einem Glaukom vergesellschaftet.

Histopathologie. Histopathologisch bilden in der *nicht teratoiden Form* die Zellzüge wenig differenzierter neuroepitheler Zellen ein- oder mehrschichtige Kanälchen oder Stränge. Die Bildung eines primitiven Glaskörpers und einer Membrana limitans externa zeigt, wie gegensätzlich die Gewebsdifferenzierung erfolgen kann. In der *teratoiden Form* findet man zusätzlich dem Ziliarkörper fremdes Gehirn-, Knorpel-, oder Muskelgewebe. Bei beiden Formen gelten als Kriterien für Bösartigkeit: die Bildung undifferenzierter Zellen, ähnlich den Retinoblasten, gehäufte Mitosen, Polymorphie, Infiltration des uvealen Stromas, Auswachsen aus dem Ziliarkörper heraus. 10% der Fälle verlaufen tödlich.

XXIII.1.1b Adulte Tumoren
Abgesehen vom banalen Fuchsschen "Adenom", das eine Epithelhyperplasie beim älteren Menschen darstellt, handelt es sich um Adenome oder Adenokarzinome, die aus kuboiden oder zylindrischen, papillen- oder kanälchenförmig angeordneten Zellen mit unterschiedlicher Pigmentierung bestehen. Die oben beschriebenen vier letzteren Bösartigkeitskriterien gelten auch hier.

XXIII.1.2 Tumoren des pigmentierten Ziliarepithels

Diese Geschwülste sind, abgesehen von den sehr zahlreich auftretenden Pigmentgranula, den vorausgegangenen analog. Die Zytoplasmavakuolen enthalten ein auf Neuraminidase empfindlich reagierendes Sialomuzin, was die Unterscheidung zwischen Primär- und Metastasenadenokarzinomen erleichtert. Bei den zytologisch bösartigen Formen wurde keinerlei Ausbreitung außerhalb des Auges beobachtet.

PLATE 46 PLANCHE 46 TAFEL 46

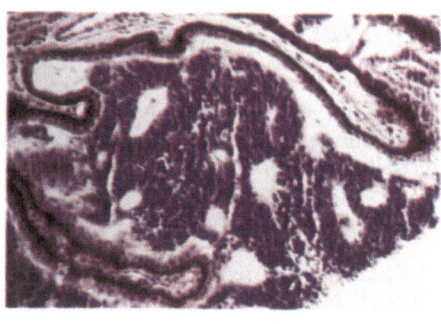

a

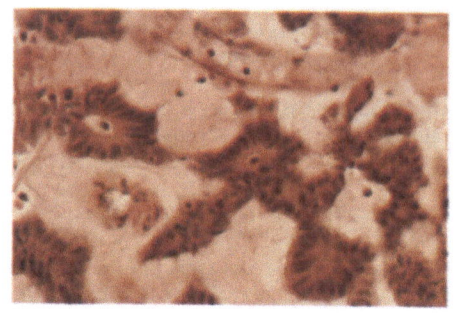

b

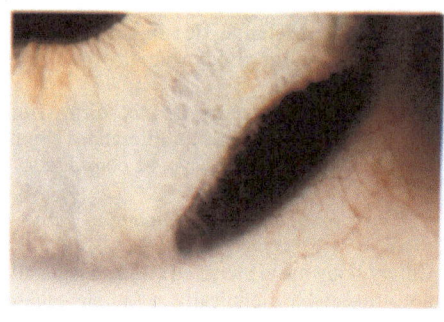

c

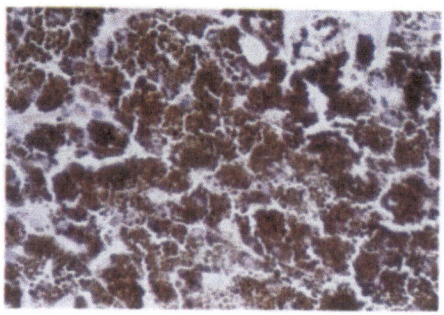

d

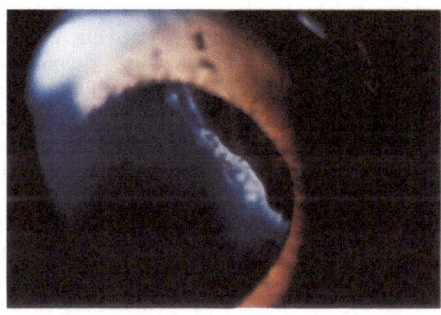

e

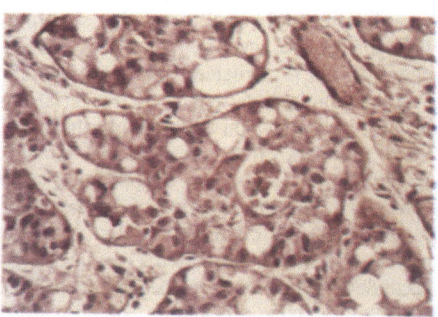

f

Fig. a. Diktyoma: histopathology.
Ciliary body tumour with intricate ribbons of cylindric cells enclosing lumina of various shapes.

Fig. b. Diktyoma: histopathology, showing within an amorphous stroma, a rosette-like arrangement of tumour cells.

Fig. c. Clinical aspect of an adenoma of the ciliary body pigment epithelium.
The tumour, growing into the anterior chamber angle, is heavily pigmented.

Fig. d. Histopathology (same tumour).
The tumour is composed of polyhedral cells with a heavy content of large pigment granules; some cells are vacuolated (containing a hyaluronidase-sensitive sialomucin).

Fig. e. Clinical aspect of pigmented ciliary body adenocarcinoma.

Fig. f. Histopathological features of ciliary body "adenocarcinoma" (bleached section): numerous vacuoles and cellular atypia.

Fig. a. Diktyome: histopathologie.
Tumeur du corps ciliaire avec des rubans de cellules cylindriques hautes entourant des espaces de forme variable.

Fig. b. Diktyome: histopathologie. Au sein d'un stroma amorphe, disposition en rosettes des cellules tumorales.

Fig. c. Aspect clinique d'un adénome de l'épithélium pigmentaire ciliaire.
La tumeur, très pigmentée, pénètre dans la chambre antérieure au niveau de l'angle camérulaire.

Fig. d. Histopathologie (de la même tumeur).
Cellules polyédriques fortement chargées en larges granules pigmentaires. Certaines cellules sont vacuolisées (contenant une sialomucine sensible à l'hyaluronidase).

Fig. e. Aspect clinique d'un adénocarcinome pigmenté du corps ciliaire.

Fig. f. Aspect histopathologique d'un adénocarcinome du corps ciliaire (coupe dépigmentée): nombreuses vacuoles, atypies cellulaires.

Abb. a. Diktyom: Histopathologie.
Tumor des Ziliarkörpers mit Streifen hoher Zylinderzellen, die unterschiedlich geformte Zwischenräume umschlingen.

Abb. b. Diktyom: Histopathologie. In einem amorphen Stroma sind die Tumorzellen rosettenförmig angeordnet.

Abb. c. Klinischer Aspekt eines Adenoms des Ziliarpigmentepithels.
Der stark pigmentierte Tumor dringt auf der Höhe der Kammerbucht in die vordere Kammer ein.

Abb. d. Histopathologie (desselben Tumors).
Stark mit pigmentierten, breiten Granula beladene polyedrische Zellen. In manchen Zellen befinden sich Vakuolen (die ein auf Hyaluronidase empfindliches Sialomuzin enthalten).

Abb. e. Klinischer Aspekt eines pigmentierten Adenokarzinoms des Ziliarkörpers.

Abb. f. Histopathologischer Aspekt eines Adenokarzinoms des Ziliarkörpers (depigmentierter Schnitt): zahlreiche Vakuolen, atypische Zellen.

PLATE 47 PLANCHE 47 TAFEL 47

XXIII.2 Melanocytic tumours of the ciliary body stroma

Most of these tumours do not differ from other uveal melanocytic proliferations. Some unique features will however be considered.

XXIII.2.1 Benign tumours

Ciliary body naevi are rare (2%) and generally not detectable clinically. Among these, melanocytomas (magnocellular naevi), although rare, are of interest owing to their reported tendency to undergo necrosis, spontaneously or following trauma. Subsequent pigment migration can induce secondary glaucoma.

XXIII.2.2 Ciliary body melanomas

Clinical features. These tumours are often diagnosed late, when they extend centrally, inducing lens displacement, deformity or opacification and visual loss. Other signs may be episcleral and conjunctival vascular engorgement or unilateral relative hypotony. A transillumination defect on the sclera is usually noticed when illuminating the pupil. These tumours often spread to the iris root, inducing an apparent iridodialysis, and secondarily to the anterior chamber. Some tumours extend circumferentially i.e.: ring melanomas which are often complicated by secondary glaucoma. Gonioscopy reveals an irregular nodular thickening of the angle elements. Increased intra-ocular pressure may result from 1) infiltration of aqueous outflow structures, 2) anterior displacement of the iris root and angle closure, 3) trabecular blockade by tumour cells carried by the aqueous circulation, 4) macrophages containing phagocytized tumour necrotic debris i.e. melanomalytic glaucoma. Extra-ocular extension, which may be detected clinically as an episcleral nodule, must be distinguished from a conjunctival melanoma, melanocytosis, scleral thinning, haematoma or cellular blue naevus.
These tumours share the *pathologic features* of choroidal melanomas, as do the *metastatic tumours* (Chapter XXIV.1.4, Plates 50–52).

XXIII.2 Tumeurs mélaniques du stroma ciliaire

Beaucoup de ces tumeurs sont semblables aux autres tumeurs mélanocytiques uvéales. Certains cas particuliers seront envisagés ici.

XXIII.2.1 Tumeurs bénignes

Les naevi ciliaires sont rares (2%) et rarement vus cliniquement. Parmi ceux-ci les mélanocytomes (naevi magnocellulaires) quoique rares, sont dignes d'intérêt du fait de leur tendance à la nécrose spontanée ou post-traumatique. La migration pigmentaire secondaire peut provoquer un glaucome.

XXIII.2.2 Mélanomes

Cliniquement ces tumeurs sont souvent décelées tard, lorsque leur extension vers le centre provoque une déformation, un déplacement ou des opacités cristalliniennes, et une baisse de vision. D'autres symptômes peuvent être une dilatation vasculaire conjonctivale et épisclérale, une hypotonie unilatérale. Un défaut de transillumination sclérale est généralement noté en éclairant la pupille. Ces tumeurs s'étendent souvent à la racine de l'iris, peuvent provoquer une apparente iridodialyse, et pénètrent secondairement dans la chambre antérieure. Certaines tumeurs, appelées mélanomes annulaires, sont circonférencielles et souvent compliquées de glaucome secondaire. La gonioscopie révèle alors un épaississement irrégulier et nodulaire des structures de l'angle. Une hypertonie peut traduire une infiltration tumorale des émonctoires, un déplacement de la racine irienne avec fermeture de l'angle, un blocage trabéculaire par des cellules tumorales ou par des macrophages chargés de débris tumoraux nécrotiques (glaucome mélanolytique). L'extension extra-oculaire sous la forme d'un nodule épiscléral ne doit pas être confondue avec un mélanome conjonctival, une mélanose, un staphylome, un hématome, un naevus cellulaire bleu.
L'*histopathologie* des mélanomes et des métastases (Chapitre XXIV.1.4, Planches 50–52) ciliaires est analogue à celle des localisations choroïdiennes.

XXIII.2 Melanotische Tumoren des Ziliarstromas

Viele dieser Geschwülste gleichen anderen melanotischen Tumoren der Uvea. Einige Sonderfälle seien hier erwähnt.

XXIII.2.1 Gutartige Tumoren

Ziliarnaevi sind selten (2%) und werden klinisch selten beobachtet. Unter ihnen ziehen die wenngleich seltenen Melanozytome (magnozelluläre Naevi) das Interesse auf sich, weil sie spontan oder nach einer Verletzung zur Nekrose neigen. Eine sekundäre Pigmentausschwemmung kann ein Glaukom verursachen.

XXIII.2.2 Maligne Melanome

Klinisch werden diese Geschwülste oft spät entdeckt, wenn ihr Wachstum ins Bulbusinnere eine Verformung, Verlagerung oder Trübungen der Linse und eine Einbuße des Sehvermögens zur Folge hat. Andere mögliche Symptome sind konjunktivale und episklerale Gefäßerweiterung, einseitige Hypotonie. Im allgemeinen kann eine sklerale Verschattung bei Transillumination durch die Pupille festgestellt werden. Diese Geschwülste erfassen die Iriswurzel, wo sie eine scheinbare Iridiodialyse bewirken, und wachsen sekundär in die Vorderkammer ein. Manche (Ringmelanome genannt) breiten sich ringförmig aus, häufig mit einem Sekundärglaukom das als Komplikation hinzukommt. Die Gonioskopie zeigt dann eine unregelmäßige Verdickung der Winkelstrukturen und Knötchen. Eine Hypertonie kann auf eine tumorale Infiltration der abführenden Gefäße, ein Verschieben der Iriswurzel mit Winkelverschluß, einen Trabekelblock durch Tumorzellen oder durch mit nekrotischem Tumormaterial beladene Makrophagen (melanolytisches Glaukom) hinweisen. Die extraokulare Ausweitung in Form eines episkleralen Knötchens darf nicht mit einem Melanom der Konjunktiva, einer Melanose, einem Staphylom, einem Hämatom oder einem blauen Zellnaevus verwechselt werden. Die *Histopathologie* der malignen Melanome und *Metastasen* (Kapitel XXIV.1.4, Tafel 50–52) im Ziliarkörper kommt der entsprechenden in der Aderhaut gleich.

PLATE 47 PLANCHE 47 TAFEL 47

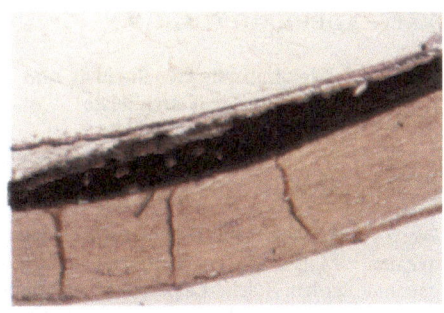

a

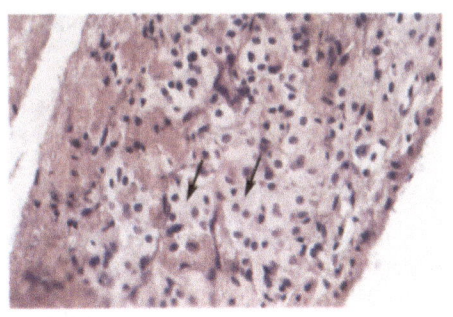

b

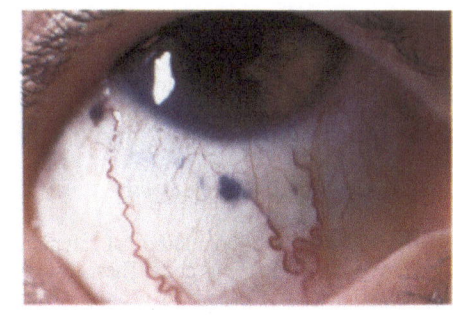

c

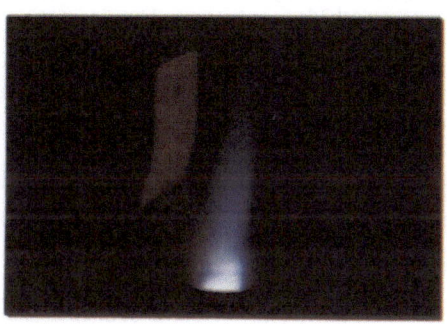

d

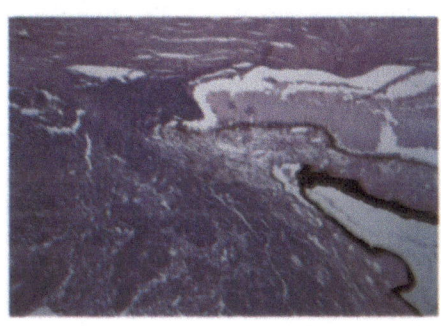

e

f

Fig. a. Melanocytoma of the ciliary body (pars plana): histopathology.
Densely pigmented diffuse tumour. Bleached preparations are necessary to analyse cellular details (Fig. b).

Fig. b. Melanocytoma of ciliary body (bleached section): histopathology.
Large, plump polyhedral cells with central, round nuclei and rarer spindle-shaped cells (→).

Fig. c. Clinical aspect of the transscleral extension of a ciliary body melanoma.

Fig. d. Clinical aspect (same patient).
The tumour invades and enlarges the anterior chamber angle (appearance of iridodialysis).

Fig. e. Annular ciliary body melanoma.

Fig. f. Histopathology of a massive ciliary body metastasis from lung carcinoma invading the trabecular meshwork and growing into the anterior chamber.

Fig. a. Mélanocytome du corps ciliaire (pars plana): histopathologie.
Tumeur diffuse très pigmentée. Des préparations dépigmentées sont nécessaires à l'analyse des détails cellulaires (Fig. b).

Fig. b. Section dépigmentée du cas précédent: histopathologie.
Volumineuses cellules polyédriques à noyau central arrondi avec de plus rares cellules fusiformes (→).

Fig. c. Aspect clinique de l'extériorisation transsclérale d'un mélanome du corps ciliaire.

Fig. d. Aspect clinique (même patiente).
La tumeur envahit et élargit l'angle camérulaire (aspect d'iridodialyse).

Fig. e. Mélanome annulaire du corps ciliaire.

Fig. f. Histopathologie d'une volumineuse métastase d'un carcinome pulmonaire dans le corps ciliaire envahissant le trabéculum et s'infiltrant dans la chambre antérieure.

Abb. a. Stark pigmentierter, undeutlich abgegrenzter Tumor des Ziliarkörpers (pars plana): Histopathologie.
Nur auf depigmentierten Schnitten ist die Zellstruktur deutlich erkennbar (Abb. b).

Abb. b. Melanozytom des Ziliarkörpers (depigmentierter Schnitt): Histopathologie.
Voluminöse polygonale Zellen mit rundlichem zentralen Kern und seltene Spindelzellen (→).

Abb. c. Klinischer Aspekt des Durchbruchs eines Ziliarkörpermelanoms durch die Sklera.

Abb. d. Klinischer Aspekt (dieselbe Patientin).
Der Tumor dringt in die Kammerbucht ein und erweitert diese (Aussehen einer Iridodialyse).

Abb. e. Ringförmiges Melanom des Ziliarkörpers.

Abb. f. Histopathologie: voluminöse Metastase eines Lungenkarzinoms im Ziliarkörper, die auf das Trabekel weiter übergreift und die vordere Kammer infiltriert.

PLATE 48 PLANCHE 48 TAFEL 48

XXIV. CHOROIDAL TUMOURS

XXIV.1 Melanocytic tumours and other neural crest-derived-tumours

XXIV.1.1 *Choroidal naevi*

These tumours are composed of atypical melanocytes called naevus cells. These lesions are common (10%) except in negroes. They must be looked for in patients with dysplastic naevus syndrome.

Clinical features. Most naevi are asymptomatic and are discovered during systematic examination. Some of them induce a visual field defect. They appear as slate grey variably pigmented tumours, with defined limits, not exceeding 2 mm in thickness. Changes in the overlying retina include drusen, serous detachment, subretinal neovascularization. The presence of orange pigment, a diameter greater than 5 disc diameters, a thickness superior to 2 mm should arouse the suspicion of a malignant lesion. Such tumours should be followed up with fundus photographs every 6 months.

Histopathology. Naevus cells are larger than normal and may be classified into 4 types: 1) plump polyhedral with a small central nucleus, typically seen in melanocytomas; 2) spindle-shaped; 3) intermediate; 4) balloon cells, with abundant foamy cytoplasm, seen in halo naevi. The occurrence of naevus-like structures along the base of a choroidal melanoma is no longer interpreted as an argument for the predisposing nature of naevi.

XXIV.1.2 *Choroidal tumours in neurofibromatosis*

These tumours, deriving also from the neural crest, include: 1) melanocytic tumours, more common; 2) neurofibromas, composed of Schwann cells, nerve axons, fibroblasts and connective tissue; 3) Schwannomas, more often solitary, encapsulated, composed of spindle-shaped cells arranged into areas of high and low cellularity (Antoni A and B); 4) ganglioneuromas, exceptional.

XXIV. TUMEURS CHOROÏDIENNES

XXIV.1 Tumeurs mélaniques et autres tumeurs dérivées de la crête neurale

XXIV.1.1 *Naevi choroïdiens*

Ces tumeurs sont formées de mélanocytes uvéaux anormaux appelés cellules naeviques. Ces lésions sont fréquentes (10%) sauf chez le noir. Elles doivent être recherchées dans le syndrome des naevi dysplasiques.

Clinique. La plupart des naevi sont asymptomatiques et de découverte fortuite. Un déficit périmétrique peut être présent. Ils apparaissent comme des tumeurs grisâtres, à bords définis, de moins de 2 mm d'épaisseur, de pigmentation variable, associés parfois à des altérations rétiniennes en regard: druses, décollements séreux, néovaisseaux sous-rétiniens. La présence de pigment orange, un diamètre supérieure à 5 diamètres papillaires, une épaisseur supérieure à 2 mm, caractérisent les naevi "suspects". Ces derniers doivent être suivis par des photographies tous les 6 mois.

Histopathologie. Les cellules naeviques, anormalement grandes, sont divisées en 4 types: 1) gonflées, polyédriques à petit noyau central, typiques des mélanocytomes; 2) fusiformes; 3) intermédiaires; 4) ballonisées, à cytoplasme spumeux, typiques des naevi en halo.
Une structure naevique ou pseudo-naevoïde peut être observée à la base de nombreux mélanomes, sans préjuger du caractère prédisposant de cette lésion.

XXIV.1.2 *Tumeurs choroïdiennes dans la neurofibromatose*

Ces tumeurs, dérivant aussi embryologiquement de la crête neurale, comprennent: 1) les tumeurs mélaniques, plus fréquentes; 2) les neurofibromes, composés de cellules de Schwann, d'axones, de fibroblastes et de tissu conjonctif; 3) les schwannomes, le plus souvent solitaires, encapsulés, composés de cellules fusiformes agencées en aires de haute ou de faible cellularité (Antoni A ou B); 4) les ganglioneuromes, exceptionnels.

XXIV. ADERHAUTTUMOREN

XXIV.1 Melanotische Geschwülste und andere von der Neuralleiste ausgehende Geschwülste

XXIV.1.1 *Aderhautnaevi*

Diese Geschwülste bilden sich aus anormalen uvealen Melanozyten, die Naevuszellen genannt werden. Solche Läsionen treten außer bei Schwarzhäutigen häufig auf (10%). Nach ihnen ist im Zusammenhang mit dem Syndrom der dysplastischen Naevi zu forschen.

Klinik. Die meisten Naevi sind klinisch asymptomatisch und werden zufällig entdeckt. Das Gesichtsfeld kann eingeschränkt sein. Sie treten als gräuliche, fest umrissene Geschwülste von weniger als 2 mm Dicke und unterschiedlicher Pigmentierung in Erscheinung; gleichzeitig können gegenüberliegend Netzhautschäden auftreten: Drusen, seröse Ablösungen, Gefäßneubildung unter der Netzhaut. Ein orangefarbenes Pigment, ein Durchmesser von mehr als 5 Papillendurchmessern, eine Dicke von mehr als 2 mm charakterisieren "verdächtige" Naevi. Diese müssen alle 6 Monate photographisch kontrolliert werden.

Histopathologie. Histopathologisch werden die anormal großen Naevizellen in vier Typen unterteilt: 1) geschwollene, polygonale mit kleinem zentralem Kern, typisch für Melanozytome; 2) spindelförmige; 3) Zwischenformen; 4) aufgeblähte mit schaumigem Zytoplasma, typisch für Halo-Naevi. Eine Naevus- oder Pseudonaevus-Struktur kann an der Basis von zahlreichen Melanomen beobachtet werden, ohne daß jedoch eine solche Läsion prädisponierend wäre.

XXIV.1.2 *Aderhauttumoren bei Neurofibromatose*

Zu diesen embryologisch ebenfalls von der Neuralleiste ausgehenden Geschwülsten zählen: 1) die am häufigsten vorkommenden, pigmentierten melanotischen Tumoren; 2) Neurofibrome, aus Schwannzellen, Axonen, Fibroblasten und Bindegewebe bestehend; 3) die meist einzeln auftretenden Schwannome mit Kapsel, bestehend aus Spindelzellen, die in zellreichen oder zellarmen Formen anzutreffen sind (Antoni A und B); 4) die außerordentlich seltenen Ganglioneurome.

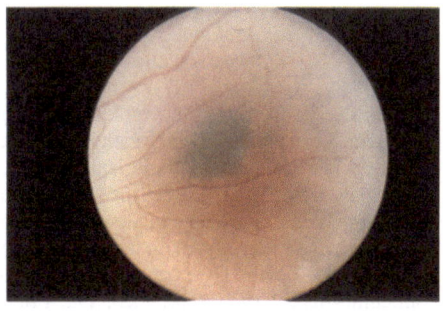

a

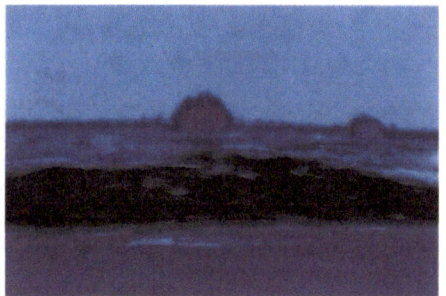

b

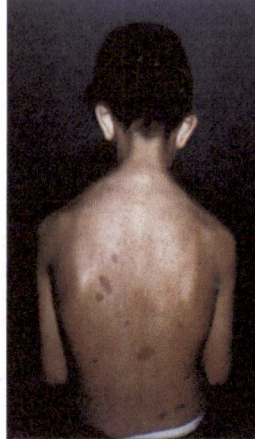

c

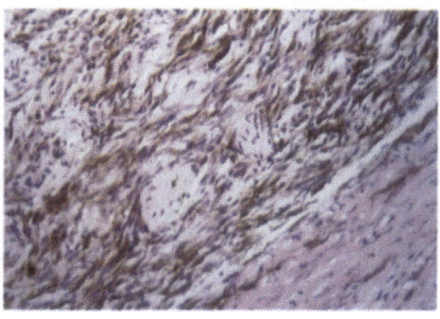

d

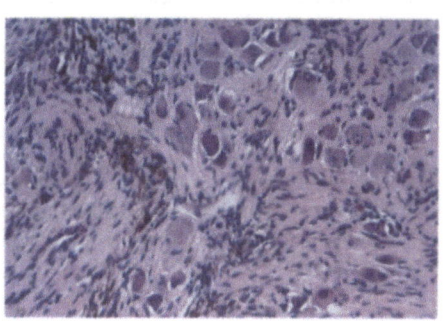

e

Fig. a. Clinical appearance of choroidal naevus.

Fig. b. Histopathology: choroidal naevus composed of spindle-shaped cells, with focal narrowing of choriocapillaris, and overlying drusen.
The neurosensory retina is artefactuously detached.

Fig. c. "Café-au-lait" spots in Von Reckling-hausen's neurofibromatosis.

Fig. d. Histopathology: Von Recklinghausen's neurofibromatosis.
Choroidal thickening by bundles of spindle-shaped cells. Ovoid bodies are seen (concentric lamellae of Schwann cells encircling central, unmyelinated axons).

Fig. e. Histopathology: ganglioneuroma in neuro-fibromatosis.
Bundles of spindle-shaped cells, numerous ganglion cells. Some melanocytes are present.

Fig. a. Aspect clinique d'un naevus choroïdien.

Fig. b. Histopathologie: le naevus choroïdien est composé de cellules fusiformes, entraînant un amin-cissement de la choriocapillaire et la formation de druses.
La rétine neurosensorielle est artificiellement décollée.

Fig. c. Taches "café au lait" dans la neuro-fibromatose de Von Recklinghausen.

Fig. d. Histopathologie: neurofibrome de Von Reck-linghausen.
Épaississement choroïdien par des faisceaux de cel-lules fusiformes avec corps ovoïdes (lamelles con-centriques de cellules de Schwann entourant des axones centraux non myélinisés).

Fig. e. Histopathologie: ganglioneurome dans la neurofibromatose.
Faisceaux de cellules fusiformes. Nombreuses cel-lules ganglionnaires à large noyau avec nucléoles bien visibles. Quelques mélanocytes sont présents.

Abb. a. Klinischer Aspekt eines Naevus der Ader-haut.

Abb. b. Histopathologie: der Aderhautnaevus be-steht aus Spindelzellen und zieht eine Verdünnung der Choriokapillaris und die Bildung von Drusen nach sich.
Die neurosensorische Netzhaut ist künstlich abgelöst.

Abb. c. "Café au lait"-Flecken bei Reckling-hausenscher Neurofibromatose.

Abb. d. Histopathologie: Von Recklinghausen Neu-rofibrom.
Verdickung der Aderhaut durch Bündel von Spindel-zellen mit ovoiden Körperchen (konzentrische Lamellen von Schwannzellen, die die nicht myelinisierten zentralen Axone umgeben).

Abb. e. Histopathologie: Ganglioneurom bei Neuro-fibromatose.
Spindelzellenbündel. Zahlreiche Ganglienzellen. An-wesenheit einiger Melanozyten mit großem Kern und gut erkennbaren Nukleolen.

PLATE 49　　　　　　　PLANCHE 49　　　　　　　TAFEL 49

XXIV.1.3 Melanosis oculi and naevus of Ota

Clinical features. Melanosis oculi is a congenital condition due to the presence in the episclera, sclera and uvea of large numbers of normal dendritic melanocytes. It is generally unilateral and, when ipsilateral congenital melanosis of the eyelid occurs, the association is named Naevus of Ota (Naevus fusco-caeruleus ophtalmo-maxillaris). The prevalence is about 0.038% in whites, 0.014% in negroes, and up to 0.84% in Japanese. Orbital, meningeal and brain involvement have also been reported. Clinically it appears as a diffuse, grey-blue cutaneous coloration, in the distribution area of one of the three branches of the trigeminal nerve. The episclera shows flat, grey to brown areas. The uveal pigmentation may be diffuse, appearing as a heterochromia, or limited to one sector. In 4.6% of reported cases a malignant transformation occurred, but this figure is probably far above the actual transformation potential in this condition.

Histopathology. Histopathology demonstrates dermal and scleral infiltration by heavily pigmented dendritic melanocytes. Uveal infiltration may extend behind the lamina cribrosa. A melanocytoma of the optic disc may be associated.

XXIV.1.3 Melanosis oculi et naevus de Ota

Clinique. La mélanose oculaire congénitale est liée à la présence dans l'épisclère, la sclère et l'uvée, de nombreux mélanocytes dendritiques normaux. Elle est généralement unilatérale et, lorsqu'une mélanose congénitale homolatérale des paupières est associée, le terme de Naevus de Ota (Naevus fusco-caeruleus ophtalmo-maxillaris) est employé. La prévalence est estimée à 0,038% chez les blancs, 0,014% chez les mélanodermes et près de 0,84% chez les Japonais. Une mélanose orbitaire, méningée et/ou cérébrale est rarement associée. Cliniquement, l'aspect est celui d'une coloration diffuse, bleu-grisâtre cutanée dans le territoire de distribution d'une des branches du trijumeau. On note au niveau épiscléral des zones grisâtres ou brunes. La pigmentation uvéale peut être diffuse, prenant l'aspect d'une hétérochromie, ou sectorielle. Dans 4,6% des cas publiés, une transformation maligne est signalée. Cependant le potentiel malin de cette mélanose est ici probablement artificiellement élevé.

Histopathologie. Sur le plan histopathologique, le derme, la sclère sont infiltrés de mélanocytes dendritiques très pigmentés. L'infiltration uvéale peut s'étendre en arrière de la lame criblée. Un mélanocytome papillaire peut être associé.

XXIV.1.3 Melanosis oculi und Naevus von Ota

Klinik. Die kongenitale Augenmelanose hängt mit dem Vorhandensein zahlreicher normaler dentritischer Melanozyten in Episklera, Sklera und Uvea zusammen. Sie ist im allgemeinen einseitig. Wenn eine kongenitale gleichseitige Melanose der Lider hinzukommt, so wird von einem Ota-Naevus (Naevus fusco-caeruleus ophtalmo-maxillaris) gesprochen. Die Prävalenz beträgt schätzungsweise bei den Weißen 0,038%, bei den Dunkelhäutigen 0,014% und ca. 0,84% bei den Japanern. Eine orbitale, meningeale und/oder zerebrale Melanose kommt selten hinzu. Das *klinische* Bild ist das einer blaugrauen diffusen kutanen Färbung im Bereich eines der Trigeminusäste. Auf der Episklera sind gräuliche oder braune Zonen festzustellen. Die Pigmentierung der Uvea kann diffus sein und wie eine Heterochromie aussehen, oder sektoriell sein. In 4,6% der veröffentlichten Fälle stellte sich im weiteren Verlauf Malignität ein. Wahrscheinlich ist jedoch das Bösartigkeitspotential dieser Melanose in diesen Fällen künstlich zu hoch.

Histopathologie. In histopathologischer Hinsicht sind Dermis und Sklera von dendritischen, stark pigmentierten Melanozyten infiltriert. Die Infiltration der Uvea kann sich hinter die Lamina cribrosa ausdehnen. Ein Melanozytom der Papille kann hinzukommen.

PLATE 49   PLANCHE 49   TAFEL 49

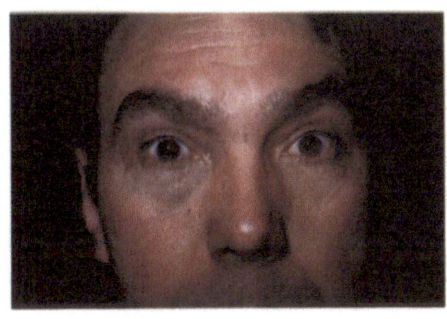

a

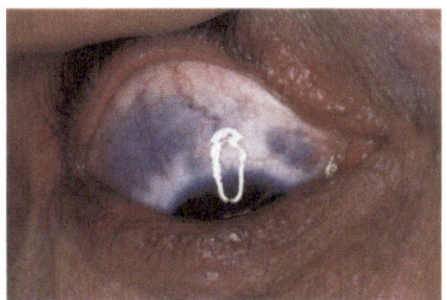

b

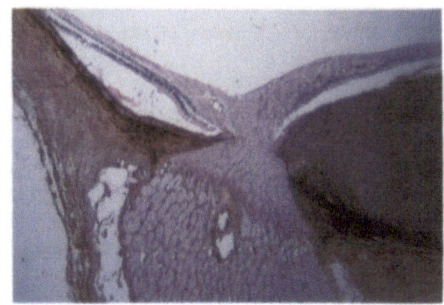

c

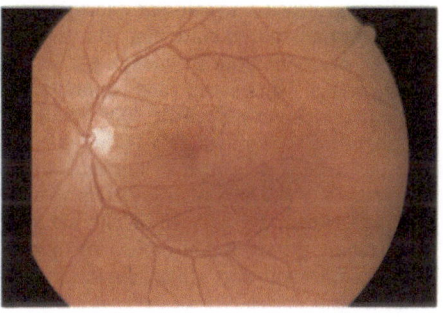

d

e

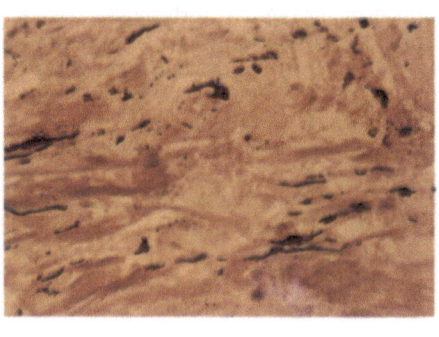

f

Fig. a. Naevus of Ota.
Facial view showing unilateral periocular cutaneous pigmentation around right eye.

Fig. b. Continued (same case as Fig. a).
Episcleral pigmentation of right eye.

Fig. c. Choroidal melanoma in patient with oculodermal melanocytosis.
Note diffuse choroidal pigmentation, and scleral pigmentation.

Fig. d-e. Fundus heterochromia in patient with ocular melanocytosis of right eye.

Fig. f. Histopathology: Dermal melanocytes in oculodermal melanocytosis (Fontana).

Fig. a. Naevus de Ota.
Photographie montrant une hyperpigmentation cutanée péri-oculaire droite.

Fig. b. Suite (même cas que Fig. a).
Pigmentation épisclérale de l'oeil droit.

Fig. c. Mélanome choroïdien chez un patient porteur d'une mélanocytose oculo-dermique ou naevus de Ota.
A noter la pigmentation choroïdienne diffuse et la pigmentation sclérale.

Fig. d-e. Hétérochromie du fond d'oeil chez un patient porteur d'une mélanocytose oculaire droite.

Fig. f. Histopathologie: mélanocytes dermiques au cours de la mélanocytose oculo-dermique (Fontana).

Abb. a. Naevus von Ota.
Photographie einer kutanen Hyperpigmentierung im Bereich des rechten Auges.

Abb. b. Fortsetzung (derselbe Fall wie Abb. a).
Episklerale Pigmentierung des rechten Auges.

Abb. c. Aderhautmelanom bei einem Patienten mit okulo-dermalen Melanozytose.
Zu beachten ist die diffuse Aderhautpigmentierung und die Lederhautpigmentierung.

Abb. d-e. Heterochromie des Fundus bei einem Patienten mit okularer Melanozytose rechts.

Abb. f. Histopathologie: Dermismelanozyten bei einer okulo-dermalen Melanozytose (Fontana).

105

PLATE 50 PLANCHE 50 TAFEL 50

XXIV.1.4 Choroidal melanomas

Uveal melanomas are the most common primary ocular malignant tumours. The average age of onset is about 50 years, with a peak in the seventh decade; childhood onset is exceptional. Naevi, melanocytosis, dysplastic cutaneous naevus syndrome, and neurofibromatosis represent predisposing conditions.

Clinical features. Visual symptoms only occur when the tumour involves the macular area. Small macular melanomas may be detected early. Observation of these lesions to document significant growth is widely advocated. A high rate of accurate diagnosis (up to 99%) is now achieved through 1) fundus examination with indirect ophthalmoscopy and Goldmann contact lens; 2) scleral transillumination to rule out a liquid lesion, e.g. uveal effusion syndrome; 3) angiography, demonstrating typically early mottling fluorescence, shadowing by orange pigment overlying the tumour, progressive staining and multiple pinpoint leaks; a double circulation pattern illustrates breaks in Bruch's membrane and retinal invasion; 4) ultrasonography demonstrating acoustic hollowness, choroidal excavation, orbital shadowing, helping to differentiate melanomas from haemangiomas and metastases.

Careful examination and follow-up in the case of small tumours allow elimination of pseudomelanomas: choroidal naevi, disciform retinal degeneration, hematomas, hypertrophy of retinal pigment epithelium, haemangiomas, metastases. Metastatic assessment including at least physical examination, routine blood checkups, chest X rays, liver enzyme measurement and liver echograms is positive in only 2% of patients at the time of the ophthalmological diagnosis.

XXIV.1.4 Mélanomes choroïdiens

Les mélanomes de la choroïde sont les plus fréquentes tumeurs intra-oculaires primitives. Ce sont le plus souvent des tumeurs de l'adulte, apparaissant autour de 50 ans, avec un pic vers la soixantaine. Les naevi, les mélanoses, le syndrome des naevi dysplasiques et la neurofibromatose sont des affections prédisposantes.

Clinique. Les symptômes visuels surviennent seulement lorsque la tumeur atteint l'aire maculaire. De petits mélanomes maculaires peuvent être décelés précocement. Dans ce cas, une surveillance clinique pour détecter une croissance tumorale est souvent recommandée. Un taux élevé de précision diagnostique (près de 99%) est aujourd'hui obtenu grâce 1) à l'examen rétinien en biomicroscopie et en opthalmoscopie indirecte; 2) à la transillumination pour éliminer une lésion liquidienne, effusion uvéale par exemple; 3) à l'angiographie qui montre une fluorescence précoce en mottes, un masquage par le pigment orange sus-jacent, une imprégnation progressive et des points de fuite multiples; l'aspect de double circulation traduit une rupture de la lame de Bruch et l'envahissement rétinien; 4) à l'échographie qui objective un vide acoustique, une excavation choroïdienne, une ombre portée sur l'orbite, distinguant ainsi les mélanomes des hémangiomes et des métastases.

Ces différents examens et la surveillance clinique en présence de petites tumeurs permettent d'éliminer: naevi choroïdiens, dégénérescence disciforme, hématomes, hypertrophie de l'épithélium pigmentaire rétinien, hémangiomes, métastases. Le bilan d'extension, qui doit comprendre au minimum examen clinique, bilan hématologique, radiographie pulmonaire, échographie et enzymologie hépatique, n'est positif que dans 2% des cas au moment du diagnostic ophtalmologique.

XXIV.1.4 Maligne Melanome der Aderhaut

Die Melanome der Aderhaut sind die häufigsten intraokularen Primärgeschwülste. Es handelt sich meist um Tumoren des Erwachsenen, die im Alter um 50 in Erscheinung treten und um 60 am häufigsten sind. Naevi, Melanosen, das Syndrom der dyplastischen Naevi und Neurofibromatose sind prädisponierende Affektionen.

Klinik. Sehstörungen treten erst auf, wenn der Tumor den Maculabereich erreicht hat. Kleine Maculamelanome können frühzeitig bemerkt werden. In diesem Fall wird oft eine klinische Überwachung zum Feststellen eines Tumorwachstums empfohlen. Ein hoher Präzisionsgrad der Diagnose (99%) wird heute 1) durch Netzhautuntersuchung mit der Spaltlampe und mit indirekter Ophthalmoskopie erreicht; 2) durch Transillumation, um eine Flüssigkeitsansammlung, beispielsweise eine uveale Effusion, auszuschließen; 3) durch Angiographie, die eine frühzeitige fleckigschollige Fluoreszenz, ein Maskierung durch das darübergelagerte orangefarbene Pigment, eine progressive Anfärbung und multiple Leckstellen zeigt; ein doppelter Kreislauf bedeutet den Durchbruch durch die Bruch-Membran und die Invasion der Retina; 4) durch Echographie, mit der sich ein Schallvakuum, ein Hohlraum in der Aderhaut, ein auf die Orbita fallender Schatten objektivieren lassen, worin sich Melanome von Hämangiomen und Metastasen unterscheiden.

Mit diesen verschiedenen Untersuchungen und mit der Beobachtung kleiner Tumoren können Aderhautnaevi, disziforme Degenerationen, Hämatome, Hypertrophien des Pigmentepithels der Netzhaut, Hämangiome, Metastasen ausgeschlossen werden. Die Allgemeinuntersuchung, die zumindest eine klinische Untersuchung, einen hämatologischen Status, Lungenradiographie, Echographie und Leberenzymologie einschließen sollte, erweist sich zum Zeitpunkt der ophthalmologischen Diagnose nur in 2% der Fälle als positiv.

PLATE 50   PLANCHE 50   TAFEL 50

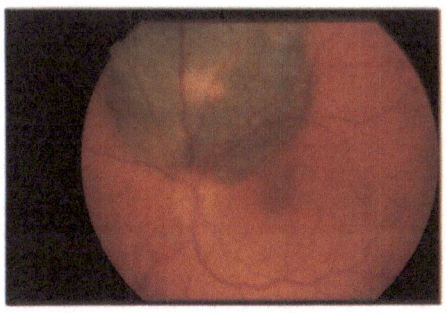

a

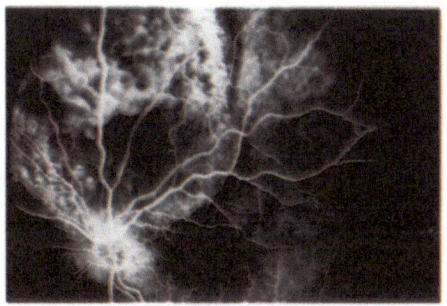

b

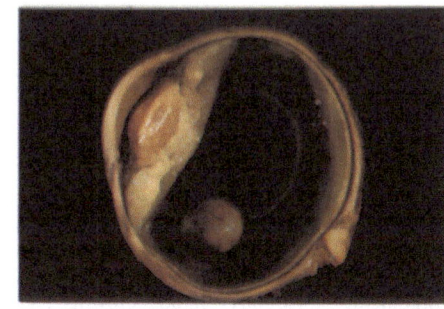

c

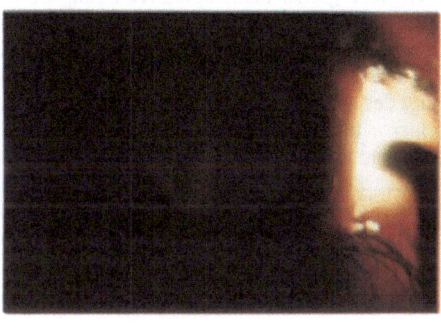

d

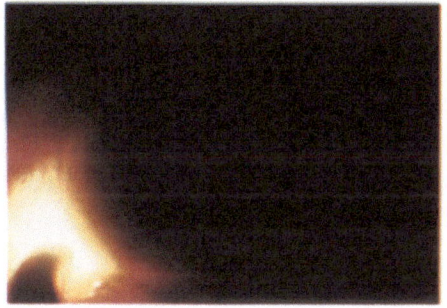

e

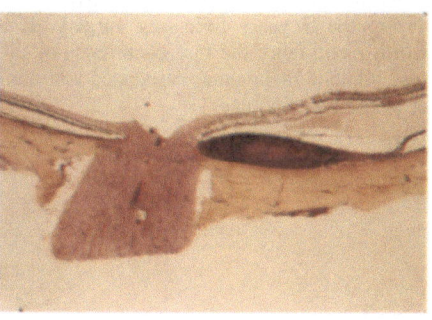

f

Fig. a. Fundus photograph.
Large pigmented choroidal melanoma above the optic disk. Note abundant orange pigment (lipofuscin) in the overlying retina. Optic nerve invasion should be suspected in this variant.

Fig. b. Fluorescein angiogram of same tumour.
Mottled fluorescence, multiple leakage pinpoints, hypofluorescence in areas of orange pigment deposits.

Fig. c. Gross picture.
This nodular choroidal melanoma has grown directly through Bruch's membrane into the subretinal space. Vascular congestion at the top of the tumour.

Fig. d-e. Transillumination through normal (d) and tumoral (e) area. Nasally located pigmented tumour of the left eye.

Fig. f. Uveal melanoma spreading out in the plane of the choroid as a slightly elevated discoid tumour.

Fig. a. Photographie du fond d'oeil.
Important mélanome choroïdien pigmenté situé au-dessus de la papille. A noter l'abondance de pigment orange (lipofuscine) en surface. L'extension au nerf optique doit être suspectée dans cette forme topographique.

Fig. b. Angiographie fluorescéïnique de la même tumeur.
Fluorescence en mottes, multiples points de fuite en tête d'épingle, masquage dans les zones de dépôts de pigment orange.

Fig. c. Macroscopie.
Le mélanome choroïdien nodulaire a traversé directement la lame de Bruch pour se développer dans l'espace sous-rétinien. Congestion vasculaire au sommet de la tumeur.

Fig. d-e. Transillumination à travers un tissu normal (d) ou tumoral (e). Tumeur pigmentée nasale de l'oeil gauche.

Fig. f. Mélanome choroïdien s'étendant dans le plan de la choroïde comme une tumeur discoïde peu surélevée.

Abb. a. Photographie des Augenhintergrundes.
Oberhalb der Papille gelegenes, großes pigmentiertes Aderhautmelanom. Zu beachten ist das sehr reichlich an der Oberfläche vorhandene orangefarbene Pigment (Lipofuszin). Bei einer solchen Lokalisation besteht der Verdacht einer Infiltration des Sehnervs.

Abb. b. Fluoreszein-Angiographie desselben Tumors.
Fleckig-schollige Fluoreszenz, vielfache stecknadelkopfähnliche Leckstellen; die Zonen mit orangefarbener Pigmentablagerung wirken abdeckend.

Abb. c. Makroskopisch.
Das knotige Aderhautmelanom hat die Bruch-Membran durchbrochen und sich in den subretinalen Raum eingewachsen. Weitgestellte Gefäße an der Tumorspitze.

Abb. d-e. Transillumation durch ein normales (d) oder Tumorgewebe (e). Pigmentierter Tumor nasal im linken Auge.

Abb. f. Aderhautmelanom, das sich wie ein scheibenförmiger, kaum erhabener Tumor innerhalb der Aderhaut ausdehnt.

PLATE 51 PLANCHE 51 TAFEL 51

Choroidal melanomas (continued)

Mélanomes choroïdiens (suite)

Maligne Melanome der Aderhaut (Fortsetzung)

Uveal melanoma *growth* follows an exponential curve with a doubling time of two months to several years. Small melanomas first grow inward, with a discoid shape, displacing Bruch's membrane. When the latter is disrupted, the tumour occupies the subretinal space with a mushroom shape. Vascular engorgement, apparently rapid growth and vitreous haemorrhage may occur. Changes in the overlying tissues include drusen formation, orange pigmentation, neurosensory retinal detachment or invasion. Scleral invasion along ciliary vessels, nerves, or vortex veins, which is a factor of unfavourable prognosis, must be detected at the time of surgery. This is more likely to occur in large or diffuse melanomas. The latter induce a slight thickening of the choroid and may remain unsuspected until extra-ocular extension occurs. Most metastases are found in the liver, often during the 5 years following surgery. It is worth mentioning the rare occurrence of diffuse bilateral melanomas associated with lung or ovarian carcinomas.

La *croissance* des mélanomes uvéaux suit une courbe exponentielle avec un temps de doublement variant de 2 mois à plusieurs années. Les petits mélanomes s'accroissent d'abord de manière discoïde puis vers l'intérieur en déplaçant la lame de Bruch, la traversant ensuite vers l'espace sous-rétinien, prenant alors une configuration en champignon. Une dilatation vasculaire, une apparente accélération de croissance, une hémorragie intra-vitréenne peuvent apparaître. Les modifications des tissus sus-jacents comprennent la formation de druses, de pigment orange, un décollement ou un envahissement rétiniens. L'envahissement scléral le long des vaisseaux ciliaires, des nerfs ou des veines vortiqueuses, facteur de mauvais pronostic, doit être recherché dès la procédure chirurgicale. Cette extériorisation survient surtout dans les tumeurs volumineuses ou diffuses. Dans ce dernier cas le discret épaississement choroïdien peut être méconnu jusqu'à ce qu'une extension extra-oculaire survienne. Les métastases se font le plus souvent vers le foie, dans les 5 ans qui suivent l'énucléation. Signalons l'existence de rares mélanomes diffus bilatéraux associés à des carcinomes bronchiques ou ovariens.

Das *Wachstum* der Melanome der Uvea verläuft exponentiell mit einer Verdoppelungszeit, die zwischen 2 Monaten und mehreren Jahren liegen kann. Kleine Melanome vergrößern sich zuerst scheibenförmig und dann nach innen, wobei sie die Bruch-Membran vor sich herschieben und danach zum subretinalen Raum hin durchwachsen und dabei ein pilzartiges Aussehen annehmen. Es kann zur Gefäßerweiterung, einer offenkundigen Wachstumsbeschleunigung, einer Blutung innerhalb des Glaskörpers kommen. Zu den darüberliegenden Gewebsveränderungen zählen die Bildung von Drusen, des orangefarbenen Pigments, eine Netzhautablösung oder eine Netzhautinfiltration. Nach einem Einwachsen in die Sklera entlang den Ziliargefäßen, den Nerven oder Vortexvenen ist als Faktor einer schlechten Prognose gleich beim operativen Eingriff zu suchen. Diese Ausbreitung kommt vor allem bei voluminösen oder diffusen Tumoren vor. Im letzteren Fall kann eine diskrete Verdickung der Aderhaut übersehen werden, bis es zu einer transskleralen extraokularen Ausbreitung kommt.

Metastasen bilden sich zumeist innerhalb 5 Jahren nach der Enukleation in der Leber. Es sei noch auf die seltenen diffusen bilateralen Melanome hingewiesen, die mit Bronchial- oder Ovarialkarzinomen einhergehen.

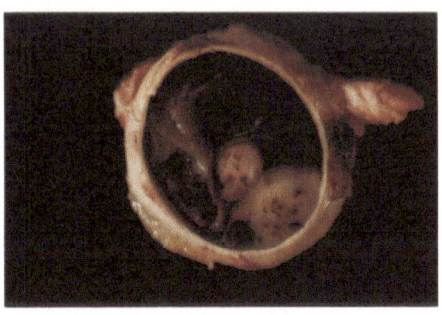

a

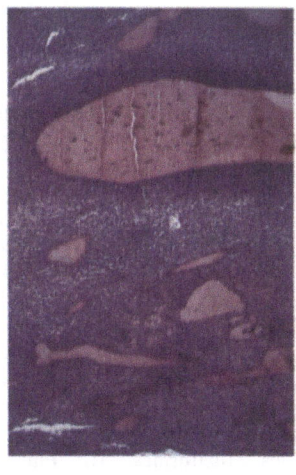

b

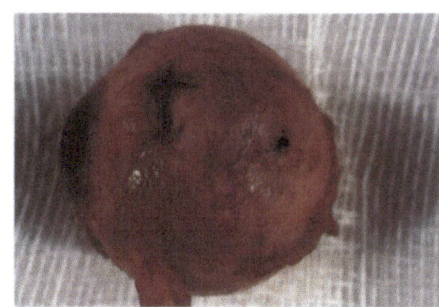

c

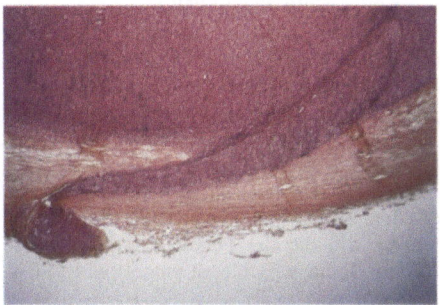

d

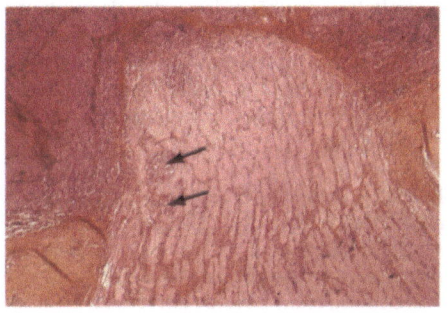

e

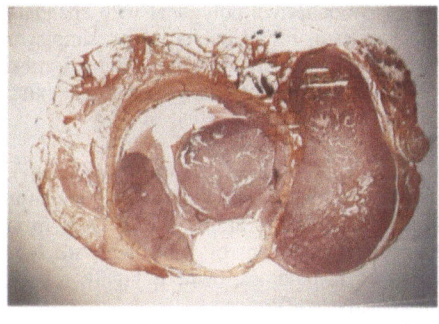

f

Fig. a. Gross picture.
Venous congestion in the tumour due to "tourniquet effect" of Bruch's membrane at sites where melanomas pass through it. Subsequent haemorrhagic necrosis and bleeding.

Fig. b. "Knapp-Rönne" type of choroidal melanoma.
Vascular engorgement due to "tourniquet effect". Intravitreal haemorrhage is associated in this variety.

Fig. c. Extra-scleral extension should be looked for at the time of surgery.

Fig. d. Histopathology: extension through expanded scleral canal all the way out to the episcleral surface, giving rise to an encapsulated epibulbar nodule.

Fig. e. Histopathology: juxtapapillary melanoma infiltrating into the optic papilla and nerve (→). A long piece of optic nerve should be cut during the enucleation.

Fig. f. Macrophotography: massive extra-ocular extension into the orbit of a uveal melanoma. Such extension can occur from flat, diffuse choroidal melanomas, and may be detected late.
late.

Fig. a. Macroscopie.
Congestion veineuse dans la tumeur du fait de l'étranglement tumoral lors de la traversée de la lame de Bruch, entraînant une nécrose hémorragique et un saignement.

Fig. b. Mélanome choroïdien du type Knapp-Rönne.
Engorgement vasculaire dû à l'"effet tourniquet" de la lame de Bruch. Une hémorragie intravitréenne est associée dans cette forme.

Fig. c. L'extension extra-sclérale doit être recherchée sur la table opératoire.

Fig. d. Histologie: extension à travers un canal scléral dilaté vers la surface épisclérale sous forme d'un nodule encapsulé épibulbaire.

Fig. e. Histopathologie: mélanome juxtapapillaire infiltrant la papille et le nerf optique (→). Le nerf optique doit être sectionné à bonne distance du globe.

Fig. f. Macrophotographie: extension extra-oculaire massive dans l'orbite d'un mélanome uvéal. De telles extensions peuvent survenir derrière des mélanomes plats et diffus, au diagnostic tardif.

Abb. a. Makroskopisch.
Venöse Hyperämie im Tumor, verursacht durch die Tumoreinschnürung beim Durchstoßen der Bruch-Membran, was eine hämorrharische Nekrose und ein Blutung zur Folge hat.

Abb. b. Aderhautmelanom vom Typ Knapp-Rönne. Gefäßerweiterung durch "Stauschlauch"-Effekt der Bruch-Membran. Bei dieser Form kommt es zur Blutung in dem Glaskörper.

Abb. c. Nach einem transskleralen Durchbruch sollte auf dem Operationstisch gesucht werden.

Abb. d. Histologie: entlang einem erweiterten Skleralkanal zur episkleralen Oberfläche hin erfolgte Ausbreitung in Form eines eingekapselten halbkugelförmigen Knötchens.

Abb. e. Histopathologie: neben der Papille gelegenes Melanom, das Papille und Sehnerv infiltriert (→). Der Sehnerv ist in ausreichendem Abstand vom Bulbus abzutrennen.

Abb. f. Makrophotographie: massive extraokulare Ausbreitung eines Uvea-Melanoms in die Orbita. Eine solche Ausbreitung kann hinter einem flachen und diffusen, spät diagnostizierten Melanom vorkommen.

Choroidal melanomas (continued)

The vital prognosis is closely related to both the largest tumour diameter and to the cytologic type.

Histopathology. The cytological classification established by Callender in 1931 and recently reviewed, includes the following categories:
- Spindle A cells. Uniform, cohesive cells with a spindle-shaped nucleus showing a nuclear longitudinal fold. The nucleoli are inconspicuous. Mitoses are rare. Some of these cells are now considered as naevic;
- Spindle B cells. Plumper, cohesive, spindle-shaped cells with larger, ovoid nuclei, distinct nucleoli, mitotic figures. Criteria for malignancy of spindle cells include: invasiveness, size of the tumour, large, hyperchromatic nuclei with mitotic activity;
- Epithelioid cells are larger, pleomorphic, poorly cohesive, polygonal with abundant cytoplasm, round nuclei, large, simple or multiple nucleoli, abundant mitotic figures. Two varieties of epithelioid cells exist: small and large.

Balloon cells, similar to those found in naevi, may be present. In many tumours, numerous lymphoid infiltrates are observed. Thus, from the cytological point of view there are four types of melanomas, with a highly related prognostic significance:
- Spindle A, 95% survival at 5 years, 85% at 15 years;
- Spindle B, 85% survival at 5 years, 80% at 15 years;
- Mixed (epithelioid and spindle), 83% survival at 5 years, 46% at 15 years;
- Epithelioid, 60% survival at 5 years, 34% at 15 years.

According to their size, choroidal melanomas are classified as follows:
- small: diameter less than 10 mm, thickness less than 2 mm;
- medium: diameter less than 15 mm, thickness less than 5 mm;
- large: diameter above 15 mm, thickness above 5 mm.

In order to provide an objective way to assess cell types and prognosis, Gamel and Mac Lean have described a computerized method aimed at evaluating the inverse of the standard deviation of the nucleolar area (ISDNA), and have derived a prognostic assessment taking into account both this value and largest tumour diameter.

Mélanomes choroïdiens (suite)

Le pronostic est étroitement lié à la taille de la tumeur (plus grand diamètre) et au type cellulaire.

Histopathologie. La classification cytologique établie par Callender en 1931 et récemment adaptée, comprend les catégories suivantes:
- Cellules fusiformes A. Uniformes, cohésives à noyau fusiforme porteur d'un pli longitudinal. Les nucléoles sont inapparents, les mitoses rares. Certaines de ces cellules sont aujourd'hui considérées comme naeviques;
- Cellules fusiformes B. Plus larges, cohésives, fusiformes à grand noyau ovoïde, nucléoles apparents avec quelques mitoses. Les critères de malignité des cellules fusiformes comprennent: tendance invasive, taille de la tumeur, gros noyaux hyperchromatiques, activité mitotique;
- Cellules épithélioïdes: de deux types (grandes ou petites), pléomorphiques, peu cohésives, polygonales à cytoplasme abondant, noyaux ronds, gros nucléoles parfois multiples, importante activité mitotique.

D'autres cellules, ballonisées, similaires à celles des naevi, des infiltrats lymphoïdes, sont fréquemment associés. Selon la cytologie, on distingue ainsi quatre types:
- Fusiformes A, 95% de survivants à 5 ans, 85% à 15 ans;
- Fusiformes B, 85% de survivants à 5 ans, 80% à 15 ans;
- Mixtes (épithélioïdes et fusiformes), 83% de survivants à 5 ans, 46% à 15 ans;
- Epithélioïdes, 60% de survivants à 5 ans, 34% à 15 ans.

On classe aussi les mélanomes choroïdiens en:
- petits: moins de 10 mm de diamètre et de 2 mm d'épaisseur;
- moyens: moins de 15 mm de diamètre et de 5 mm d'épaisseur;
- grands: plus de 15 mm de diamètre et de 5 mm d'épaisseur.

Pour fournir un mode standardisé de prédiction du type et du pronostic, Gamel et Mac Lean ont décrit une méthode informatisée prenant en compte l'Inverse de la Déviation Standard de l'Aire Nucléolaire (ISDNA), et le plus grand diamètre de la tumeur.

Maligne Melanome der Aderhaut (Fortsetzung)

Die Prognose hängt eng mit der Größe des Tumors (größter Durchmesser) und mit dem Zelltyp zusammen.

Histopathologie. Die von Callender 1931 aufgestellte und kürzlich überarbeitete Klassifizierung enthält folgende Kategorien:
- Spindelzelltyp A. Uniforme, eng aneinander liegende Zellen mit spindelförmigem Kern, der eine Längsfalte aufweist. Nukleolen treten nicht in Erscheinung, Mitosen sind selten. Manche dieser Zellen werden heute als Naevi-Zellen betrachtet;
- Spindelzelltyp B. Breitere, eng zusammenhängende, spindelförmige Zellen mit großem, eiförmigem Kern, sichtbaren Nukleolen und einigen Mitosen. Zu den Bösartigkeitskriterien der Spindelzellen zählen: Neigung zur Ausbreitung, Größe des Tumors, große hyperchromatische Kerne, Mitosenaktivität;
- Epitheloidzelltyp. Zweierlei Zelltypen (groß oder klein), pleomorph, wenig zusammenhängend, polygonal mit reichlichem Zytoplasma, runden Kernen, großen, manchmal multiplen Nukleolen, starke Mitosenaktivität.

Andere Zellen sind oft mit vorhanden: Ballonzellen wie die der Naevi, lymphatische Infiltrate. Je nach Zytologie unterscheidet man 4 Typen:
- A-spindelförmige, 95% überlebende nach 5 Jahren, 85% nach 15 Jahren;
- B-spindelförmige, 85% überlebende nach 5 Jahren, 80% nach 15 Jahren;
- Gemischte (epitheloide und spindelförmige), 83% überlebende nach 5 Jahren, 46% nach 15 Jahren;
- Epitheloide, 60% überlebende nach 5 Jahren, 34% nach 15 Jahren.

Melanome der Aderhaut werden somit eingestuft in:
- kleine: unter 10 mm Durchmesser und 2 mm Dicke;
- mittlere: unter 15 mm Durchmesser und 5 mm Dicke;
- große: über 15 mm Durchmesser und 5 mm Dicke.

Zur Erstellung einer Standardmethode für Typbestimmung und Prognose haben Gamel und Mac Lean eine EDV-Methode beschrieben, bei der die Relation Zellkern/Nukleolen (ISDNA) und der größte Durchmesser des Tumors berücksichtigt werden.

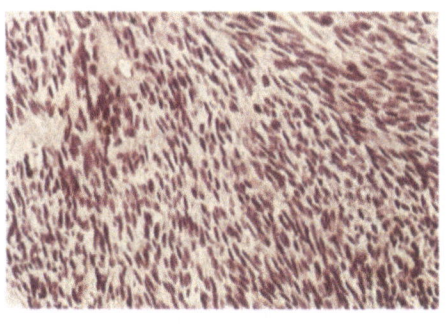

a

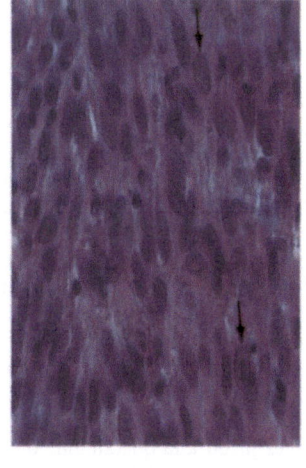

b

c

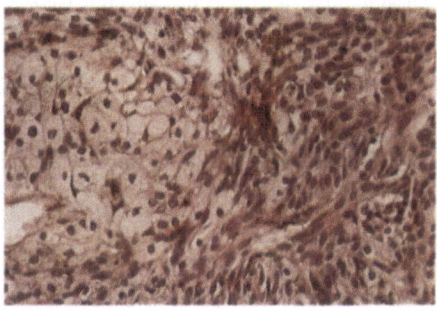
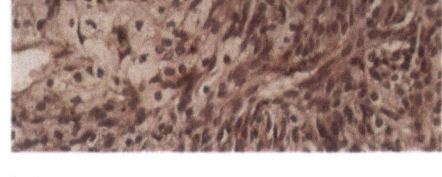

d

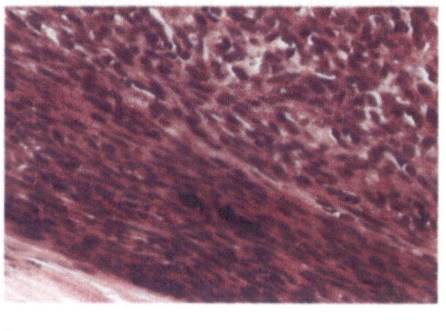

e

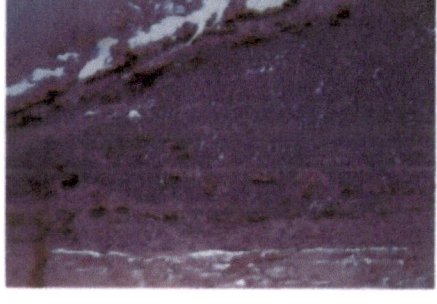

f

Fig. a. Spindle A cells.
These cells are elongated and cohesive, with ill-defined cell borders. The nuclei contain folds appearing as dark stripes.

Fig. b. Spindle A and B cells.
Spindle B cells (→) are plumper and cohesive, with ill-defined cell borders. Nucleoli are distinct.

Fig. c. Epitheloid cell type.
The cells are not cohesive, they have distinct borders and vary in size. Nuclei are large, oval, often monstrous, and contain prominent nucleoli (→)

Fig. d. Balloon cell transformation in a choroidal melanoma.
These tumour cells are larger, clearer and contain lipids or glycogen (Xanthomatous pattern). They represent a degenerative change in tumour cells, of possible immunological origin.

Fig. e. Naevic configuration at the base of uveal melanoma (see text: naevi page 102).

Fig. f. Lymphoid infiltrates in choroidal melanomas.
Such findings are quite common, but their significance is not clear.

Fig. a. Cellules fusiformes A.
Elles sont allongées, à limites imprécises. Les noyaux comportent des lignes sombres dans l'axe longitudinal, correspondant à des indentations.

Fig. b. Cellules fusiformes A et B.
Ces dernières (→) sont cohésives, plus volumineuses, à limites imprécises. Les nucléoles sont apparents.

Fig. c. Cellules épithélioïdes.
Ces cellules sont non cohésives, à limites nettes, et de taille variable. Les noyaux sont larges, ovalaires, souvent monstrueux (→) et contiennent de gros nucléoles.

Fig. d. Transformation en cellules ballonisées dans un mélanome choroïdien.
Les cellules tumorales sont plus grandes, claires et contiennent des lipides ou du glycogène (aspect spumeux). Elles traduisent une dégénérescence des cellules tumorales, d'origine immunologique possible.

Fig. e. Configuration naevique à la base d'un mélanome uvéal (voir le texte: naevus page 102).

Fig. f. Infiltrats lymphoïdes dans un mélanome choroïdien.
Cette constatation est fréquente mais de signification mal définie.

Abb. a. Spindelzellen vom Typ A.
Sie sind länglich, unscharf abgegrenzt. Die Kerne enthalten dunkle Linien entlang der Längsachse, die Falten entsprechen.

Abb. b. Spindelzellen vom Typ A und B.
Diese letzteren (→) sind voluminöser, haften stark aneinander, sind undeutlich abgegrenzt. Die Nukleolen sind sichtbar.

Abb. c. Epithelioide Zellen.
Diese Zellen haften nicht aneinander, sind deutlich abgegrenzt und von unterschiedlicher Größe. Die Kerne sind breit, oval, oft mißgebildet (→) und enthalten große Nukleolen.

Abb. d. Umwandlung in Ballonzellen in einem Aderhautmelanom.
Die Tumorzellen sind größer, heller und enthalten Lipide oder Glycogen (schaumiges Aussehen). Sie zeigen eine Degeneration der Tumorzellen, möglicherweise immunologisch bedingt.

Abb. e. Naevusstrukturen an der Basis eines Melanoms der Uvea (siehe Text: Naevus Seite 102).

Abb. f. Lymphatische Infiltrate in einem Aderhautmelanom.
Diese werden häufig festgestellt, ihre Bedeutung ist wenig bekannt.

PLATE 53 PLANCHE 53 TAFEL 53

XXIV.2 Vascular tumours

XXIV.2.1 Haemangiomas

Clinical features. These vascular hamartomas may occur in two types:
- a localized, isolated, orange red tumour, often located in the macular area, sometimes complicated by leakage into the subretinal space, cystoid macular edema, and proliferative changes in the overlying retinal pigment epithelium;
- a diffuse thickening of the choroid, in patients with Sturge-Weber syndrome.

They are usually asymptomatic until middle age or found incidentally in the third decade. Angiography is often helpful when showing 1) early injection of large vascular channels; 2) widespread leakage at the surface of the tumour; 3) pooling in the outer retina. Indocyanin green angiography is accepted as a useful diagnostic tool. Ultrasonography shows a characteristic high reflectivity pattern with no choroidal excavation. In Sturge-Weber angiomatosis (see Plate 32), ipsilateral glaucoma is frequently associated. The risk of secondary retinal detachment is high.

Histopathology. Histopathology most often shows large, thin walled vessels (cavernous haemangiomas).

XXIV.2 Tumeurs vasculaires

XXIV.2.1 Hémangiomes

Clinique. Ces hamartomes vasculaires peuvent revêtir deux aspects:
- une tumeur rouge-orange, non pigmentée, isolée, souvent localisée à l'aire maculaire, se compliquant parfois de fuites sous-rétiniennes, d'oedème maculaire cystoïde, de prolifération de l'épithélium pigmentaire;
- un épaississement choroïdien diffus, chez des patients atteints de syndrome de Sturge-Weber.

Ces tumeurs sont généralement asymptomatiques jusqu'à la quarantaine ou décelées par hasard vers la trentaine. L'angiographie est souvent utile, montrant 1) une injection précoce de larges espaces vasculaires; 2) une diffusion étendue à toute la surface tumorale; 3) une accumulation liquidienne dans les couches externes de la rétine. L'angiographie au vert d'Indocyanine est considérée comme un apport diagnostique utile. L'échographie montre une hyperréflectivité typique sans excavation choroïdienne. Dans l'angiomatose de Sturge-Weber (voir Planche 32), un glaucome homolatéral est souvent associé. Le risque de décollement rétinien est, aussi, élevé.

Histopathologie. Ces tumeurs sont composées le plus souvent de larges vaisseaux à fines parois (hémangiomes caverneux).

XXIV.2 Gefäßtumoren

XXIV.2.1 Hämangiome

Klinik. Diese Gefäßhamartome können in zweierlei Form auftreten:
- eine rot-orangene, pigmentlose, einzelne, oft in der Maculagegend lokalisierte Geschwulst, zu der manchmal noch eine subretinale Exsudation, ein zystoides Maculaödem und Wucherung des Pigmentepithels hinzukommen können;
- eine diffuse Aderhautverdickung bei Patienten mit dem Sturge-Weber-Syndrom.

Diese Geschwülste sind im allgemeinen asymptomatisch bis zum Alter von etwa vierzig Jahren oder werden um die dreißig durch Zufall bemerkt. Eine Angiographie ist oft von Nutzen, da sie 1) eine frühzeitige Injektion weiter Gefäßräume; 2) eine unscharf abgegrenzte Farbstoffdiffusion an der ganzen Tumoroberfläche; 3) eine Flüssigkeitsansammlung innerhalb der äußeren Netzhaut Schichten ausweisen kann. Die Angiographie mit Indocyanin Grün wird als für die Diagnose sinnvoll erachtet. Die Echographie zeigt eine typische Hyperreflektivität ohne Hohlraumbildung der Aderhaut. Bei der Sturge-Weber-Angiomatose (siehe Tafel 32) kommt oft ein gleichseitiges Glaukom hinzu. Auch besteht ein hohes Risiko der Netzhautablösung.

Histopathologie. Histophatologisch bestehen diese Geschwülste meistens aus breiten, meist feinwandigen Gefäßen (kavernöse Hämangiome).

XXIV.3 Choroidal osteomas

Clinical features. Choroidal osteomas are recently recognized tumours composed of compact bone occupying the juxtapapillary and macular region. They appear in young females as discrete, slightly elevated tumours with an orange or creamy colour and well defined geographic borders. Choroidal neovascularization may occur.

Histopathology. The exact nature of these tumours (choristomas or reactive osseous proliferation) is unknown. They contain compact bone lying between the choriocapillaris and the outer choroidal vessels. Channels through the bone allow communications between both circulations. Changes in the overlying retinal pigment epithelium and neuroepithelium are common.

XXIV.3 Ostéomes choroïdiens

Clinique. Récemment individualisés, les ostéomes choroïdiens sont composés d'os compact occupant la région maculaire et juxta-papillaire. Ils surviennent, chez la jeune femme, comme des tumeurs orangées ou crème, légèrement surélevées à contours géographiques nets. Une néovascularisation choroïdienne peut survenir.

Histopathologie. Leur pathogénie est inconnue (choristomes ou ossification réactive). Ils sont formées d'os compact situé entre la choriocapillaire et les vaisseaux choroïdiens externes. Des canaux trans-osseux permettent les communications entre les deux circulations. Des altérations de l'épithélium pigmentaire et du neuro-épithélium sont fréquentes.

XXIV.3 Osteom der Aderhaut

Klinik. Die kürzlich beschriebenen Osteome der Aderhaut bestehen aus kompaktem, in der Makulagegend oder dicht bei der Papille gelegenem Knochen. Sie treten bei der jungen Frau als orange- oder cremefarbene, leicht erhöhte Geschwülste mit deutlichen geographischen Konturen auf. Eine Neovaskularisierung der Aderhaut kann eintreten. Ihre Pathogenese ist unbekannt (Choristom oder reaktive Ossifikation).

Histopathologie. Histologisch werden solche Geschwülste aus kompaktem Knochen gebildet, der zwischen der Choriokapillaris und den äußeren Aderhautgefäßen angesiedelt ist. Den Knochen durchquerende Kanäle schaffen eine Verbindung zwischen den beiden Zirkulationen. Alterationen des Pigmentepithels und des Neuroepithels treten häufig auf.

PLATE 53 PLANCHE 53 TAFEL 53

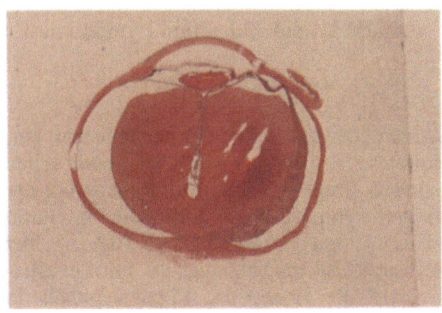

a

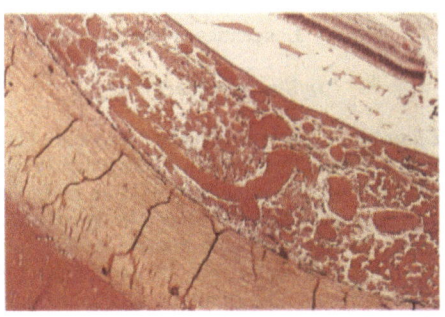

b

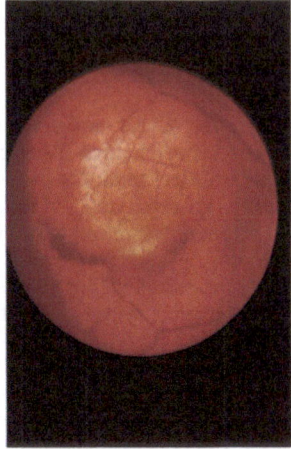

c

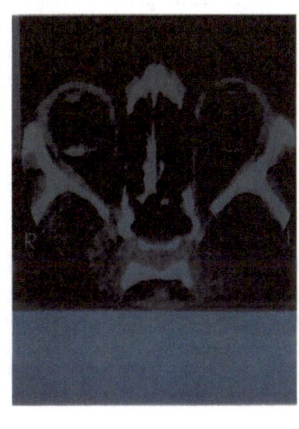

d

e

Fig. a. Choroidal haemangioma. Gross picture: diffuse choroidal haemangioma with subretinal haemorrhage and total retinal detachment.

Fig. b. Choroidal haemangioma: histopathology. Haemangioma occurring in a patient with Sturge-Weber syndrome. The haemangioma is not demarcated from the choroidal vasculature.

Fig. c. Osseous choristoma of choroid: clinical appearance.
Irregular, elevated yellow-white macular lesion. Small spiderlike vascular tufts are present on the tumour surface. Inferior haemorrhagic retinal detachment suggest an associated choroidal neovascularization.

Fig. d. Same case: CT scan showing the X-Ray opaque osteoma.

Fig. e. Choroidal osteoma: histopathology. Intra-choroidal mass containing numerous bone trabeculae.

Fig. a. Hémangiome choroïdien. Aspect macroscopique d'un hémangiome choroïdien diffus avec hémorragies sous-rétiniennes et décollement rétinien total.

Fig. b. Hémangiome choroïdien: histopathologie. Hémangiome choroïdien dans un syndrome de Sturge-Weber-Krabbe. L'hémangiome n'est pas distinct de la circulation choroïdienne.

Fig. c. Aspect clinique d'un choristome osseux choroïdien.
Lésion maculaire irrégulière, surélevée, blancjaunâtre. De petites spicules vasculaires sont présentes à la surface. Un décollement rétinien hémorragique inférieur traduit la présence de néovaisseaux choroïdiens.

Fig. d. Même cas: démonstration tomodensitométrique de l'ostéome, radio-opaque.

Fig. e. Ostéome choroïdien: histopathologie. Masse intra-choroïdienne contenant de nombreuses travées osseuses.

Abb. a. Makroskopischer Aspekt eines diffusen Hämangioms der Aderhaut mit Blutungen unter der Netzhaut und totaler Nethautablösung.

Abb. b. Hämangiom der Aderhaut bei einem Sturge-Weber-Krabbe-Syndrom: Histopathologie. Das Hämangiom setzt sich nicht von der Aderhautzirkulation ab.

Abb. c. Klinischer Aspekt eines Knochenchoristoms der Aderhaut.
Unregelmäßige, erhabene, weißgelbliche, in der Macula-Gegend lokalisierte Läsion. Kleine Gefäß-Spiculae befinden sich an der Oberfläche. Eine mit Blutung einhergehende untere Netzhautablösung weist auf das Vorhandensein neugebildeter Aderhautgefäße hin.
Abb. d. Derselbe Fall: Tomodensitometrische Darstellung des radio-opaken Osteoms.

Abb. e. Osteom der Aderhaut: Histopathologie. Im Innern der Aderhaut befindliche Masse, die zahlreiche Knochenbälklein enthält.

113

XXIV.4 Leukaemias and lymphomas

Leukaemic infiltrates

Clinical features. Uveal involvement, although present histopathologically in 50% to 90% patients with leukaemia, is rarely detectable clinically. In acute lymphoid leukaemia, choroidal infiltration produces a localized or diffuse tumour, a shallow serous retinal detachment secondary to pinpoint leaks in the pigment epithelium, pigment epithelium alterations.
In myeloid leukaemia, uveal or orbital granulocytic sarcoma (formerly called "chloroma") may be revealing. A maskerade inflammatory aspect may induce diagnostic delay.

Histopathology. The histopathological diagnosis can be made on orbital tissue before blood disorders occur, through histochemical staining procedures (Leder stain) or immunohisto-chemistry (Lysozyme). The prognosis is poor.

Lymphoid infiltrates – small cell lymphoplasmacytic lymphomas (former reactive lymphoid hyperplasia)

Clinical features. In this site, as well as in the orbit, immunohistochemical studies have shown that these tumours, presenting clinically as diffuse melanomas, are most often monoclonal. Response to corticosteroids may be a diagnostic tool.

Malignant cerebro-retinal lymphoma (histiocytic lymphoma, non-hodgkin lymphoma, former reticulum cell sarcoma

Clinical features. These are "large cell" lymphomas involving both the central nervous system, the uveal tract, retina and vitreous. The most common clinical aspect is severe chronic vitritis, with multiple yellowish, placoïd, sharply demarcated, infiltrates with pigment clumping. Vitreous aspiration may show tumour cells and lead to oculocerebral radiation therapy.

XXIV.5 Metastatic carcinomas

Clinical features. They represent the more common uveal tumours. Clinically they are often multiple, lightly pigmented, slightly elevated and often associated with mottled pigmentation and overlying retinal serous detachment. The primary cancer is most frequently found in the breast in females and in the lung in males.

XXIV.4 Leucémies et lymphomes

Infiltrats leucémiques

Clinique. L'atteinte uvéale, présente histologiquement chez 50 à 90% des patients, est rarement décelée cliniquement. Elle revêt, le plus souvent dans la leucémie lymphoïde aiguë, la forme d'une tumeur diffuse ou localisée, d'un soulèvement séreux rétinien lié à des points de fuite au niveau de l'épithélium pigmentaire, de remaniements de cet épithélium.
Dans les leucémies myéloïdes, un sarcome granulocytaire (ex chlorome) uvéal ou orbitaire peut être inaugural. Un tableau inflammatoire peut égarer cliniquement.

Histopathologie. Le diagnostic précis, avant même que les anomalies sanguines ne surviennent, peut être établi grâce à des colorations histochimiques (Leder) ou immunohistochimiques (Lysozyme). Le pronostic est mauvais.

Infiltrats lymphoïdes – lymphomes lymphoplasmocytiques à petites cellules (ancien hyperplasie lymphoïde réactionnelle)

Clinique. Comme dans l'orbite, l'étude immunohistochimique a montré que ces tumeurs, dont l'aspect clinique est celui des mélanomes diffus, sont le plus souvent monoclonales. Le test aux corticoïdes peut représenter une épreuve diagnostique.

Lymphome malin cérébro-rétinien (lymphome histiocytique ou non hodgkinien, ancien réticulosarcome)

Clinique. Ce sont des lymphomes à grandes cellules touchant l'uvée, la rétine, le vitré, le système nerveux central. L'aspect clinique est celui d'une uvéite torpide sévère, avec multiples placards jaunâtres saupoudrés de pigment, à bords nets.
Une ponction aspiration vitréenne peut montrer des cellules tumorales et conduire à une irradiation oculocérébrale.

XXIV.5 Carcinomes métastatiques

Clinique. Ce sont les plus fréquentes des tumeurs uvéales. Cliniquement ces tumeurs, souvent multiples, peu pigmentées, peu élevées, sont souvent associées à une pigmentation en mottes et à un soulèvement séreux susjacents. Le carcinome primitif est retrouvé le plus souvent au niveau mammaire chez la femme, pulmonaire chez l'homme.

XXIV.4 Leukämien und Lymphome

Leukämische Infiltrate

Klinik. Die bei 50 bis 90% der Patienten eingetretene Schädigung der Uvea wird selten klinisch festgestellt; sie tritt zumeist bei der akuten lymphatischen Leukämie in Form eines diffusen oder lokalisierten Tumors, einer serösen Netzhautabhebung, die mit Leckstellen auf der Ebene des Pigmentepithels in Zusammenhang steht, sowie reaktiven Veränderungen dieses Epithels auf.
Bei den myeloischen Leukämien kann ein granulozytäres Sarkom (Ex-Chlorom) der Uvea oder der Orbita das erste Anzeichen sein. Ein entzündlicher Zustand kann klinisch irreführen.

Histopathologie. Eine präzise Diagnose noch vor dem Auftreten von Blutanomalien kann mit histochemischen (Leder) oder immunhistochemischen Färbungen (Lysozyme) erzielt werden. Die Prognose ist schlecht.

Lymphatische Infiltrate – "lymphoplasmozytäre Kleinzellenlymphome" (früher reaktive lymphoide Hyperplasie)

Klinik. Wie bei der Orbita hat die immunhistochemische Untersuchung gezeigt, daß diese Tumoren, deren klinischer Aspekt dem der diffusen Melanome entspricht, meist monoklonal sind. Der Kortikoidtest kann diagnostische Hinweise geben.

Malignes Zerebro-retinales Lymphom (Histiozyten- oder non Hodgkinsches Lymphom, früher Retikulosarkom)

Klinik. Dies sind großzellige Lymphome, von denen die Uvea, die Netzhaut, der Glaskörper, das zentrale Nervensystem betroffen sein können. Das klinische Bild ist das einer schweren torpiden Uveitis mit vielfachen gelblichen, deutlich geränderten, pigmentübersäten Feldern. Mit einer Punktion und Aspiration des Glaskörpers können Tumorzellen nachgewiesen werden und zu einer okular-zerebralen Bestrahlung veranlassen.

XXIV.5 Metastasen

Klinik. Dies sind die häufigsten Uveatumoren. Klinisch gehen die oft multiplen, wenig pigmentierten, kaum erhabenen Geschwülste meist mit einer darüberliegenden fleckig-scholligen Pigmentierung und serösen Erhebung einher. Das Primärkarzinom befindet sich bei der Frau zumeist in der Brust, beim Mann in der Lunge.

PLATE 54 PLANCHE 54 TAFEL 54

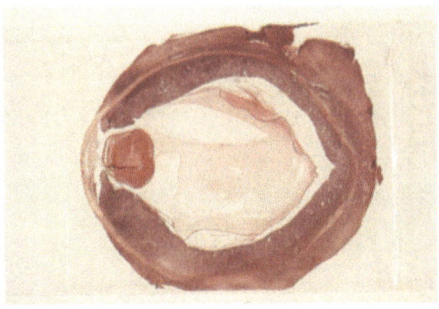

a

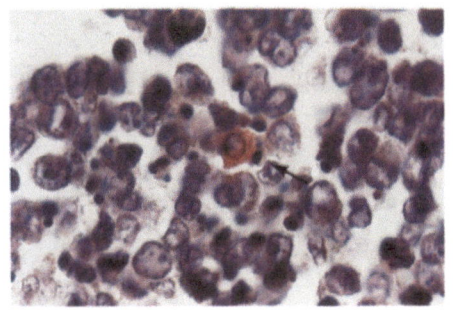

b

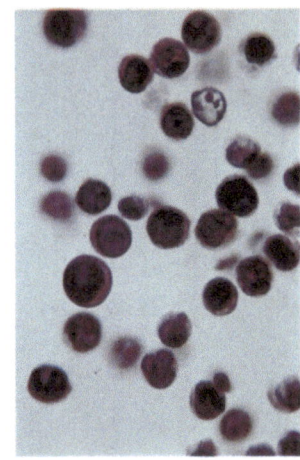

c

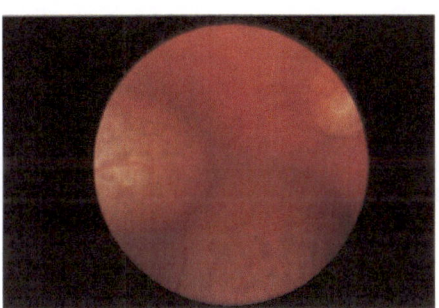

d

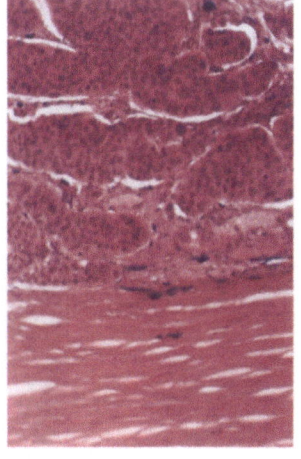

e

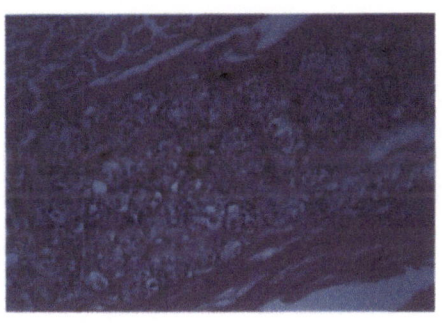

f

Fig. a. Granulocytic sarcoma of the uvea.
Massive diffuse uveal thickening with tumour cell infiltrates.

Fig. b. Continued.
Eosinophilic myelogenous leukemic cells are stained red with Leder's method (Naphtol ASD Chloracetate) (→).

Fig. c. Malignant oculocerebral lymphoma (reticulum cell sarcoma).
Vitreous aspirate: large cells with scanty cytoplasm and pleomorphic atypical, round, slightly indented nuclei with coarse chromatin and distinct nucleoli.

Fig. d. Fundus photograph.
Multiple choroidal metastases from lung adenocarcinoma.

Fig. e. Histopathology: Metastatic pulmonary adenocarcinoma.
Malignant epithelial cells with ill-defined borders, nuclear atypia and arrangement in lobules. Normal melanocytes are compressed at the base of the tumour.

Fig. f. Histopathology: metastatic breast carcinoma.
Adenomatous features with acinar like structures.

Fig. a. Sarcome granulocytaire uvéal.
Infiltration uvéale diffuse et massive par les cellules tumorales.

Fig. b. Suite.
Cellules leucémiques de la lignée éosinophile se colorant en rouge par la méthode de Leder (Naphtol ASD Chloracétate) (→).

Fig. c. Liquide d'aspiration vitréenne.
Lymphome malin cérébro-rétinien (ex. réticulo-sarcome). Grandes cellules à cytoplasme peu abondant, noyaux arrondis, légèrement indentés, pléomorphiques, à chromatine dense et nucléole visible.

Fig. d. Fond d'oeil.
Métastases choroïdiennes diffuses d'un adénocarcinome pulmonaire.

Fig. e. Histopathologie: adénocarcinome pulmonaire métastatique.
Cellules épithéliales malignes à limites imprécises, avec atypies nucléaires et arrangement en lobules. Les mélanocytes normaux sont comprimés à la base de la tumeur.

Fig. f. Histopathologie: carcinome mammaire métastatique.
Aspect adénomateux avec structures pseudo-acineuses.

Abb. a. Granulozytäres Sarkom der Uvea.
Diffuse und massive Tumorzelleninfiltration in der Uvea.

Abb. b. Fortsetzung.
Leukämiezellen der eosinophilen Reihe, die sich mit der Leder-Methode (Naphtol ASD Chlorazetat) rot färben (→).

Abb. c. Aspirierte Glaskörperflüssigkeit.
Bösartiges zerebro-retinales Lymphom (früher Retikulosarkom). Große Zellen mit spärlichem Zytoplasma und rundlichem Kern, pleomorph, mit dichtem Chromatin. Die Kernmembran ist häufig eingekerbt.

Abb. d. Augenhintergrund.
Diffuse Aderhautmetastasen eines Lungenadenokarzinoms.

Abb. e. Histopathologie: Metastatisches Lungenadenokarzinom.
Bösartige epitheliale Zellen, ungenau abgegrenzt und Kernatypien, lappenförmig angeordnet. Die normalen Melanozyten sind an der Tumorbasis zusammengepreßt.

Abb. f. Histopathologie: Metastatisches Brustkarzinom.
Adenomatöses Aussehen mit pseudo-azinären Strukturen.

D

Tumours of the retina and the optic disc

*

Tumeurs de la rétine et de la papille optique

*

Geschwülste der Netzhaut und der Papille

PLATE 55   PLANCHE 55   TAFEL 55

XXV. MALIGNANT TUMOUR RETINOBLASTOMA

Clinical features. This rare tumour found in small children (one case in 20000 viable new-born infants) is sometimes bilateral. Provided that its detection and treatment are early, its prognosis is relatively favourable (85% survival rate after five years). Leucocoria behind a transparent lens or monocular strabismus are the most frequent primary clinical features. Certain clinical varieties deserve a special mention, in spite of their rarity:

- retinoblastoma in the older child, with its diffuse type of growth and with a pseudohypopyon;
- a type with massive spontaneous necrosis resulting in phthisis bulbi: histologically, viable tumour cells are surrounded by areas of necrosis. Such a possibility makes enucleation of phthisis bulbi without obvious etiology essential in early childhood;
- regressive retinoblastoma is sometimes discovered in parents of affected children during a routine examination;
- exceptionally a bilateral retinoblastoma can be associated with a pinealoma ("trilateral retinoblastoma").

In the anterior segment of the eye, rubeosis or pseudohypopyon can make the diagnosis difficult. Glaucoma, sometimes with buphthalmos, can be the consequence of rubeosis or of the presence of tumour cells in the trabeculum. The tumour can spread into the vitreous body, forming large spherical whitish seedlings which are easily seen with the slit lamp and are very different from the opacities of the vitreous body in uveitis; these "snowballs" are pathognomonic of retinoblastoma. This tumour may also extend to the optic nerve. Clinically, CAT is indispensable and may then show an enlargement of the retrobulbar optic nerve. During enucleation, the nerve must always be sectioned far behind the globe. The pathologist cuts the nerve right behind the sclera and performs transversal sections for histology. If invasion of the optic nerve is present and goes farther than the surgical section, additional treatment is necessary. Massive invasion of the choroid is rare; it also makes the prognosis worse and requires a change in therapy.

XXV. TUMEUR MALIGNE RÉTINOBLASTOME

Aspects cliniques. Tumeur maligne de la première enfance, peu fréquente (1 sur 20000 naissances viables) le rétinoblastome, souvent bilatéral, doit être dépisté et traité précocément. A cette condition son pronostic est relativement bon (85% de survie après 5 ans). La leucocorie derrière un cristallin clair, le strabisme monoculaire, sont les signes d'appel les plus fréquents. Diverses formes cliniques, bien que rares, méritent d'être connues:

- une forme du grand enfant à croissance diffuse avec pseudo-hypopyon;
- une forme avec nécrose massive spontanée aboutissant à l'atrophie du globe. L'histologie montre la présence de cellules tumorales encore viables entourées de plages de nécrose. Une phtise oculaire inexpliquée du petit enfant doit donc être énucléée;
- la forme régressive, rare, observée chez l'adulte lors d'enquêtes familiales;
- une forme exceptionnelle associant une atteinte oculaire bilatérale à une localisation à la glande pinéale (rétinoblastome "trilatéral").

Dans le segment antérieur la tumeur peut provoquer un rubeosis ou encore un pseudo-hypopyon par dépôt de cellules tumorales qui peut prêter à confusion avec une uvéite si les milieux sont troubles. Un glaucome, avec buphtalmie parfois, peut être la conséquence du rubeosis ou de l'encombrement du trabéculum par les cellules néoplasiques. La tumeur peut essaimer dans le vitré sous forme de masses sphéroïdes blanchâtres, ("snowballs") bien visibles à la lampe à fente, très différentes du trouble du vitré accompagnant une uvéite, et tout-à-fait pathognomoniques. Elle peut envahir le nerf optique dont l'épaississement peut être recherché en tomodensitométrie. A l'intervention le nerf doit toujours être sectionné loin du globe. Au laboratoire il est coupé au ras du globe, puis examiné en coupes transversales. L'envahissement au-delà du point de section impose un traitement complémentaire à la chirurgie. L'envahissement massif de la choroïde, rare, aggrave également le pronostic.

XXV. BÖSARTIGE GESCHWÜLSTE DER NETZHAUT RETINOBLASTOM

Klinik. Das Retinoblastom, eine eher seltene (1 von 20000 lebensfähigen Geburten), oft beidseitig auftretende bösartige Geschwulst des Kleinkindes, muß frühzeitig erkannt und behandelt werden. Unter dieser Voraussetzung ist die Prognose verhältnismäßg günstig (85% Überlebenschancen nach 5 Jahren). Leukokorie hinter einer hellen Linse, einseitiger Strabismus sind die häufigsten Signale. Verschiedene, wenngleich seltene klinische Formen bedürfen besonderer Erwähung:

- auftreten beim älteren Kind, diffus wachsend, mit Pseudo-hypopyon;
- eine Form mit spontaner massiver Nekrose, die zu einer Atrophie des Bulbus führt. Die Histologie zeigt das Vorhandensein noch lebensfähiger, von Nekrosefeldern umgebener Tumorzellen. Bei einer unklaren Phthisis bulbi bei einem Kleinkind ist deshalb eine Enukleation notwendig;
- die seltene regressive Form, die beim Erwachsenen anläßlich Familienuntersuchungen beobachtet wird;
- außergewöhnliche Fälle, wo zu der beidseitigen Augenerkrankung ein pineales Retinoblastom hinzukommt ("trilaterales" Retinoblastom).

Im vorderen Segment kann der Tumor eine Rubeosis oder ein Pseudohypopyon durch Tumorzellablagerung hervorrufen, was mit einer Uveitis verwechselt werden kann, wenn die Medien trübe sind. Die Rubeosis oder die Trabekelüberschwemmung mit neoplastischen Zellen kann ein Glaukom – manchmal mit Buphtalmus – zur Folge haben. Die Geschwulst kann in Form weißlicher, mit der Spaltlampe gut sichtbarer rundlicher Massen ("snowballs") in den Glaskörper ausschwärmen; diese sind von einer mit einer Uveitis einhergehenden Trübung des Glaskörpers völlig verschieden und ganz und gar pathognomonisch. Sie kann auf den Nervus opticus übergreifen, bei dem per Tomodensitometrie nach einer Verdickung zu suchen ist. Bei der Operation muß der Nerv stets weit vom Bulbus abgetrennt werden. Im Labor wird er direkt am Bulbus abgeschnitten und in Querschnitten untersucht. Eine Ausdehnung über den Durchtrennungsschnitt hinaus macht neben der Chirurgie eine zusätzliche Behandlung erforderlich. Das seltene massive Eindringen in die Aderhaut verschlechtert die Prognose ebenfalls.

PLATE 55　　　　　　　PLANCHE 55　　　　　　　TAFEL 55

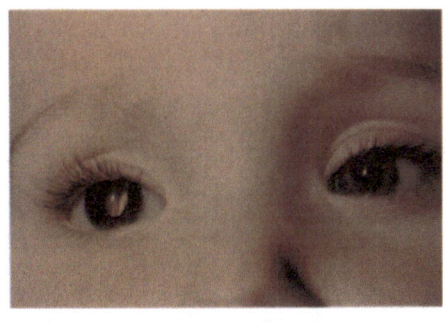

a

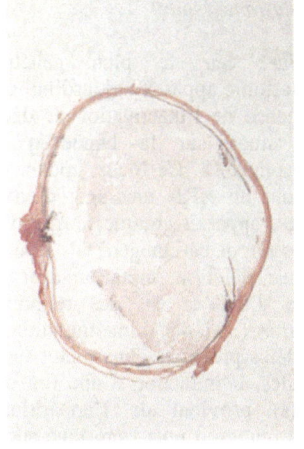

b

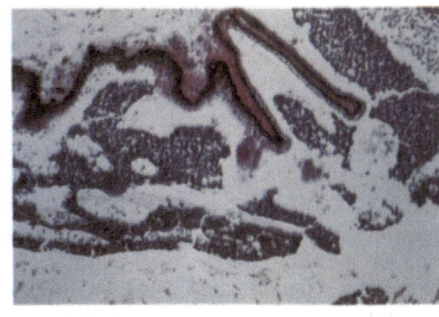

c

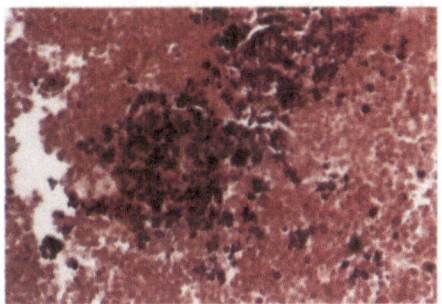

d

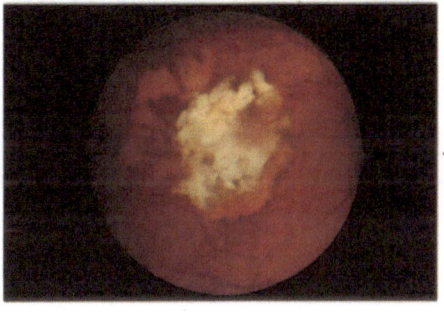

e

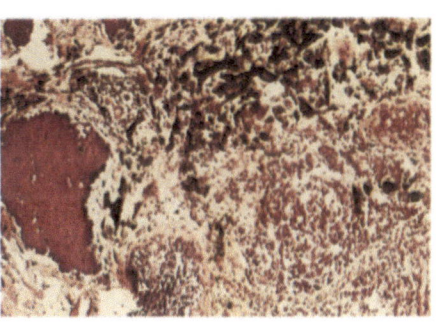

f

Fig. a. Leucocoria with a whitish vascularized tumour recognizable behind the lens.

Fig. b. Diffuse variety, with a flat type of growth and mimicking an anterior uveitis with hypopyon. These two features combine to make the diagnosis all the more difficult.

Fig. c. Histopathology of this diffuse variety in the area of the ciliary body.
It is worth noticing that the invasion of the optic nerve is also possible in this type.

Fig. d. Phthisis bulbi. Tumour cells surrounded by an area of necrotic tissue. It is remarkable that this can happen in phthisis bulbi, but never in microphthalmia.

Fig. e. The regressive type is clinically similar to the scar of a retinoblastoma which has been treated by irradiation: area of atrophic tissue with more or less abundant deposits of calcium.

Fig. f. Histopathology of regressive retinoblastoma. Tumour cells and areas of calcification.

Fig. a. Leucocorie avec masses blanches vascularisées rétrolentales.

Fig. b. Forme diffuse de rétinoblastome, évoluant à plat, accompagnée d'un pseudohypopyon, deux raisons pour en rendre le diagnostic difficile.

Fig. c. Aspect histopathologique au niveau du corps ciliaire d'une forme diffuse.
Il faut noter qu'au pôle postérieur l'envahissement du nerf optique est possible dans cette forme, malgré une évolution lente.

Fig. d. Dans un globe en phtise, présence de tissu de nécrose au sein duquel on découvre des cellules de rétinoblastome. Notons que cette tumeur, par contre, ne se développe jamais sur un oeil microphtalme.

Fig. e. La forme régressive se présente cliniquement comme une cicatrice de rétinoblastome traité par irradiation: plage d'atrophie plus ou moins calcifiée.

Fig. f. Rétinoblastome régressif.
Plages calcifiées et cellules tumorales.

Abb. a. Leukokorie mit weißen vaskularisierten, retrolentalen Massen.

Abb. b. Diffuse Retinoblastom-Form, die sich flach ausdehnt, begleitet von einem Pseudo-Hypopyon, zwei Gründe, die die Diagnose erschweren können.

Abb. c. Histopathologischer Aspekt einer diffusen Form auf Höhe des Ziliarkörpers.
Zu beachten ist, daß bei dieser Form trotz langsamer Entwicklung am hinteren Pol eine Invasion des Sehnervs möglich ist.

Abb. d. In einem phthisischen Bulbus vorhandenes Nekrosegewebe, in dem Retinoblastomzellen anzutreffen sind. Hier muß gesagt werden, daß sich dieser Tumor nie auf einem Mikrophthalmus entwickelt.

Abb. e. Die regressive Form stellt sich klinisch wie eine Retinoblastomnarbe nach Bestrahlung dar: mehr oder weniger kalzifiziertes Atrophiefeld.

Abb. f. Regressives Retinoblastom.
Kalzifizierte Felder und Tumorzellen.

Retinoblastoma (continued)

Genetic aspects. Retinoblastoma appears today as the consequence of the inactivation of both alleles of a gene located on the q 1.4 band of chromosome 13. This locus, encoding in normal situations a RNA messenger of about 4,7 kilobases, is seen as a "cancer suppressor gene". It can be inactivated by deletion or mutation with loss of function. In hereditary retinoblastoma (30% to 40%) a mutation in one of the two allele loci is present in all germinal cells. Induction of one (or more) tumour(s) stems from the occurrence of a second postzygotic mutation on the allele locus in one (or more) somatic cell(s) (i.e. retinoblasts). In non-hereditary retinoblastoma both mutations occur at the somatic level in the same cell. For this reason, such tumours are unique (one focus, one eye) and exceptional.

Rétinoblastome (suite)

Génétique. Sur le plan génétique, le rétinoblastome apparaît aujourd'hui comme la conséquence de l'inactivation de deux gènes allèles situés sur la bande q 1.4 des chromosomes 13. Ce locus, codant normalement pour un ARN messager d'environ 4,7 kilobases, apparaît comme le site d'un gène "suppresseur de carcinogénèse". Il peut être inactivé par délétion, mutation avec perte de fonction. Dans le cas des rétinoblastomes héréditaires (30 à 40%) une mutation d'un des deux allèles préexiste dans toutes les cellules germinales. L'induction d'une (ou plusieurs) tumeur(s) provient de l'apparition d'une seconde mutation post-zygotique sur le locus allèle d'une (ou plusieurs) cellule(s) somatique(s) (rétinoblastes). Dans la forme non héréditaire les deux mutations surviennent au niveau somatique dans une même cellule. Pour cette raison, de telles tumeurs sont uniques (un foyer, un seul oeil) et exceptionnelles.

Retinoblastom (Fortsetzung)

Genetik. In genetischer Hinsicht wird heute das Auftreten des Retinoblastoms als Folge der Inaktivierung von zwei Allel-Genen angesehen, die auf dem Band q 1,4 der Chromosomen 13 lokalisiert sind. Diese Stelle, normalerweise für eine RNS von 4,7 Kilobasen kodiert, gilt als Standort für ein "Karzinogenese-Repressor-Gen". Sie kann durch Deletion, – Mutation mit Funktionsverlust – inaktiviert werden. Bei vererbten Retinoblastomen (30 bis 40%) präexistiert eine Mutation eines der beiden Allele in sämtlichen Keimzellen. Die Induktion eines Tumors (oder mehrerer Tumoren) kommt zustande, indem auf dem Allel-Standort eine zweite postzygotische Mutation einer (oder mehrerer) somatischer Zelle(n) (Retinoblasten) stattfindet. Bei der nicht hereditären Form erfolgen die beiden Mutationen auf somatischer Ebene in ein und derselben Zelle. Deshalb treten solche Tumoren einzeln (ein Herd, ein einziges Auge) und nur ausnahmsweise auf.

PLATE 56 PLANCHE 56 TAFEL 56

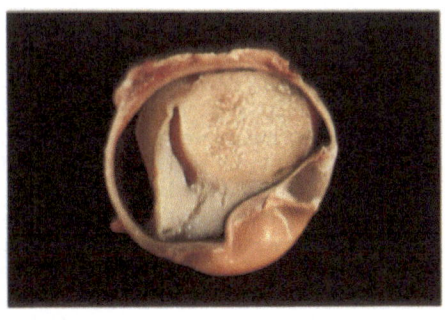

a

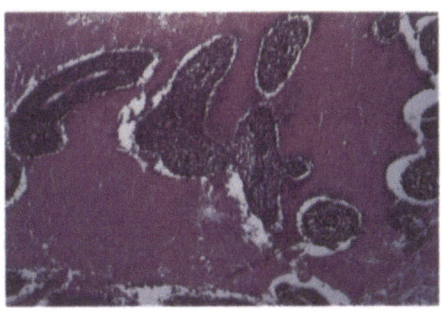

b

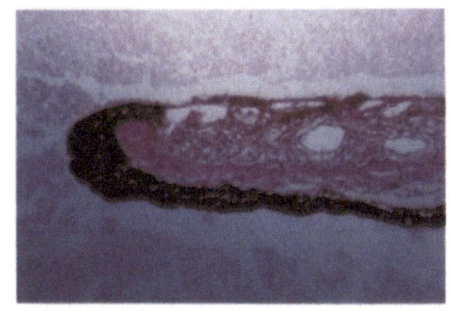

c

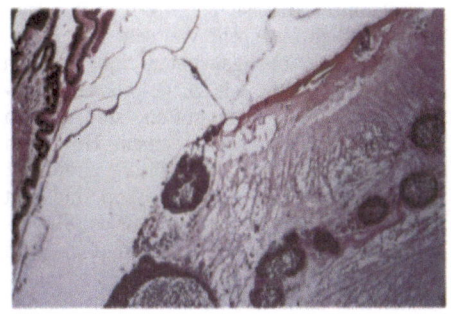

d

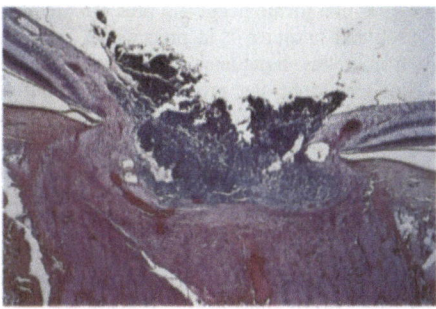

e

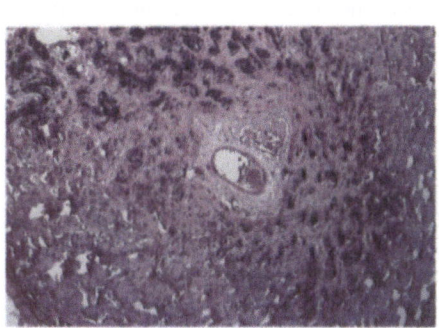

f

Fig. a. Gross examination. Yellowish tumour, of granular consistency, showing scattered deposits of calcium, which are almost constant.

Fig. b. At low power, perivascular growth, with necrosis at some distance from the vessels.

Fig. c. Usual signs of rubeosis iridis: Neovascularization of the anterior limiting layer, ectropion uveae due to peripheral anterior synechiae. This is one of the causes of glaucoma, and of the corneal oedema which can make the diagnosis difficult.

Fig. d. Histopathological aspect of the spherical intra-vitreous floaters which are easily recognizable with the slit lamp, and pathognomonic.

Fig. e. The posterior extension is sometimes restricted to the optic disc.

Fig. f. If the invasion of the optic nerve (seen here on a perpendicular section), goes farther than the surgical section, there is a great risk of extension to the orbit and distant metastases.

Fig. a. Examen macroscopique. Masse jaunâtre, de consistance grumeleuse, parsemée de dépôts calcaires, quasi constants.

Fig. b. Au faible grossissement, disposition périthéliale caractéristique; nécrose à distance des vaisseaux.

Fig. c. Le rubeosis s'accompage de ses signes habituels: Vascularisation de la face antérieure de l'iris, ectropion de l'uvée, par synéchies antérieures périphériques. Il est l'une des causes du glaucome (avec buphtalmie parfois), dont l'opacité cornéenne peut cacher la tumeur.

Fig. d. Aspect histopathologique des masses intra-vitréennes bien visibles à la lampe à fente et pathognomoniques.

Fig. e. L'extension postérieure peut se limiter à la papille.

Fig. f. Lorsqu'elle touche le nerf optique (vu ici en coupe transversale), au-delà de son point de section, elle est le prélude à l'envahissement de l'orbite et à la généralisation.

Abb. a. Bei makroskopischer Untersuchung gelbliche Masse von krümeliger Konsistenz, praktisch immer mit Kalkablagerungen übersät.

Abb. b. Bei schwacher Vergrößerung charakteristische peritheliale Anordnung; Nekrose in Abstand von den Gefäßen.

Abb. c. Die Rubeosis geht mit den gewohnten Anzeichen einer: Vaskularisierung der Irisvorderseite, Ectropium uveae, durch periphere vordere Synechien. Sie ist eine der Ursachen des Glaukoms (manchmal mit Buphthalmus), dessen Hornhauttrübung die Geschwulst verdecken kann.

Abb. d. Histopathologischer Aspekt der an der Spaltlampe deutlich sichtbaren und ganz und gar pathognomonischen Massen im Innern des Glaskörpers.

Abb. e. Die Ausdehnung nach hinten kann sich auf die Papille beschränken.

Abb. f. Wenn der Nervus opticus (hier im Querschnitt gesehen) über die Durchtrennungsstelle hinaus erfaßt ist, so steht die Invasion der Orbita und die Generalisierung bevor.

121

PLATE 57   PLANCHE 57   TAFEL 57

Retinoblastoma (continued)

Histopathology. Gross examination shows a tumour of a creamy colour, usually presenting white spots, which are actually small deposits of calcium: the latter can be detected beforehand by medical imaging, and are thus of great diagnostic importance, especially if the media have lost their transparency. In the sections these deposits are seen under low power in a tumour with a predominantly perivascular growth, and which becomes necrotic at some distance from the vessels.

Three *cytological* varieties of retinoblastoma are described:
- the undifferentiated type is formed of cells with strongly basophilic nuclei, a scanty cytoplasm, and presenting some mitotic activity;
- a more differentiated type characterized by spherical structures with clear centres, the so-called Flexner-Wintersteiner rosettes;
- a much rarer type is mostly seen in association with the preceding one: it shows small bunches of elongated cells, which end in a relatively large cavity or are arranged in an arc of circle (Tso's "Fleurettes"). Electron microscopy shows the characteristic anatomical features of the photoreceptors.

Unfortunately it is not possible so far to define a precise relationship between these cytological varieties and the prognosis. The latter depends more on early detection and treatment, and on the possible invasion of the optic nerve and/or the choroid.

Differential diagnosis. The diagnosis of retinoblastoma needs differentiation from other diseases which may give rise to a white mass in the pupil behind a transparent lens: retrolental fibroplasia, mostly bilateral and usually linked to oxygenotherapy in case of prematurity; severe uveitis followed by total retinal detachment; congenital retinal dysplasia, which is usually bilateral, and often associated with several systemic syndromes; hyperplastic primary vitreous, unilateral, mostly in a microphthalmic eye; morning glory syndrome, congenital abnormality of the optic disc in which the glial proliferation in front of the disc may sometimes mimic a tumour. But the presence of a cataractous lens does not exclude the diagnosis of retinoblastoma.

Rétinoblastome (suite)

Histopathologie. L'examen macroscopique montre une tumeur de teinte crémeuse contenant presque toujours des points blancs. Ces calcifications sont repérables préalablement grâce à l'imagerie médicale: elles ont de ce fait une grande importance diagnostique, surtout lorsque les milieux sont troubles. On les retrouve au microscope où le faible grossissement montre une tumeur à disposition périthéliale, mais se nécrosant à distance des vaisseaux.

Sur le plan cytologique, trois formes sont connues:
- une forme indifférenciée formée de cellules à petits noyaux fortement basophiles, au cytoplasme peu abondant, et présentant des mitoses;
- une forme plus différenciée caractérisée par la présence de formations sphériques à centre clair, les rosettes de Wintersteiner;
- enfin une forme beaucoup plus rare, le plus souvent associée à la précédente, où l'on trouve des bouquets de cellules très allongées dont les prolongements aboutissent à une cavité ou se disposent en arc de cercle ("Fleurettes" de Tso); en microscopie électronique on y retrouve les éléments caractéristiques des cellules visuelles.

Malheureusement rien ne permet actuellement d'affirmer qu'il existe une relation entre ces variétés cytologiques et le pronostic. Ce dernier est lié surtout à la précocité du diagnostic et du traitement, et à l'état du nerf optique et de la choroïde.

Diagnostic différentiel. Le diagnostic différentiel se pose surtout avec d'autres leucocories, atteintes rétiniennes ou rétino-vitréennes sévères derrière un cristallin clair: fibroplasie rétrolentale, bilatérale, liée le plus souvent à l'oxygénothérapie du prématuré; uvéite grave ayant abouti à un décollement total de la rétine; dysplasie rétinienne congénitale, bilatérale dont diverses variantes sont connues; persistance avec hyperplasie du vitré primitif, unilatérale, sur un oeil souvent microphtalme; morning glory syndrome, anomalie congénitale de la papille dans laquelle une masse gliale prépapillaire peut parfois simuler une tumeur. Cependant la présence d'une cataracte ne permet pas d'écarter le diagnostic de rétinoblastome.

Retinoblastom (Fortsetzung)

Histopathologie. Bei der makroskopischen Untersuchung zeigt sich ein cremefarbener Tumor, der fast immer weiße Punkte enthält. Diese Kalzifizierungen sind zuvor schon auf dem bildtechnischen Material erkennbar: Sie sind daher von großer Bedeutung für die Diagnose, besonders wenn die Augenmedien trübe sind. Sie sind wieder unter dem Mikroskop anzutreffen, wo bei schwacher Vergrößerung ein perithelialer Tumor, der in Gefäßentfernung nekrotisch wird, zu sehen ist.

In zytologischer Hinsicht sind drei Formen bekannt:
- eine undifferenzierte Form, bestehend aus Zellen mit kleinen, stark basophilen Kernen, spärlichem Zytoplasma, die Mitosen aufweisen;
- eine differenziertere Form, die durch das Vorhandensein kugeliger Gebilde mit hellem Zentrum, den Wintersteiner-Rosetten, gekennzeichnet ist;
- schließlich eine sehr viel seltenere Form, die mit der obengenannten einhergeht, in der Zellsträuße mit ausgesprochen länglichen Zellen anzutreffen sind, deren Verlängerungen bis zu einem Hohlraum reichen oder sich bogenförmig anordnen; unter dem Elektronenmikroskop sind dort die charakteristischen Elemente der Sinneszellen zu erkennen ("Fleurettes" nach Tso).

Leider läßt bisher nichts den Schluß zu, daß ein Zusammenhang zwischen diesen zytologischen Formen und der Prognose besteht. Diese letztere hängt hauptsächlich von der frühzeitig gestellten Diagnose und unternommenen Behandlung, sowie vom Zustand des Sehnervs und der Aderhaut ab.

Differential Diagnose. Die Differentialdiagnose wird hauptsächlich zwischen anderen Leukokorien, schweren Netzhaut- oder Netzhaut-Glaskörpererkrankungen hinter einer hellen Linse gestellt; retrolentale Fibroplasie, die meist bilateral und auf Sauerstofftherapie bei Frühgeborenen zurückzuführen ist; schwere Uveitis, die zu einer völligen Netzhautablösung geführt hat; kongenitale bilaterale Netzhautdysplasie, von der verschiedene Varianten bekannt sind; Persistenz mit Hyperplasie des primären Glaskörpers, einseitig, auf einem oft mikrophthalmischen Auge; Morning glory-Syndrom, kongenitale Anomalie der Papille, in der eine präpapilläre Gliamasse manchmal einen Tumor vortäuschen kann. Jedoch läßt das Vorhandensein einer Linsentrübung ein Retinoblastom nicht ausschließen.

PLATE 57 PLANCHE 57 TAFEL 57

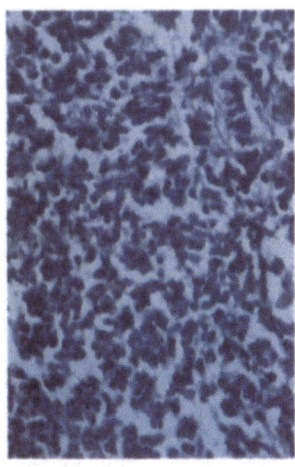

a

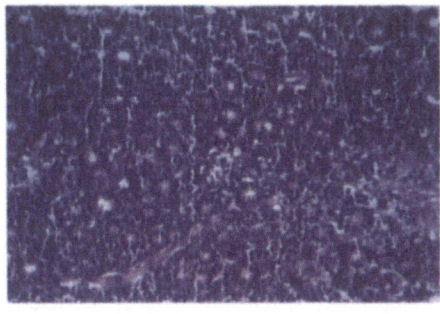

b

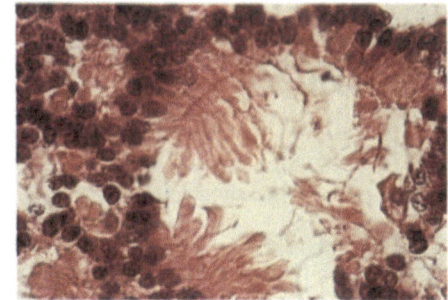

c

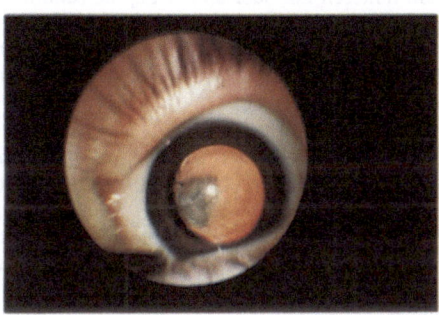

d

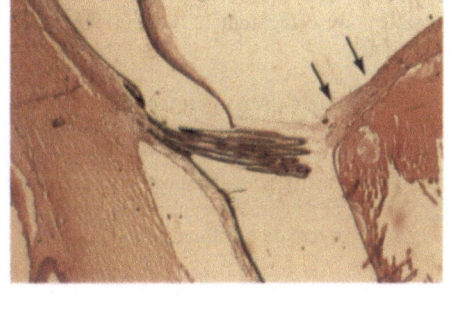

e

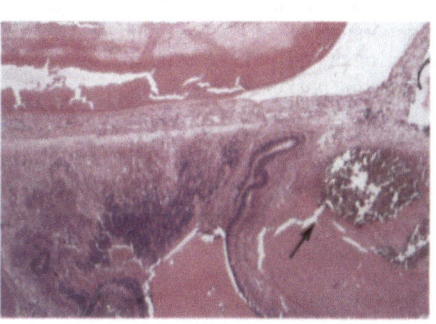

f

Fig. a. Undifferentiated variety.
Marked basophilia of the nuclei; scarcity of the cytoplasm.

Fig. b. Flexner-Wintersteiner rosettes.
The aspect under low power has been compared to a flower bed. They differ from Homer-Wright rosettes, which present a fibrillar centre and are less distinctive.

Fig. c. Clusters of well differentiated visual cells (Tso's "fleurettes").
The outer segments of the photoreceptors converge towards large cavities.

Fig. d. Retro-illumination from the fundus in persistant hyperplastic vitreous.
The retrolental mass is visible, and also one elongated ciliary process (at nine o'clock), which is characteristic of the presence of retractile retrolental tissue.

Fig. e. Histopathology of hyperplastic primary vitreous.
Equator of the lens to the right. Retrolental tissue (⇉) and elongated ciliary process.

Fig. f. Norrie's disease – Retinal detachment with dysplasia (the lens is at the top of the picture).
Retinal folds; pseudo-rosettes with quasi-normal retinal layers. The pseudocystic cavity on the right (→) is the result of a haemorrhage, a frequent complication in this disease.

Fig. a. Forme indifférenciée.
Noyaux fortement basophiles, cytoplasme réduit.

Fig. b. Rosettes de Flexner-Wintersteiner.
Les Rosettes donnent au faible grossissement l'aspect en "parterre de fleurs". Elles se distinguent des rosettes de Homer-Wright, moins caractéristiques, dépourvues de cavité centrale.

Fig. c. Bouquets de cellules visuelles fortement différenciées ("fleurettes" de Tso).
Articles externes convergeant par leur extrémité vers de larges formations cavitaires.

Fig. d. Lueur pupillaire dans une persistance du vitré primitif.
On aperçoit la masse rétrolentale, et un procès ciliaire étiré (sur l'axe de 9 H).

Fig. e. Image histopathologique d'une persistance de vitré primitif.
On aperçoit l'équateur du cristallin à droite, et la masse rétrolentale (⇉), attirant les procès ciliaires.

Fig. f. Maladie de Norrie – Décollement rétinien avec dysplasie (cristallin en haut).
Plissements rétiniens; pseudo-rosettes. La formation pseudokystique à droite (→) est un épanchement de sang, fréquent dans cette variété de dysplasie rétinienne.

Abb. a. Undifferenzierte Form.
Stark basophile Kerne, spärliches Zytoplasma.

Abb. b. Flexner-Wintersteiner-Rosetten.
Die schwache Vergrößerung ergibt ein "blumenbeetartiges" Aussehen. Sie unterscheiden sich von den weniger bezeichnenden Homer-Wright-Rosetten, die keinen zentralen Hohlraum besitzen.

Abb. c. Sträuße stark differenzierter Sinneszellen (Tso-"Fleurettes").
Die äußeren Glieder laufen mit ihren Enden zu weiten Hohlgebilden zusammen.

Abb. d. Pupillenleuchten bei persistierendem primärem Glaskörper.
Man bemerkt die retrolentale Masse und einen (im 9-Meridian) ausgezogenen Ziliarfortsatz.

Abb. e. Histopathologisches Bild bei einem persistierenden primären Glaskörper.
Rechts der Linsenäquator, die retrolentale Masse (⇉), welche die Ziliarfortsätze an sich heranzieht.

Abb. f. Norrie-Krankheit – Netzhautablösung mit Dysplasie (Linse oben).
Netzhautfalten, Pseudorosetten. Das pseudozystische Gebilde rechts (→) ist ein Bluterguß, wie er bei dieser Art von Netzhautdysplasie häufig vorkommt.

PLATE 58 PLANCHE 58 TAFEL 58

XXVI. GLIAL TUMOURS OF THE RETINA AND THE OPTIC DISC

XXVI.1 Astrocytoma (Phakomatoses)

Clinical features. Tuberous sclerosis (Bourneville, 1880) is one of the phako-matoses. It is congenital and hereditary, and remarkable for the development of multiple tumours of the skin, the brain, several viscera, the kidney mostly. The most striking clinical features are mental deficiency, epilepsy, and small tumours of the face which are angio-fibromas (the former "sebaceous adenomas" of Pringle, a terminology recalling the simultaneous hyperplasia of the dermal sebaceous glands). Death by cerebral tumour occurs usually before 25. Ophthalmoscopy may show, on the posterior retina or on the optic disc, hemispherical, white or greyish tumours, sometimes with a mulberry-like sur-face, of the size of the optic disc or slightly larger: the phakomas.

Histopathology. These lesions are superfi-cially located, at the level of the nerve fibre layer. They are glial tumours, made of spindle-shaped or globular astrocytes and they usually present foci of calcification.

The *true glioma of the retina* is usually an astrocytoma; it is extremely rare and is mostly observed in children. On occasion the tumour can be confused with a retinoblastoma and lead to enucleation. It is sometimes an isolated tumour but may also develop together with the systemic involvement of a phakomatosis, neurofibromatosis or tuberous sclerosis.
Histologically the retinal astrocytoma presents the same characteristics as the cerebral astrocytoma. The evolution of this tumour is slow, and it does not metastasize.

XXVI. TUMEURS GLIALES DE LA RÉTINE ET DE LA PAPILLE

XXVI.1 Astrocytome (Phacomatoses)

Clinique. La sclérose tubéreuse (Bourneville, 1880) est classée parmi les phacomatoses. Congénitale, héréditaire, elle se caractérise par le développement de tumeurs multiples de la peau, du cerveau, de divers viscères, le rein le plus souvent. Les traits cliniques les plus frappants sont le déficit mental, l'épilepsie, et de petites tumeurs de la face qui sont des an-giofibromes (anciens "adénomes sébacés" de Pringle, terminologie fondée sur l'hyperplasie simultanée des glandes sébacées). L'évolution est habituellement fatale avant 25 ans par tumeur cérébrale. Le fond d'oeil peut montrer au pôle postérieur ou à la papille des tumeurs arrondies, de teinte blanche ou grisâtre, à surface parfois muriforme, de la taille d'une papille ou légèrement supérieure: les phacomes.

Histopathologie. Au microscope ces lésions sont superficielles, au niveau de la couche des fibres nerveuses. Ce sont des tumeurs gliales, formées d'astrocytes d'aspect fusiforme ou globuleux et se caractérisent par la quasi con-stance de foyers de calcification.

Le *gliome vrai de la rétine*, astrocytome le plus souvent, est extrêmement rare. Il s'observe surtout chez l'enfant, et peut con-duire à l'énucléation par confusion avec un rétinoblastome. Il peut être isolé ou entrer dans le cadre d'une phacomatose, maladie de Recklinghausen ou de Bourneville.
Histopathologiquement l'astrocytome rétinien ressemble aux tumeurs cérébrales de même nom. D'évolution très lente, cette tumeur ne métastase pas.

XXVI. GLIAGESCHWÜLSTE DER NETZHAUT UND DER PAPILLE

XXVI.1 Astrozytom (Phakomatosen)

Klinik. Die tuberöse Sklerose (Bourneville, 1880) gehört zu den Phakomatosen. Sie ist kongenital, hereditär; charakteristisch für sie ist die Entwicklung von Geschwülsten in der Haut, im Gehirn, in verschiedenen Viszera, zumeist der Niere. Die auffälligsten klinischen Anzeichen sind Schwachsinn, Epilepsie, kleine Gesichtsgeschwülste (Angiofibrome, früher Pringlesche "Talgdrüsenadenome", wobei diese Bezeichnung von der gleich-zeitigen Hyperplasie der Talgdrüsen herrührt). Die Krankheit verläuft meist vor dem Alter von 25 Jahren tödlich aufgrund eines Gehirntumors. Der Augenhintergrund kann am hinteren Pol oder an der Papille rundliche Geschwülste von weißlicher oder gräulicher Farbe mit manchmal brombeerähnlicher Oberfläche in Papillengröße oder leicht größer aufweisen: Phakome.

Histopathologie. Unter dem Mikroskop liegen diese Läsionen oberflächlich, im Bereich der Nervenfaserschicht. Es sind Gliatumoren, bestehend aus Astrozyten mit spindel- oder kugelförmigen Aussehen; typisch sind die fast stets vorhandenen Kalzifizierungsherde.

Das *echte Netzhautgliom*, zumeist Astro-zytom, kommt außerordentlich selten vor. Es ist vor allem beim Kind zu beobachten und kann auf Grund der Verwechslung mit einem Retinoblastom zur Enukleation veranlassen. Es kann vereinzelt oder im Rahmen einer Phakomatose, Recklinghausen- oder Bourne-ville-Krankheit auftreten.
Das Netzhaut-Astrozytom ähnelt den gleich-namigen Gehirntumoren. Diese sich sehr langsam entwickelnde Geschwulst bildet keine Metastasen.

PLATE 58 PLANCHE 58 TAFEL 58

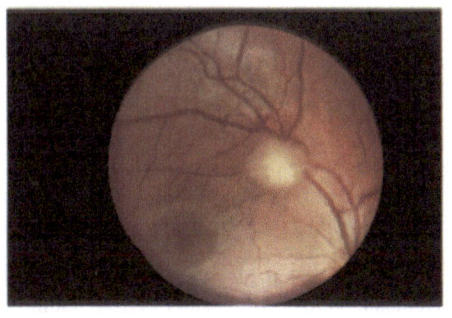

a

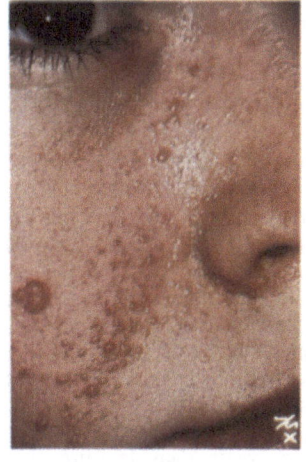

b

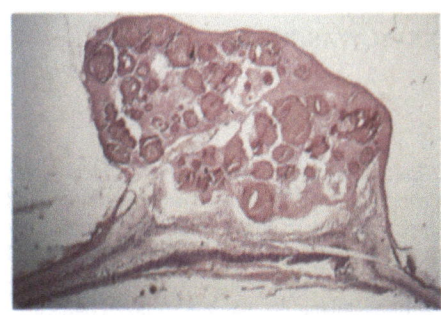

c

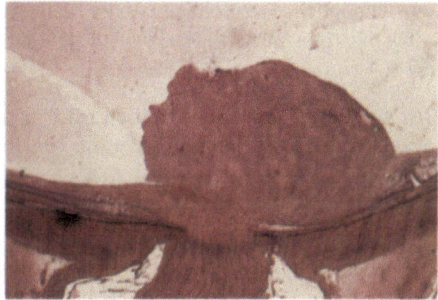

d

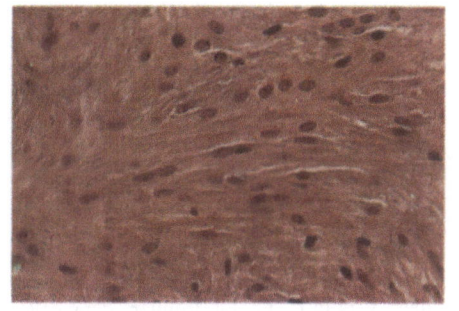

e

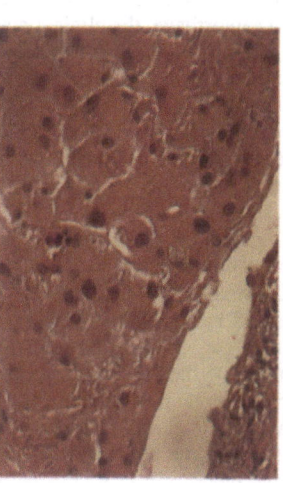

f

Fig. a. Tuberous sclerosis (Bourneville).
This superficial, unpigmented tumour is a common example of retinal involvement.

Fig. b. Tuberous sclerosis (Bourneville).
Small hemispherical skin tumours of the face with a "butterfly" distribution. They were formerly considered as sebaceous adenomas, but are actually angiofibromas.

Fig. c. Tuberous sclerosis (Bourneville).
Characteristic features of the retinal glial tumours; the foci of calcification are easily recognized.

Fig. d. Clinically the astrocytoma is a solitary, unilateral, flat tumour.
It is located on or around the optic disc. It can be observed in a microphthalmic eye (which is not the case with retinoblastoma).

Fig. e. Usual histopathological aspect of the retinal astrocytoma: spindle-shaped, long, irregular cells with long cytoplasmic processes which intermingle in bundles. Pseudo-rosettes may be observed, resulting from the grouping of the cells around capillaries.

Fig. f. Globular astrocytes as in this figure, are less common.

Fig. a. Sclérose tubéreuse (Bourneville).
Aspect clinique fréquent d'un phacome rétinien. Tumeur superficielle non pigmentée.

Fig. b. Sclérose tubéreuse (Bourneville).
Petites tumeurs cutanées de la face, arrondies, à disposition "en papillon" considérées autrefois comme des adénomes sébacés. Ce sont en fait des angiofibromes.

Fig. c. Sclérose tubéreuse (Bourneville).
Aspect caractéristique des tumeurs gliales rétiniennes avec leurs foyers de calcification bien reconnaissables.

Fig. d. L'astrocytome réalise en clinique une tumeur unique, unilatérale, peu saillante, papillaire ou péripapillaire.
Contrairement au rétinoblastome il peut s'observer sur un oeil microphtalme.

Fig. e. Aspect histopathologique le plus courant de l'astrocytome rétinien. Cellules fusiformes, allongées, irrégulières, aux longs prolongements cytoplasmiques qui s'entrelacent en faisceaux; le stroma est abondant, de structure fibrillaire. Les cellules sont parfois groupées autour de capillaires, donnant des aspects de pseudorosettes.

Fig. f. Aspect plus rare: astrocytes globuleux.

Abb. a. Tuberöse Sklerose (Bourneville).
Häufiger klinischer Aspekt eines Netzhautphakoms. Oberflächlicher, nicht pigmentierter Tumor.

Abb. b. Tuberöse Sklerose (Bourneville).
Kleine Gesichtshauttumoren, rundlich, in "Schmetterlings-Anordnung", die früher für Talgdrüsenadenome gehalten wurden. Es handelt sich faktisch um Angiofibrome.

Abb. c. Tuberöse Sklerose (Bourneville).
Charakteristisches Erscheinungsbild der Netzhaut-Gliageschwülste mit ihren gut erkennbaren Kalzifizierungsherden.

Abb. d. Klinisch bildet das Astrozytom einen einzigen, einseitigen, wenig vorstehenden, papillären oder peripapillären Tumor.
Im Gegensatz zum Retinoblastom kann es in einem Mikrophthalmus beobachtet werden.

Abb. e. Häufigster histopathologischer Aspekt eines Netzhaut-Astrozytoms. Spindelförmige, längliche, unregelmäßige Zellen mit langen Zytoplasmaausläufern, die sich in Bündeln durchflechten; das Stroma ist reichlich, von fibrillärer Struktur. Die Zellen sind manchmal um Kapillaren angeordnet und ergeben so das Bild von Pseudorosetten.

Abb. f. Eine seltenere Erscheinung: kugelige Astrozyten.

PLATE 59 PLANCHE 59 TAFEL 59

XXVII. VASCULAR TUMOURS

XXVII.1 Coats disease

Clinical features. The disease which Coats described in 1908 is of unknown etiology and appears in the young. Its characteristic feature is a more or less extensive exudative retinal detachment with various vascular abnormalities (telangiectases, micro-aneurysms, saccular dilatations of the veins, areas of non-perfusion and areas of leakage). The dominant clinical picture can either be that of the vascular abnormalities or that of their consequence: exudates and haemorrhages. If the details of the fundus are not blurred by vitreous haemorrhage, the clinical diagnosis is most of the time easy, particularly the distinction from the other types of leucocoria of infancy. Nevertheless enucleation has sometimes been necessary, because a retinoblastoma could not be excluded, or due to a neovascular glaucoma.

Histopathology. Histopathology shows the two prominent features of the disease: the vascular abnormalities and their consequences, exudates and haemorrhages. The vascular abnormalities are predominant in the veins (thickening of the vascular walls, hyaline degeneration, organized thrombosis, telangiectases), and in the capillaries of the peripheral retina. Through the altered endothelial layer, plasma and blood cells cross the vascular wall towards the retina. Here, lipidic exudates, haemorrhages, oedema, degenerative lesions, a proliferation of macrophages containing lipids or pigment and cholesterol cristals can be found. The latter may also be met with in the subretinal fluid. The affected eye may worsen progressively and become blind by total exudative retinal detachment. An adequate photocoagulation or cryo-application can sometimes slow down the course of localized lesions.

XXVII. TUMEURS VASCULAIRES

XXVII.1 Maladie de Coats

Clinique. La maladie décrite par Coats en 1908, d'étiologie inconnue, généralement unilatérale, survient chez le sujet jeune. Elle se caractérise par un décollement rétinien exsudatif plus ou moins étendu avec des anomalies vasculaires diverses (vaisseaux télangiectasiques, micro-anévrysmes, dilatations veineuses sacculaires, zones de non perfusion et zones de fuite). Selon les cas, le facteur anomalie vasculaire ou ses conséquences, exsudats et hémorragies dominent le tableau. Sauf hémorragie dans le vitré cachant les détails, le diagnostic est généralement aisé, en particulier avec les autres leucocories du jeune enfant. Cependant dans certains cas il a fallu énucléer, devant l'impossibilité d'exclure un rétinoblastome, ou du fait d'un glaucome néovasculaire douloureux.

Histopathologie. On retrouve, associées dans des proportions variables, les deux caractéristiques de la maladie: les anomalies vasculaires et leurs conséquences exsudatives et hémorragiques. Les premières prédominent aux capillaires de la rétine périphérique (télangiectasies, épaississement des parois, dégénérescence hyaline, thrombose organisée). A travers un endothélium altéré, plasma et cellules traversent la paroi vasculaire vers la rétine. On trouvera dans celle-ci: exsudats souvent lipidiques, hémorragies, oedème, dégénérescence; une importante prolifération de macrophages contenant des lipides ou du pigment, ainsi que des cristaux de cholestérol, qui fusent dans le liquide sous-rétinien. Le globe atteint de maladie de Coats peut évoluer vers la cécité par décollement total. Une photocoagulation ou une cryo-application adéquates peuvent parfois aider à limiter des formes localisées.

XXVII. GEFÄSSTUMOREN DER NETZHAUT

XXVII.1 Morbus Coats

Klinik. Die von Coats 1908 beschriebene Krankheit unbekannter Ätiologie tritt meist einseitig beim Jugendlichen auf. Sie ist durch eine exsudative, mehr oder weniger ausgedehnte Netzhautablösung mit verschiedenen Gefäßanomalien (telangiektasische Gefäße, sackartige Venenerweiterungen, fokale Perfusionsausfälle und Abschnitte mit vermehrter Durchlässigkeit) gekennzeichnet. Je nach Fall dominiert bei dem Krankheitsbild der Gefäßanomaliefaktor oder seine Auswirkungen, Exsudate und Blutungen. Außer bei einer die Einzelheiten verdeckenden Blutung im Glaskörper ist die Diagnose im allgemeinen einfach, insbesondere im Vergleich zu anderen Leukokorien des Kleinkindes. In manchen fällen mußte jedoch eine Enukleation vorgenommen werden, da ein Retinoblastom unmöglich auszuschließen oder weil ein schmerzhaftes neovaskuläres Glaukom vorhanden war.

Histopathologie. Histopathologisch trifft man in unterschiedlichen Proportionen die beiden Charakteristika der Krankheit wieder an: Gefäßanomalien und ihre Folgen in Form von Exsudaten und Blutungen. Die ersteren treten vorwiegend an den Venen auf (verdickte Wände, hyaline Degeneration, organisierte Thrombose, Telangiektasien, vor allem an den peripheren Kapillaren). Durch eine krankhaft verändertes Endothel durchsetzen Serum und Blutzellen die Gefäßwand zur Netzhaut hin. In dieser finden sich (meist lipidreiche) Exsudate, Hämorrhagien, Ödem, Degenerationserscheinungen; eine Proliferation von Makrophagen, die Lipide oder Pigment enthalten, sowie Cholesterolkristalle, die sich in der subretinalen Flüssigkeit ausbreiten. Der an dem Morbus Coats erkrankte Bulbus kann durch völlige Netzhautablösung erblinden. Lichtkoagulation oder eine richtig angewandte Kryokoagulation können manchmal helfen, lokalisierte Formen in Grenzen zu halten.

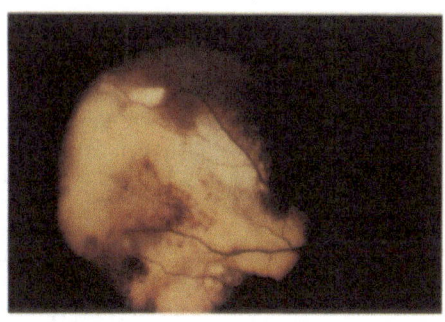

a

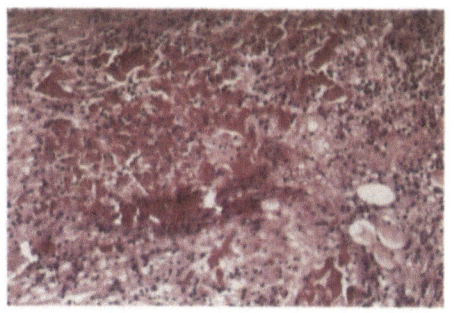

b

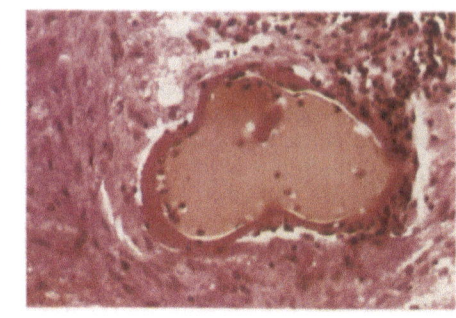

c

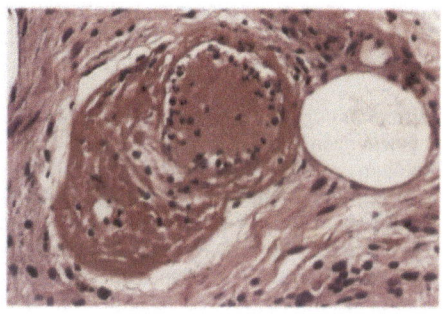

d

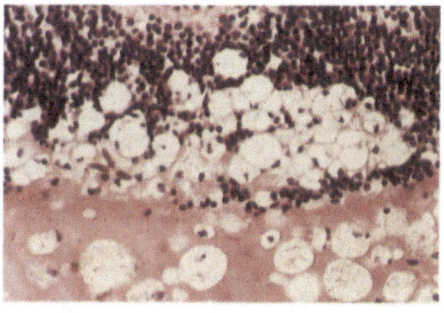

e

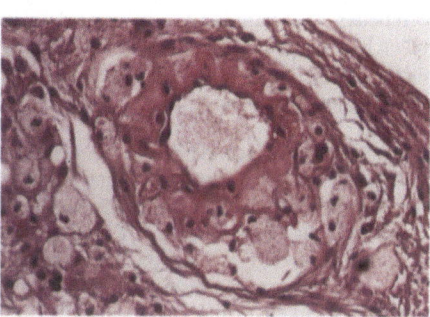

f

Fig. a. Coats disease.
Ophthalmoscopical aspect of the fundus, with exudative retinal detachment, haemorrhages and vascular abnormalities.

Fig. b. Histopathology: exudative areas are better seen after staining with PAS.

Fig. c. Telangiectasis and thickening of vascular wall.

Fig. d. Telangiectasis.
Leaking of vascular wall; perivascular exudates.

Fig. e. Lipid-containing macrophages.
Foam cells in the retina and in the subretinal fluid.

Fig. f. Perivascular foam cells.

Fig. a. Maladie de Coats.
Aspect clinique du décollement exsudatif avec hémorragies et anomalies vasculaires.

Fig. b. Histopathologie: plages exsudatives mieux visibles après coloration au PAS.

Fig. c. Télangiectasie et épaississement de la paroi vasculaire.

Fig. d. Télangiectasie.
Exsudats périvasculaires.

Fig. e. Macrophages contenant des lipides.
Cellules spumeuses dans la rétine et dans le liquide sous-rétinien.

Fig. f. Cellules spumeuses périvasculaires.

Abb. a. Morbus Coats.
Ophthalmoskopisches Aussehen des Augenhintergrundes. Exsudative Netzhaut-Ablösung, Blutungen, Gefäßanomalien.

Abb. b. Histopathologie: exsudative Zonen sind besser erkennbar nach Färbung mit PAS.

Abb. c. Telangiektasie und Verdickung der Gefäßwand.

Abb. d. Telangiektasie.
Perivaskuläres Exsudat.

Abb. e. Lipidreiche Makrophagen.
Schaumzellen in der Netzhaut und in der subretinalen Flüssigkeit.

Abb. f. Perivaskuläre Schaumzellen.

127

PLATE 60   PLANCHE 60   TAFEL 60

XXVII.2 Von Hippel's disease

Clinical features. The capillary haemangiomas of the retina develop close to the optic disc or at the periphery of the fundus. They appear de novo in a healthy retina and grow progressively. In their more common endophytic variety they present the shape of a sessile globular formation with wide and sinuous afferent and efferent vessels the colour of arterial blood. Their exophytic variety is mostly located in the vicinity of the optic disc; it is difficult to diagnose without the help of angiofluorography. Progressively the vessels become leaky, leading to the formation of lipidic exudates, circinate retinopathy, retinal oedema, exudative retinal detachment, superficial retinal neovascularization with haemorrhages and retinovitreal traction. These complications are often unavoidable in spite of early treatment. Lindau's disease is one of the phakomatoses. It is hereditary and usually characterized by a cerebellar haemangioma, associated with other localizations. When the retina is one of them, the condition is referred to as Von Hippel-Lindau's disease.

Histopathology. Histopathological examination is mostly performed in late stages, when complications such as painful haemorrhagic glaucoma, or a suspicion of intra-ocular tumour have led to enucleation. The proliferation of newly-formed vessels, which is exceptionally observed in the early stages, is then concealed among exudates, haemorrhages, stromal cells containing lipids, retinal gliosis. The angioblastic proliferation is underlined by reticulin. Between the vascular cavities are found cells with an often foamy cytoplasm: the stromal cells of uncertain origin. It is worth noting that early treatment with photo- or cryo-coagulation can sometimes stop the retinal evolution of this disease.

XXVII.2 Maladie de Von Hippel

Clinique. Les hémangiomes capillaires de la rétine se développent près de la papille ou en périphérie. Ils apparaissent de novo dans une rétine saine et se constituent progressivement. Dans leur variété endophytique plus fréquente ils forment un ballonnet sessile avec des vaisseaux afférents et efférents larges et sinueux, de la teinte du sang artériel. La forme exophytique, surtout juxta-papillaire, est difficilement reconnue sans l'angiofluorographie. Peu à peu les vaisseaux deviennent perméables, donnant lieu à des exsudats lipidiques, une rétinopathie circinée, un oedème rétinien, un décollement exsudatif de la rétine, une néovascularisation de surface avec hémorragies et traction vitréenne. Ces complications sont souvent inévitables malgré un traitement précoce. La maladie de Lindau est une phacomatose, héréditaire, caractérisée par un hémangiome habituellement cérébelleux, associé à des localisations extra-cérébelleuses. Lorsque la rétine est atteinte on parle de maladie de Von Hippel-Lindau.

Histopathologie. Les examens histopathologiques sont pratiqués le plus souvent à un stade tardif, lorsque des complications justifient l'énucléation, pour glaucome hémorragique douloureux ou suspicion de tumeur intra-oculaire par exemple. La prolifération néovasculaire – observée exceptionnellement à ses stades de début – est alors noyée dans les exsudats, les hémorragies, les cellules stromales à contenu lipidique, la gliose rétinienne. La prolifération angioblastique est soulignée par la réticuline. Entre les cavités vasculaires on trouve des cellules à cytoplasme souvent spumeux, les cellules stromales d'origine discutée. Il faut noter qu'un traitement précoce par photo- et/ou cryocoagulation peut parfois arrêter l'évolution de cette affection.

XXVII.2 Von Hippelsche Erkrankung

Klinik. Kapillar-Hämangiome der Netzhaut entwickeln sich in der Nähe der Papille oder in der Peripherie. Sie treten de novo in einer gesunden Netzhaut auf und entwickeln sich allmählich. Bei der häufigeren endophytischen Form bilden sie eine kleine flache Erhebung mit breiten, gewundenen afferenten und efferenten Gefäßen von der Farbe arteriellen Blutes. Die vor allem juxtapapillare exophytische Form ist ohne Fluoreszenzangiographie schwer zu erkennen. Allmählich werden die Gefäße durchlässig, so daß sich Lipidexsudate, eine Retinopathia circinata, ein Netzhautödem, eine exsudative Netzhautablösung, eine Neovaskularisierung der Netzhautoberfläche mit Blutungen und Glaskörpertraktion ergeben. Solche Komplikationen sind oft trotz frühzeitiger Behandlung unvermeidbar. Die Lindausche Krankheit ist eine hereditäre Phakomatose, gekennzeichnet durch ein meist zerebelares Hämangiom, sowie extra-zerebelaren Lokalisationen. Wenn die Netzhaut dabei erkrankt, spricht man von der Von Hippel-Lindau-Krankheit.

Histopathologie. Die histopathologischen Untersuchungen werden meist in einem späten Stadium vorgenommen, wenn Komplikationen eine Enukleation wegen schmerzhaften Glaukoms oder Verdacht auf intraokularen Tumor rechtfertigen. Die – im frühen Stadium nur ausnahmsweise beobachtete – neovaskuläre Proliferation ist dann von Exsudationen, Blutungen, lipidhaltigen Stromazellen, Netzhautgliose überdeckt. Die Proliferation von Angioblasten wird in der Retikulinfärbung hervorgehoben. Zwischen den Gefäßhohlräumen finden sich Zellen mit oft schaumigem Zytoplasma: die Stromazellen fraglicher Herkunft. Eine frühzeitige Behandlung durch Licht- oder Kryokoagulation kann manchmal den Verlauf dieser Krankheit stoppen.

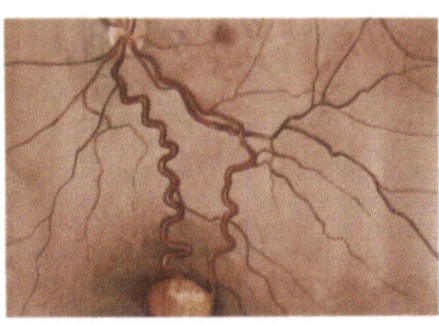

a

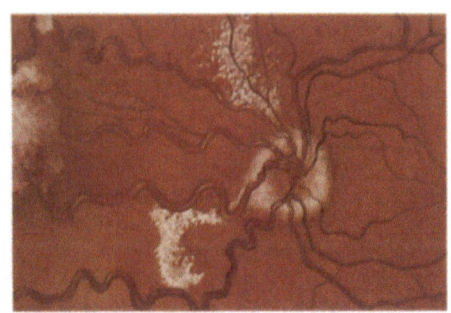

b

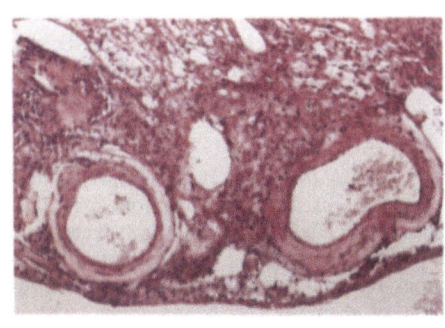

c

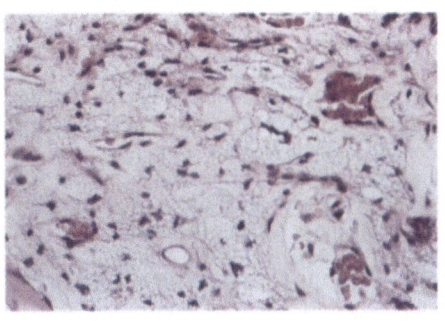

d

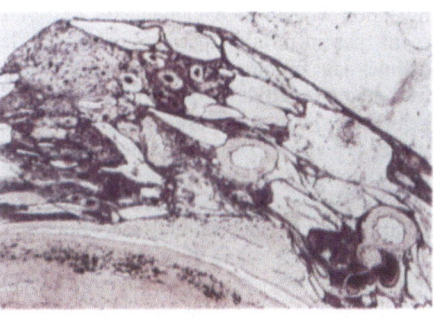

e

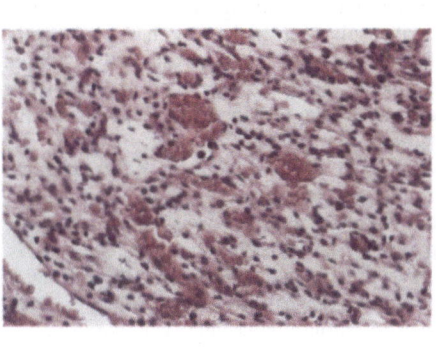

f

Fig. a. Characteristic feature of von Hippel's disease. Red globular formation in the peripheral retina, with large sinuous afferent and efferent vessels. (Collection of Dr Jacques Mawas.)

Fig. b. Another clinical aspect: the vascular abnormalities involve several vessels of the posterior retina. Globular formation surrounded by retinal gliosis. Exudates – Blurred disc. (Collection of Dr Jacques Mawas.)

Fig. c. Large feeding vessels, with thickening of the walls.

Fig. d. Cells with foamy cytoplasm.

Fig. e. In front of an altered pigment epithelium (lower part of the figure), large vessels and vascular spaces.

Fig. f. Newly formed capillaries.

Fig. a. Ballonnet caractéristique de la maladie de Von Hippel: périphérique, avec vaisseaux afférents et efférents sinueux et de gros calibre. (Collection du Dr Jacques Mawas.)

Fig. b. Autre aspect clinique: anomalies vasculaires touchant de nombreux vaisseaux du pôle postérieur. Ballonnet entouré de gliose. Exsudats – Oedème papillaire. (Collection du Dr Jacques Mawas.)

Fig. c. Vaisseaux nourriciers de gros calibre, à parois épaissies.

Fig. d. Cellules à cytoplasme spumeux.

Fig. e. Au-devant d'un épithélium pigmentaire altéré (en bas), gros vaisseaux et espaces vasculaires.

Fig. f. Capillaires néoformés.

Abb. a. Charakteristisches Knötchen der von Hippelschen Krankheit: an der Peripherie gelegen, mit gewundenen, großkalibrigen afferenten und efferenten Gefäßen. (Kollektion Dr. Jacques Mawas.)

Abb. b. Anderer klinischer Aspekt: Anomalien an zahlreichen Gefäßen des hinteren Pols.
Von Gliose umgebenes Knötchen. Exsudate – Papillenödem. (Kollektion Dr. Jacques Mawas.)

Abb. c. Großkalibrige ernährende Gefäße mit verdickten Wandungen.

Abb. d. Zellen mit schaumigem Zytoplasma.

Abb. e. Vor einem krankhaft veränderten Pigmentepithel (unten) große Gefäße und Gefäßräume.

Abb. f. Neugebildete Kapillaren.

129

PLATE 61 PLANCHE 61 TAFEL 61

XXVIII. RETINA AND DISORDERS OF THE BLOOD AND BLOOD FORMING ORGANS

Clinical features. The clinical retinal features of these diseases are manifold but lack specificity. Their distinction from neoplastic lesions of the fundus is usually easy. For obvious reasons haemorrhage is the most common of them. It can be pre-retinal with a horizontal level, retinal, flameshaped at the level of the nerve fibres, forming irregular flakes when they are deeply located. In leukaemia, the accumulation of white blood cells in the centre of the lesions may produce "shuttle" haemorrhages, with a white centre (Roth's spots). Oedema of the optic disc and exudates are other common clinical features.

Histopathology. It is acute leukaemia which provokes the most severe lesions: enlargement of the veins, sheathing of the vessels through perivascular infiltration by leukaemic cells, nodular infiltrate by the same cells, vascular occlusion, haemorrhages of the posterior retina with the possibility of bleeding into the vitreous. Infiltrates of the choroid can determine a detachment of either pigment epithelium or neuroepithelium. The infiltration by immature cells can extend to other parts to the eyeball, such as: sclera, iris, ciliary body, optic nerve and its meningeal sheaths. This happens more often in acute than in chronic leukaemia. It is worth noting that sometimes during the evolution of a case of chronic leukaemia the appearance of an exudative retinal detachment may be the first sign of a deterioration of the systemic condition.

XXVIII. RÉTINE ET MALADIES DU SANG ET DES ORGANES HÉMATOPOÏÉTIQUES

Clinique. Les manifestations cliniques de ces affections sont variées, mais peu spécifiques. Elles posent rarement des problèmes de diagnostic différentiel avec des lésions néoplasiques du fond d'oeil. L'hémorragie est le symptôme le plus banal. Elle peut être prérétinienne avec un niveau horizontal, rétinienne, en flammèche au niveau des fibres nerveuses, ou en plages dans les couches profondes. Dans les leucémies, l'accumulation des globules blancs au centre de l'hémorragie lui donne parfois l'aspect "en navette", à centre blanc (taches de Roth). D'autres manifestations cliniques fréquentes sont l'oedème papillaire et les exsudats.

Histopathologie. C'est la leucémie aiguë qui donne lieu aux atteintes les plus sévères: dilatation veineuse, engainements des vaisseaux par infiltration périvasculaire par des cellules leucémiques, infiltrats nodulaires par les mêmes cellules, occlusion vasculaire, hémorragie du pôle postérieur pouvant envahir le vitré. Des infiltrats choroïdiens peuvent entrainer un décollement de l'épithélium pigmentaire ou du neuro-épithélium. L'infiltration par des cellules immatures peut atteindre aussi la sclère, l'iris, le corps ciliaire, le nerf optique et ses gaines méningées. Elle est plus fréquente dans la leucémie aiguë que dans les formes chroniques. Cependant il faut noter que dans certaines leucoses chroniques une atteinte rétinienne sous la forme d'un décollement exsudatif doit faire craindre une aggravation de l'atteinte générale.

XXVIII. RETINA UND ERKRANKUNGEN DES BLUTES UND DER BLUT-BILDENDEN ORGANE

Klinik. Die klinischen Manifestationen dieser Krankheiten sind vielseitig, aber wenig spezifisch. Sie geben selten Anlaß zur Differentialdiagnose mit neoplastischen Läsionen des Augenhintergrundes. Die Hämorrhagie ist das banalste Symptom. Sie kann präretinal, mit oberer horizontaler Grenze, retinal, flämmchenartig zwischen den Nervenfasern oder flächenhaft in den tieferen Schichten, auftreten. Bei Leukämien ergibt die Anhäufung weißer Blutkörperchen im Zentrum der Blutung manchmal ein "schiffchenartiges" Aussehen mit weißem Zentrum (Roth-Flecken). Andere häufige klinische Anzeichen sind das Papillenödem und Exsudate.

Histopathologie. In histopathologischer Sicht hat die akute Leukämie die schwerwiegendsten Folgen: Venenerweiterung, hüllenartiger Überzug der Gefäße durch perivaskuläre Infiltration von Leukämiezellen, knötchenförmige Infiltrate durch dieselben Zellen, Gefäßverschluß, Blutungen am hinteren Pol, die sich in den Glaskörper ergießen können. Aderhautinfiltrate können eine Ablösung des Pigmentepithels oder des Neuroepithels zur Folge haben. Die Infiltration durch immature Zellen kann auf der Sklera, der Iris, im Ziliarkörper, im Sehnerv und dessen Scheiden auftreten. Sie kommt häufiger bei akuter Leukämie als bei den chronischen Formen vor. Es ist jedoch darauf zu achten, daß bei gewissen chronischen Leukosen eine Netzhautbeteiligung in Form einer exsudativen Ablösung eine Verschlechterung des Allgemeinzustandes befürchten läßt.

PLATE 61 PLANCHE 61 TAFEL 61

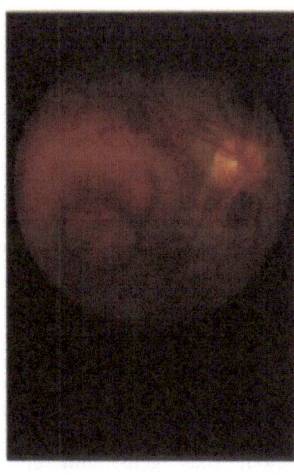

a

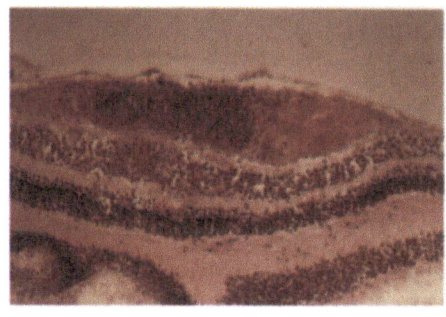

b

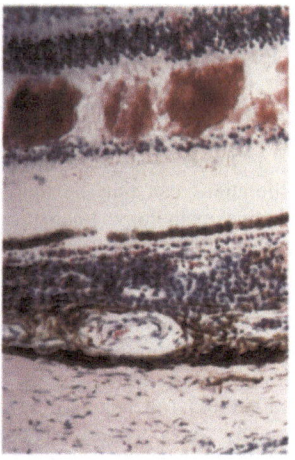

c

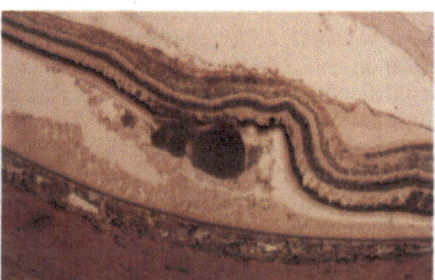

d

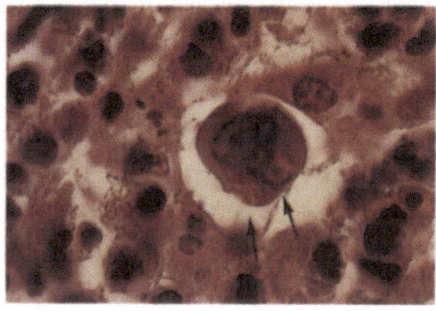

e

f

Fig. a. Ophthalmoscopic picture of a myeloid leukaemia.
Haemorrhages of various morphology. The lower temporal pseudo-tumoral mass is probably a sub-retinal infiltrate.

Fig. b. Acute leucosis.
Pre-retinal haemorrhage with central accumulation of leucocytes.

Fig. c. Retinal haemorrhages and diffuse leukaemic infiltrate of the choroid.
(The apparent separation of the retina from the choroid is due to artefact.)

Fig. d. Sub-retinal nodular leukaemic infiltrate with serous detachment of the retina.

Fig. e. Bilateral exudative retinal detachment in a Richter's syndrome.

Fig. f. Richter's syndrome.
Terminal reticulo-sarcomatous episode of a lymphoid leukaemia. Presence of large abnormal cells of Sternberg type (→).

Fig. a. Fond d'oeil lors d'une leucémie myéloïde.
Hémorragies de morphologie variée. La masse pseudo-tumorale temporale inférieure est probablement le témoin d'un infiltrat sous-rétinien.

Fig. b. Leucose aiguë.
Hémorragie prérétinienne avec accumulation de leucocytes en son centre.

Fig. c. Hémorragies intra-rétiniennes et infiltrat leucémique diffus de la choroïde.
(La séparation rétine-choroïde est un artefact.)

Fig. d. Infiltrat nodulaire leucémique sous-rétinien avec décollement séreux de la rétine.

Fig. e. Décollement rétinien exsudatif bilatéral au cours d'un syndrome de Richter.

Fig. f. Syndrome de Richter.
Épisode terminal leuco-sarcomateux d'une leucémie lymphoïde. Présence de grandes cellules anormales Sternbergoïdes (→).

Abb. a. Augenhintergrund bei einer myeloischen Leukämie.
Hämorrhagien unterschiedlicher Morphologie. Die pseudotumorale Masse temporal unten deutet wahrscheinlich auf ein subretinales Infiltrat hin.

Abb. b. Akute Leukose.
Präretinale Blutung mit Leukozytenansammlung in der Mitte.

Abb. c. Intraretinale Blutungen und diffuses leukämisches Aderhautinfiltrat.
(Die Trennung von Netzhaut und Aderhaut ist ein Artefakt.)

Abb. d. Knötchenförmiges leukämisches Infiltrat unter der Netzhaut mit seröser Netzhautablösung.

Abb. e. Bilaterale exsudative Netzhautablösung im Verlauf eines Richter-Syndroms.

Abb. f. Richter-Syndrom.
Leukosarkomatöse Endphase einer lymphoiden Leukämie. Vorhandensein großer anormaler Sternberg-ähnlicher Zellen (→).

PLATE 62 PLANCHE 62 TAFEL 62

XXIX. TUMOURS OF THE RETINAL PIGMENT EPITHELIUM

Clinical features. The pigment epithelium of the retina reacts to manifold stimulations by a localized or diffuse hyperplasia. These mostly flat proliferations can thus be found in any type of retinal pathology: traumatic, inflammatory, degenerative. But true neoplasias are rare. Sometimes they are found by chance in a globe which has been enucleated for another reason. On rare occasions, despite their black colour under ophthalmoscopy, they have led to enucleation owing to the confusion with a malignant choroidal melanoma (the colour of which usually tends towards slate-grey). A true neoplasia of the retinal pigment epithelium is clinically a darkly pigmented, sometimes polychromic mass, located in the posterior retina, often close to the optic disc.

Histopathology. The benign tumours often present an *adenomatous appearance*: strands of cells and tubular glandlike structures sometimes with a central cavity. There are also, but not as often as in hyperplasia, homogeneous, often lamellar structures, which are an accumulation of newly-formed basal membranes. E.M. shows the cytological characteristics of pigment epithelium.
The malignant tumours are *adenocarcinomas;* anaplasia, pleomorphism, increased mitotic activity distinguish them from the benign type. Invasion of the choroid is possible. But trans-scleral extension has never been observed; a few exceptional cases of death by "metastasis" lack histological confirmation.

XXIX. TUMEURS DE L'ÉPITHÉLIUM PIGMENTAIRE DE LA RÉTINE

Clinique. L'épithélium pigmentaire de la rétine répond par une hyperplasie diffuse ou localisée, à de multiples stimulations. Ces proliférations, généralement non surélevées, se constatent ainsi dans toute la pathologie rétinienne, traumatique, inflammatoire, dégénérative. Mais les véritables tumeurs sont rares. Elles peuvent être découvertes fortuitement dans un globe énucléé pour une autre raison. Malgré leur teinte très noire à l'ophtalmoscopie, elles peuvent conduire à l'énucléation par confusion avec un mélanome malin de la choroïde (qui prend généralement une teinte ardoisée). Les vraies néoplasies de l'épithélium pigmentaire se présentent donc en clinique comme une masse pigmentée très sombre, ou polychrome, à localisation plutôt postérieure, parapapillaire souvent.

Histopathologie. Les formes bénignes ont souvent une *structure adénomateuse*: cordons et formations tubulaires d'aspect glandulaire avec parfois une cavité centrale. On y trouve aussi, plus rarement que dans les hyperplasies, des structures anhistes, souvent lamellaires, accumulation de membranes basales néoformées. Au microscope électronique on retrouve les caractéristiques cytologiques de l'épithélium pigmentaire.
Les formes malignes, *les adénocarcinomes*, se distinguent des précédentes par l'anaplasie, le pléomorphisme, et l'activité mitotique augmentée. On peut trouver aussi un envahissement de la choroïde. Mais l'extension transsclérale n'a jamais été observée, et les exceptionnels décès par "métastase" n'ont jamais été vérifiés histologiquement.

XXIX. GESCHWÜLSTE DES PIGMENT-EPITHELS DER NETZHAUT

Klinik. Das Pigmentepithel der Netzhaut antwortet mit einer diffusen oder lokalisierten Hyperplasie auf vielfache Stimulierungen. Diese im allgemeinen nicht erhabenen Proliferationen sind somit in der gesamten Netzhautpathologie, gleich ob traumatisch, entzündlich oder degenerativ, anzutreffen. Aber richtige Tumoren sind selten. Sie können zufällig in einem aus einem anderen Grund enukleierten Bulbus entdeckt werden. Trotz ihrer in der Ophthalmoskopie sehr schwarzen Färbung können sie aufgrund einer Verwechslung mit einem bösartigen Aderhautmelanom (das gemeinhin eine schiefergraue Färbung annimmt) zu einer Enukleation Anlaß geben. Die echten Neoplasien des Pigmentepithels treten klinisch also wie eine sehr dunkle oder polychrome Pigmentmasse mit eher hinten, oft neben der Papille gelegener Lokalisierung in Erscheinung.

Histopathologie. Die gutartigen Formen haben oft eine *adenomatöse Struktur*: Stränge und röhrenförmige Gebilde mit drüsenartigem Aussehen, manchmal mit einem zentralen Hohlraum. Seltener als bei den Hyperplasien findet man dort auch amorphe, oft lamellenartige Strukturen, Anhäufungen neugebildeter Basalmembranen. Unter dem Elektronenmikroskop kann man die zytologischen Merkmale des Pigmentepithels erkennen.
Die bösartigen Formen, *Adenokarzinome*, unterscheiden sich von den vorausgegangenen durch Anaplasie, Pleomorphie und verstärkte Mitosentätigkeit. Man kann auch ein Einwachsen in die Aderhaut antreffen. Aber eine transsklerale Ausweitung ist noch nie beobachtet worden, und die äußerst seltenen Todesfälle durch "Metastasen" wurden histologisch nie bestätigt.

PLATE 62   PLANCHE 62   TAFEL 62

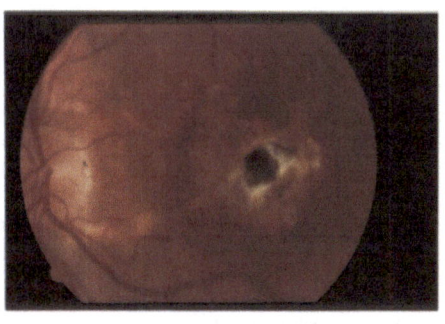

a

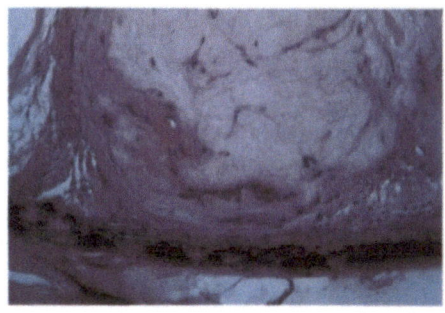

b

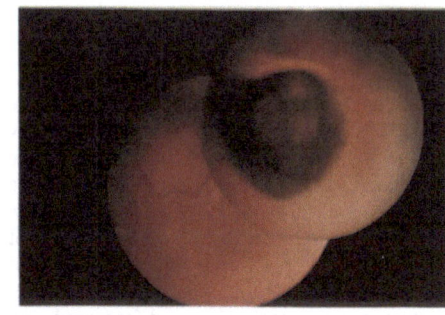

c

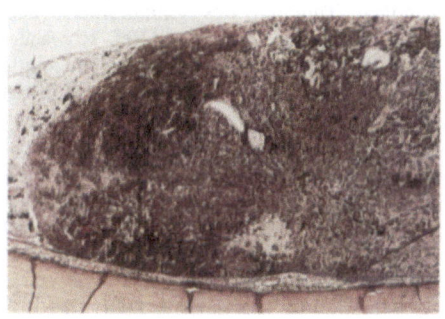

d

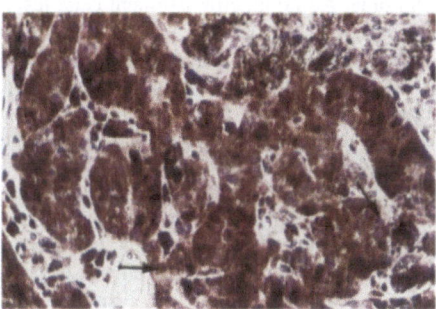

e

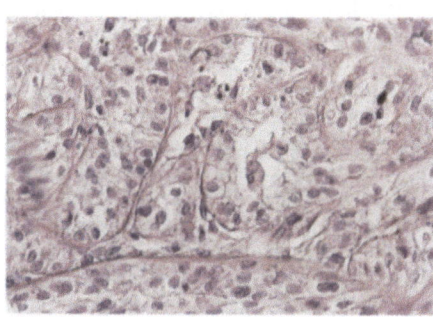

f

Fig. a. Pseudo-tumoral hyperplasia accompanying a multifocal placoid epitheliopathy.
Prominent lesion, of a dark colour, presenting also some yellow areas. No histological confrontation.

Fig. b. Histopathology of a pseudo-tumoral hyperplasia of the posterior retina.
Fortuitous discovery in an enucleated eye with absolute glaucoma. The non-pigmented homogeneous area is probably an accumulation of newly-formed basal membrane material.

Fig. c. Adenocarcinoma of pigment epithelium.
Dark pigmentation (in contrast with the slate-grey pigmentation of the malignant melanoma of the choroid).

Fig. d. Adenocarcinoma of pigment epithelium.
General view under low power. Well limited tumour mass, with sometimes a tubular structure (on the right-hand side of the figure).

Fig. e. Higher power.
The tubular structures are more easily recognizable. Cell pleomorphism, and a few mitotic figures (→).

Fig. f. Depigmented section.
The cytological details are more obvious. The adenoid structure is still visible.

Fig. a. Hyperplasie pseudo-tumorale accompagnant une épithéliopathie en plaques.
Lésion surélevée, à pigmentation très sombre à côté de plages jaunes. Pas de confrontation histologique.

Fig. b. Histopathologie d'une hyperplasie pseudo-tumorale du pôle postérieur.
Découverte fortuite dans un globe énucléé pour glaucome absolu. La partie non pigmentée, anhiste, est probablement une accumulation de basales néoformées.

Fig. c. Adénocarcinome de l'épithélium pigmentaire.
Pigmentation très sombre (contrairement à la teinte ardoisée du mélanome choroïdien).

Fig. d. Adénocarcinome.
Vue d'ensemble. Masse tumorale bien délimitée, présentant parfois des formations tubulaires (dans la moitié droite de la figure).

Fig. e. Fort grossissement.
Formations tubulaires mieux reconnaissables. Pléomorphisme cellulaire et quelques mitoses. (→).

Fig. f. Coupe dépigmentée.
Coupe dépigmentée montrant mieux les détails cytologiques. La structure adénoïde reste reconnaissable.

Abb. a. Pseudotumorale Hyperplasie, mit einer Plattenepitheliopathie einhergehend.
Erhabene Läsion mit sehr dunkler Pigmentierung neben gelben Feldern. Kein histologisches Substrat.

Abb. b. Histopathologie einer pseudotumoralen Hyperplasie am hinteren Pol.
Zufällige Entdeckung in einem wegen absoluten Glaukoms enukleierten Bulbus. Der nicht pigmentierte, amorphe Teil ist wahrscheinlich eine Anhäufung neugebildeter Basalmembranen.

Abb. c. Adenokarzinom des Pigmentepithels.
Sehr dunkle Pigmentierung (im Gegensatz zur Schieferfarbe des Aderhautmelanoms).

Abb. d. Adenokarzinom.
Gesamtansicht. Gut abgegrenzte Tumormasse, die manchmal schlauchförmige Gebilde aufweist (in der rechten Bildhälfte).

Abb. e. Starke Vergrößerung.
Die schlauchförmigen Gebilde sind deutlicher zu erkennen. Pleomorphie der Zellen und einige Mitosen (→).

Abb. f. Depigmentierter Schnitt.
Depigmentierter Schnitt, der die zytologischen Einzelheiten besser erkennen läßt. Die adenoide Struktur bleibt erkennbar.

XXX. MELANOCYTOMA OF THE OPTIC DISC

Clinical features. The melanocytoma of the optic disc is a small, jet black tumour, mostly found by chance. It is located right on the optic disc, and may extend partially along the vessels. It is always benign, but after some years small haemorrhages, an enlargement of the blind spot or, exceptionally, a decrease of visual acuity can be observed. This evolution however is extremely slow and far from being constant. Contrary to the malignant choroidal melanoma, this tumour is more common in patients with a strongly pigmented choroid, especially black people.

Histopathology. The histopathological features are known owing to the study of globes enucleated erroneously with a diagnosis of choroidal melanoma. The aspect is the same as in the homonymous tumours of the ciliary body, and occasionally of the choroid. Low power shows a strongly pigmented tumour taking up part of the optic disc, entering frequently into the lamina cribrosa, and even into the retrolaminar section of the optic nerve. The pigment-laden cells can be studied accurately only after depigmentation. They are large, polyhedral, with small, regular nuclei, and without mitoses; they are in contact with each other, without interposed stroma. The pigment is entirely intra-cellular. Owing to the benign histological aspect of this lesion D. Cogan suggested calling it magnocellular naevus. Under E.M. the pigment is obviously of the uveal type.

XXX. MÉLANOCYTOME DE LA PAPILLE

Clinique. D'un noir de jais, franchement papillaire et pouvant déborder le long des vaisseaux, le mélanocytome de la papille est une petite tumeur, le plus souvent découverte fortuitement. Toujours bénin, il peut se compliquer à la longue de petites hémorragies et s'accompagner parfois d'un élargissement de la tache aveugle, exceptionnellement d'une baisse de vision. Mais cette évolution est inconstante et extrêmement lente. Contrairement au mélanome de la choroïde cette tumeur est plus fréquente chez les sujets à choroïde fortement pigmentée, mélanodermes en particulier.

Histopathologie. L'histopathologie est connue par les cas énucléés pour suspicion de mélanome de la choroïde. L'aspect est celui qu'on trouve dans les tumeurs homonymes du corps ciliaire, exceptionnellement de la choroïde. Au faible grossissement cette lésion hyperpigmentée occupe une partie de la papille et pénètre souvent dans la lame criblée et dans la partie rétrolaminaire du nerf optique. Les cellules, noires de pigment, sont définissables seulement après dépigmentation. Elles sont polyédriques, de grande taille, contrastant avec des noyaux petits, centraux, réguliers, dépourvus de mitoses; elles sont adossées les unes aux autres, sans stroma interposé. Le pigment est entièrement intracellulaire. L'aspect histologique bénin de cette lésion a fait proposer par D. Cogan le terme de naevus magnocellulaire. Au microscope électronique le pigment est de type uvéal.

XXX. MELANOZYTOM DER PAPILLE

Klinik. Das pechschwarze, eideutig papillare Melanozytom der Papille, das sich den Gefäßen entlang fortsetzen kann, ist ein kleiner Tumor, der meist zufällig entdeckt wird. Er ist immer gutartig, kann aber auf die Dauer Komplikationen durch kleine Blutungen hervorrufen und bisweilen eine Erweiterung des blinden Flecks, ausnahmsweise auch eine Einbuße des Sehvermögens bewirken. Diese Evolution ist jedoch sehr langsam, und tritt selten auf. Im Gegensatz zum Melanom der Aderhaut ist dieser Tumor häufiger bei Personen mit stark pigmentierter Aderhaut, insbesondere Melanodermen, anzutreffen.

Histopathologie. Die Histopathologie ist durch die wegen Verdachts auf Aderhautmelanom enukleierten Fälle bekannt. Das Aussehen ist dasselbe wie bei den gleichnamigen Tumoren des Ziliarkörpers, ausnahmsweise der Aderhaut. Bei schwacher Vergrößerung nimmt diese hyperpigmentierte Läsion einen Teil der Papille ein und dringt dann häufig in die Lamina cribrosa und den hinter der Lamina gelegenen Teil des Sehnervs ein. Die von Pigment geschwärzten Zellen sind erst nach Depigmentierung definierbar. Sie sind polygonal, groß, was in Kontrast zu den kleinen zentralen, regelmäßigen nicht mitotischen Kernen steht; sie sind ohne Zwischenstroma aneinandergereiht. Das Pigment ist ausschließlich intrazellulär. Wegen des gutartigen histologischen Aspekts dieser Läsion trat D. Cogan für die Bezeichnung magnozellulärer Naevus ein. Unter dem Elektronenmikroskop ist das Pigment vom uvealen Typ.

PLATE 63   PLANCHE 63   TAFEL 63

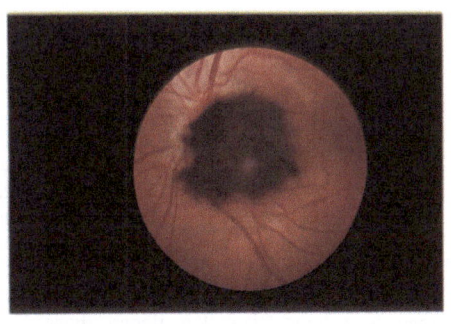

a

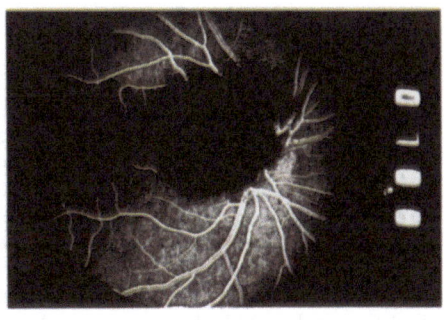

b

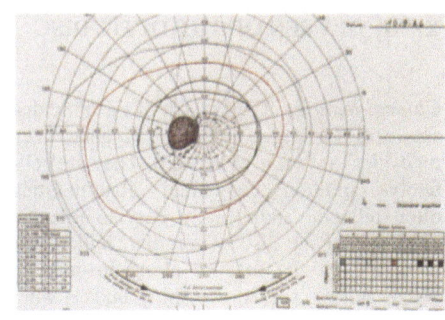

c

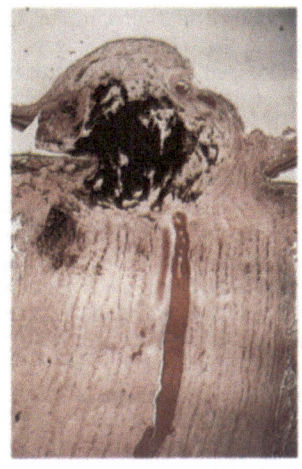

d

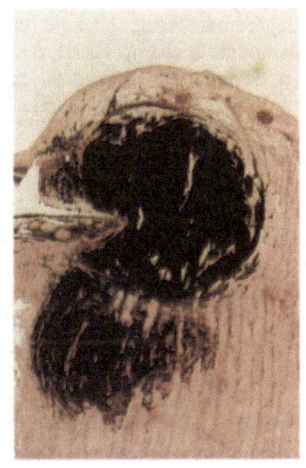

e

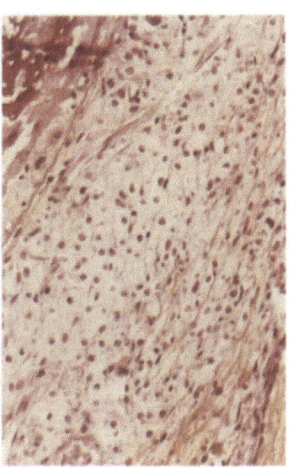

f

Fig. a. Usual clinical aspect of the melanocytoma of the optic disc.

Fig. b. As expected, the very dense pigment forms a screen under angiofluorography.

Fig. c. The enlargement of the blind spot is well-known. It does not mean malignancy.

Fig. d. Usual histopathological aspect under low power.
The retrolaminar extension is frequent.

Fig. e. Uniformly pigmented cells.
On E.M., the pigment is of the uveal type. The most likely pathogenesis is an abnormal migration of pigmented cells from the neural crest, deviating from their original uveal destination.

Fig. f. After depigmentation.
Polyhedral regular cells with small nuclei and scanty nucleoli.

Fig. a. Aspect clinique habituel du mélanocytome de la papille.

Fig. b. Comme il est prévisible le pigment très dense forme écran à l'angiofluorographie.

Fig. c. L'élargissement de la tache aveugle est connu. Il ne doit pas être considéré comme un signe de malignité.

Fig. d. Aspect habituel au faible grossissement.
L'extension rétrolaminaire est fréquente.

Fig. e. Cellules hyperpigmentées de façon uniforme.
En microscopie électronique le pigment apparaît de type uvéal. La thèse pathogénique la plus vraisemblable est une migration anormale de cellules pigmentées provenant de la crête neurale et destinées primitivement à l'uvée.

Fig. f. Après dépigmentation.
Cellules polyédriques régulières à petits noyaux centraux aux rares nucléoles.

Abb. a. Gewöhnlicher klinischer Aspekt des Melanozytoms der Papille.

Abb. b. Wie vorausgesehen bildet das sehr dichte Pigment einen Schirm auf den fluoreszenzangiograpischen Bildern.

Abb. c. Die Ausweitung des blinden Flecks ist bekannt und darf nicht als Zeichen von Bösartigkeit betrachtet werden.

Abb. d. Gewöhnliches Aussehen bei schwacher Vergrößerung.
Häufig setzt sich die Geschwulst hinter der Lamina cribrosa fort.

Abb. e. Gleichmäßig hyperpigmentierte Zellen.
Unter dem Elektronenmikroskop ist das Pigment als vom uvealen Typ zu erkennen. Die wahrscheinlichste These der Krankheitsentstehung ist eine anormale Wanderung von Pigmentzellen, die von der Neuralleiste herkommen und ursprünglich für die Uvea bestimmt waren.

Abb. f. Nach Depigmentierung.
Regelmäßige polyedrische Zellen mit kleinen zentralen Kernen und nur wenigen Nukleolen.

PLATE 64   PLANCHE 64   TAFEL 64

XXXI. DRUSEN OF THE OPTIC DISC

Clinical features. The Drusen of the optic disc are still wrongly called "Hyaline verrucosities" (at least in French). They are relatively common congenital abnormalities, often bilateral and usually easy to identify. The edge of the disc is irregular, milled, and there are on the disc or along its margins small, yellow, sometimes shiny bulges. They may accompany a blurred disc, mimicking papilloedema. Sometimes they are located deep within the disc; the only simple way to make the diagnosis in this case is to use contact lens and slit lamp; the light of the latter, much stronger than that of an ophthalmoscope, will be reflected by the deeply located drusen. These lesions may increase slightly in the adult; they may alter the visual field, provoke small haemorrhages, and exceptionally decrease visual acuity.

Histopathology. Accidental discoveries in work on enucleated eyes, have shown that they are always in front of the lamina cribrosa, in either a superficial or a deep location. They are basophilic acellular masses of varied shapes, with calcifications forming concentric lamellae. It is worth noting that the calcium is detectable by modern medical imaging, which can thus, in isolated cases, help to determine the etiology of a disc oedema.

XXXI. VERRUCOSITÉS HYALINES (DRUSES) DE LA PAPILLE

Clinique. Les druses de la papille, encore appelées à tort verrucosités hyalines, sont des anomalies congénitales banales, souvent bilatérales, généralement aisées à reconnaître. Le bord de la papille est irrégulier, crénelé, et on trouve sur la papille même ou le long de ses bords de petites surélévations jaunâtres parfois brillantes. Elles peuvent s'accompagner d'un flou de la papille évoquant un oedème. Parfois elles se trouvent en profondeur dans la papille et le seul moyen de les déceler rapidement est l'examen au verre de contact à la lampe à fente dont elles réfléchissent la lumière, plus puissante que celle de l'ophtalmoscope. Ces lésions peuvent augmenter légèrement chez l'adulte et sont à même d'amputer le champ visuel, rarement de provoquer de petites hémorragies, exceptionnellement d'abaisser l'acuité visuelle.

Histopathologie. Au microscope, découvertes de hasard sur des globes énucléés, elles se localisent en avant de la lame criblée, en profondeur ou en surface de la papille. Ce sont des amas basophiles, acellulaires de forme variée, calcifiés en lamelles concentriques. Le terme de "verrucosités hyalines" n'est donc pas justifié. (Notons que le calcium est détectable avec les techniques modernes d'imagerie médicale; exceptionnellement, il peut être utile d'y recourir pour le diagnostic étiologique d'un oedème papillaire).

XXXI. DRUSEN DER PAPILLE

Klinik. Die Drusen der Papille sind banale kongenitale, meist bilaterale Anomalien, die im allgemeinen leicht zu erkennen sind. Der Papillenrand ist unregelmäßig, eingekerbt, und auf der Papille selbst oder entlang ihren Rändern befinden sich kleine gelbliche, manchmal glänzende Erhebungen. Gleichzeitig kann die Papille ödematig verschwommen aussehen. Bisweilen liegen diese Erhebungen tief in der Papille und sind rasch nur mit Hilfe einer Kontaktlinse und der Spaltlampe zu erkennen, da deren stärkeres Licht, im Gegensatz zu dem eines Ophthalmoskops, von den Drusen reflektiert wird. Diese Läsionen können beim Erwachsenen leicht zunehmen und sind in der Lage, das Gesichtsfeld zu beeinträchtigen, seltener kleine Blutungen zu verursachen oder in Ausnahmefällen die Sehschärfe einzuschränken.

Histopathologie Unter dem Mikroskop liegen die durch Zufall in enukleierten Bulbi entdeckten Drusen vor der Lamina cribrosa, in der Tiefe oder an der Oberfläche der Papille. Es sind basophile, azelluläre Anhäufungen von unterschiedlicher Form, die in konzentrischen Lamellen kalzifiziert sind. Die Bezeichnung "hyaline Drusen" ist also nicht gerechtfertigt. (Hierzu sei noch bemerkt, daß Kalzium mit den modernen bildtechnischen Möglichkeiten nachweisbar ist; es kann ausnahmsweise angebracht sein, sich diese zur Abklärung eines Papillenödems zunutze zu machen).

PLATE 64   PLANCHE 64   TAFEL 64

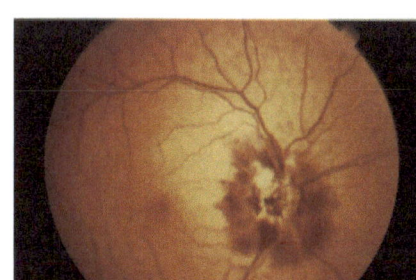

a

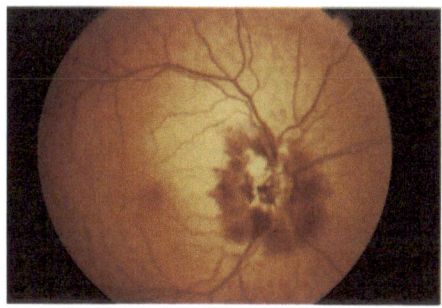

b

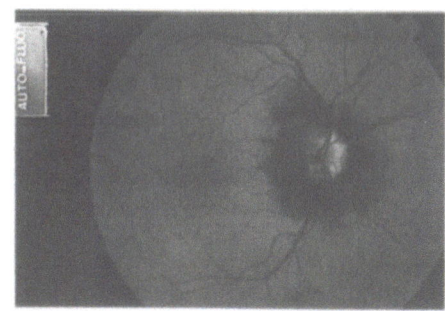

c

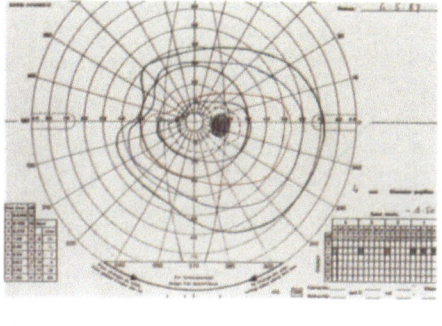

d

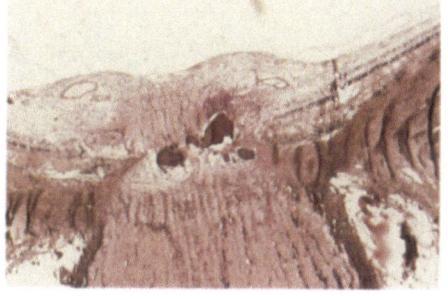

e

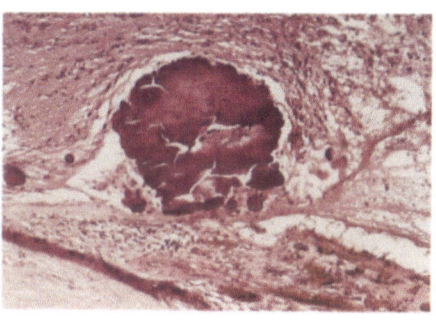

f

Fig. a. Usual aspect of the drusen.
The margin of the disc appears milled, with small shiny bulges.

Fig. b. Drusen with haemorrhages encircling and partly covering the disc. (Same case as Fig. a, fellow eye.)

Fig. c. Autofluorescence shows that drusen are present in Fig. b.

Fig. d. Example of visual field changes accompanying the presence of drusen.

Fig. e. Histopathology.
The calcified drusen are easily identified in front of the lamina cribrosa.
(The papilloedema was due here to a generalized leucosarcomatosis, cause of death.)

Fig. f. Calcified mass pushing aside the adjacent normal tissue.

Fig. a. Druses de la papille.
Aspect habituel. Bord de la papille crénelé par de petites surélévations réfringentes.

Fig. b. Druses accompagnées d'une couronne d'hémorragies péripapillaires qui les recouvrent en partie. (Même cas que la Fig. a, oeil controlatéral.)

Fig. c. L'auto-fluorescence montre la présence de druses. (Cas de la Fig. b.)

Fig. d. Exemple de modification du champ visuel accompagnant les druses de la papille.

Fig. e. Histopathologie.
Druses calcifiées en avant de la lame criblée.
(L'oedème papillaire est lié ici à une leucosarcomatose généralisée qui a entraîné le décès.)

Fig. f. Masse calcifiée refoulant les tissus voisins.

Abb. a. Drusen der Papille.
Gewöhnliches Aussehen. Papillenrand durch kleine lichtbrechende Erhebungen eingekerbt.

Abb. b. Drusen mit einem Kranz peripapillärer Blutungen, von denen sie teilweise zugedeckt sind. (Derselbe Fall wie auf Abb. a, jedoch das andere Auge.)

Abb. c. Die Eigenfluoreszenz verweist auf das Vorhandensein van Drusen. (Derselbe Fall wie auf Abb. b.)

Abb. d. Beispiel einer mit Drusen der Papille einhergehenden Gesichtsfeldveränderung.

Abb. e. Histologie.
Kalzifizierte Drusen vor der Lamina cribrosa.
(Das Papillenödem steht hier in Zusammenhang mit einer generalisierten Leukosarkomatose, die den Tod zur Folge hatte.)

Abb. f. Kalzifizierte Masse, die die benachbarten Gewebe zurückdrängt.

137

Technical appendix

In ocular oncology, close collaboration between the ophthalmologist and the pathologist is necessary if the gap between the two disciplines is not to be an obstacle. Certain technical recommendations were thus felt to be useful in both cases.

Recommendations for the ophthalmologist

1. The *fixative* normally used (10% or 15% formaldehyde, or Bouin's solution) should be available in the operating room. The volume should be 5 times that of the specimen. In certain circumstances a direct cooperation with the laboratory is indispensable. Special fixatives will thus be needed in cases such as EM studies (2% glutaraldehyde), or immunohistological labelling (4% paraformaldehyde). Extemporaneous examination requires a fragment of unfixed tissue to be brought to the laboratory in ice for cryostat section.

2. In *biopsy* or *excision*, tissue samples must be taken with a steel knife, not with the coagulator, which creates extended necrosis at the edge of the lesion, rendering difficult the evaluation of the extension and even making diagnosis impossible, in cases where the fragment is of reduced size.

3. If a valid diagnosis is to be assured, the pathologist will require a short *clinical history*, indicating the duration of the lesion. In many cases, an accompanying *diagram* will be extremely helpful in determining the configuration of the tissue and the optimum orientation for macroscopic section and inclusion. For the same reason it may be useful to mark the nasal or temporal side of the tissue with a suture.

4. *Pieces of conjunctiva* or iris frequently roll up on contact with the fixative. To prevent this, the tissue is flattened smoothly before fixation, on a piece of blotting tissue as used for hemostasis.

5. *Enucleation.*
a) Enucleation for choroidal malignant melanoma has to be followed immediately, in the operating room, by a thorough macroscopical examination of the eye in order to detect a possible trans-scleral extension. The latter is brown or black, flat or slightly bulging above the surface of the sclera, in contact with the main tumour mass.
b) Enucleation for retinoblastoma requires section of the optic nerve at 10 mm behind the globe. During the operation, traction on the nerve is easier if the oblique muscles have been severed beforehand. Section of the optic nerve must be performed with scissors and not with a loop, because the latter does not allow a long piece of nerve to be cut behind the globe. The same technique must be used in adults for the enucleation of an eye containing

Appendice technique

Certaines recommandations techniques paraissent utiles à une bonne collaboration entre deux disciplines habituellement assez éloignées l'une de l'autre, l'ophtalmologie et l'anatomie pathologique.

Recommandations pour l'ophtalmologiste

1. Le *fixateur* de routine doit être prêt (Formol à 10% ou 15%, ou liquide de Bouin) à la salle d'opération. Son volume doit être 5 fois supérieur à celui du globe.
Une collaboration directe avec le laboratoire sera indispensable dans certains cas particuliers. C'est ainsi qu'il faudra un fixateur spécial pour la microscopie électronique (glutaraldehyde à 2%), un autre pour l'immuno-histochimie (paraformaldéhyde à 4%). En cas d'examen extemporané un fragment de tissu frais sera apporté immédiatement au laboratoire, dans de la glace, pour coupe au cryostat.

2. Les *prélèvements*, biopsie ou excision, doivent se faire au bistouri d'acier plutôt qu'au bistouri électrique qui nécrose de façon étendue les bords de la lésion, empêche d'en juger l'extension et peut même, en cas de petit fragment, en gêner l'identification.

3. Une brève *histoire clinique*, précisant la durée d'évolution, est indispensable à une bonne interprétation. Il serait dans bien des cas très utile d'y annexer un *schéma* permettant d'orienter l'inclusion. La réponse de l'anatomo-pathologiste en sera plus précise. Si la pièce excisée ou la biopsie n'a pas une forme assez caractéristique, on repère le côté temporal ou le côté nasal par un fil précisé sur le schéma.

4. Les *pièces de conjonctive* ou les fragments d'iris s'enroulent facilement au contact du fixateur; il est impossible ensuite de les mettre à plat de façon à orienter correctement l'inclusion. Le mieux est de les étaler doucement avant fixation en les plaçant sur un support neutre du type éponge triangulaire d'hémostase.

5. *L'énucléation.*
a) Une énucléation pour mélanome choroïdien doit être suivie immédiatement d'un examen macroscopique du globe à la recherche d'une saillie pigmentée ou d'une tache, témoin d'une extériorisation transsclérale. Rappelons que cette perforation de la sclère se fait toujours en face de la tumeur, et non à distance.
b) L'énucléation pour rétinoblastome doit comporter une bonne partie du nerf optique intra-orbitaire (10 mm). Pour l'obtenir il suffit de sectionner les muscles obliques et de bien tirer sur le globe avant de couper le nerf aux ciseaux. (L'anse est à déconseiller, car elle ne

Technischer Anhang

Einige technische Empfehlungen sind für eine gute Zusammenarbeit zwischen zwei in der Regel recht weit voneinander entfernten Disziplinen angebracht, nämlich Ophthalmologie und Histopathologie.

Empfehlungen für den Ophthalmologen

1. Die gewohnte *Fixationslösung* (10 oder 15 %iges Formol oder Bouin-Flüssigkeit) sollte im Operationssaal bereitstehen. Sie muß 5 mal das Volumen des Augapfels haben. Eine direkte Zusammenarbeit mit dem Labor wird in bestimmten Fällen unerläßlich sein. Eine spezielle Fixation ist für Elektronenmikroskopie notwendig (2 %iges Glutaraldehyd), eine andere für Immun-Histochemie (4 %iges Paraformaldehyd). Bei Schnellschnitten wird ein Frischgewebefragment sofort auf Eis für den Kryostatschnitt ins Pathologielabor gebracht.

2. Die *Gewebsentnahme* – Biopsie oder Exzision – sollte eher mit dem Stahl- als mit dem elektrischen Skalpell erfolgen, da dieses die Läsionsränder großflächig nekrotisiert, die Feststellung ihres Ausmaßes erschwert und im Fall eines kleinen Fragments sogar die Identifizierung erschweren kann.

3. Eine kurze *Krankengeschichte* mit Angabe der Verlaufsdauer ist für eine richtige Interpretation unentbehrlich. In vielen Fällen wäre eine beigefügte *Skizze*, mit deren Hilfe die Einbettung in der richtigen Lagen erfolgen kann, von Nuzten. Dem Ophthalmo-Pathologen ermöglicht sie eine präzisere Antwort. Ist die Form der Exzision oder Biopsie nicht charakteristisch genug, wird die Schläfen- oder Nasenseite durch einen auf dem Schema angegebenen Faden markiert.

4. *Konjunktiva-Teile* oder Iris-Fragmente rollen sich beim Kontakt mit der Fixationslösung leicht zusammen; es ist danach unmöglich, sie so flachzulegen, daß die Einbettung korrekt erfolgt. Am besten werden sie vor dem Fixieren vorsichtig auf einem neutralen Träger vom Typ dreieckiger Hämostaseschwamm ausgebreitet.

5. *Enukleation.*
a) Nach einer Enukleation bei Choroidalmelanom sollte sofort eine makroskopische Augapfeluntersuchung vorgenomen werden, wobei nach einer pigmentierten Erhebung oder einem pigmentierten Fleck, die auf einen Sklera-Durchbruch hinweisen, zu suchen ist. Eine solche Perforation liegt stets über dem Tumor und nicht in Abstand von ihm.
b) Die Enukleation bei einem Retinoblastom muß einen langen Teil des intraorbitalen Sehnervs, (10 mm), mit einbeziehen. Um ihn zu erreichen, braucht man nur die schrägen Muskeln abzutrennen und kräftig an dem Bul-

a malignant choroidal melanoma in close contact with the optic disc. Here also the invasion of the orbit is possible through the extension of the tumour along the optic nerve vessels or along its meningeal sheaths.

c) In order to facilitate orientation of the eye for gross examination and section, it is useful to leave the external rectus relatively long or to mark it with a suture.

d) Section of the eye is always sagittal. Its orientation is chosen according to the site of the tumour. Specification of the latter in your request form will be of great help to the pathologist.

6. The relatively recent technique of *aspiration-biopsy* seems to be gaining favour among ophthalmic surgeons, chiefly in the field of orbital oncology. It might in certain circumstances make it possible to avoid surgical exploration and its risks.

permet pas de sectionner le nerf à distance du globe.)

La même technique doit être utilisée lors de l'énucléation d'un mélanome choroïdien surplombant la papille, car lui aussi peut atteindre l'orbite en longeant le paquet vasculaire du nerf optique.

c) D'autre part pour faciliter l'orientation, il est pratique de laisser le muscle droit externe relativement long ou de le marquer d'un fil.

d) L'axe de section du globe, toujours sagittal, sera choisi en fonction de la localisation de la tumeur intra-oculaire. Il sera bon de la préciser sur la demande d'examen.

6. Une technique récente semble se développer de plus en plus, consistant à faire des *ponctions-biopsies* orbitaires au trocart, guidées au besoin par l'imagerie médicale. Elle permettrait dans certains cas d'éviter l'exploration chirurgicale qui peut ne pas être anodine.

bus zu ziehen, um dann den Nerv mit der Schere abzuschneiden. (Von der Schlinge ist abzuraten, da damit ein vom Augapfel entferntes Abtrennen des Nervs nicht möglich ist). Dieselbe Technik sollte bei der Enukleation eines über die Papille ragenden Choroidalmelanoms angewandt werden, da auch dieses entlang dem hinteren Gefäßbündel die Augenhöhle erreichen kann.

c) Für eine leichtere Orientierung ist es im übrigen praktisch, den M. rectus externus verhältnismäßig lang zu lassen oder mit einem Faden zu markieren.

d) Die Wahl der stets sagittalen Sektionsachse des Augapfels hängt von der Lokalisation des intra-okularen Tumors ab. Man tut gut daran, letztere auf dem Untersuchungsauftrag anzugeben.

6. Eine neue Methode, der zufolge mit dem Trokar *Orbitapunktionen und -biopsien* eventuell unter Zuhilfenahme von bildgebenden Techniken durchgeführt wird, scheint immer mehr an Boden zu gewinnen. In manchen Fällen kann damit anscheinend eine eigentliche, nicht unbedingt harmlose chirurgische Orbita-Exploration vermieden werden.

Recommendations for the pathologist

Recommandations pour l'anatomo-pathologiste

Empfehlungen für den Ophthalmo-Pathologen

Satisfactory histological preparations of a complete eye are difficult to obtain, principally because of the differences in consistency of the anatomical components of the globe: the sclera and the cornea are very dense tissues and the lens becomes hard after fixation; the retina and the choroid on the other hand are thin and very fragile. To avoid folds or tearing, a special substance is necessary for the inclusion. Celloidin was used for a long time; unfortunately, the sections were too thick for a good cytological study (12μ) and, besides, the inclusion took several weeks; in addition, due to the persistence of the collodion, certain stains were impossible to obtain. It has been replaced by certain types of paraffin-wax, with a melting point at 56–58°C.

Macroscopic section of the eye is easier when its consistency is firm. Therefore it is usually carried out after dehydration.

This section is made sagitally and oriented according to the localization of the intra-ocular tumour. Even if the latter has been described by the ophthalmologist, it must be confirmed by transillumination of the eye. A pigmented tumour (or a haemorrhage) is usually opaque to a well focused light. If the pathology of the whole eye is under consideration, the best section is horizontal; this makes it possible to include on the same slide the optic disc and the macular area.

The pathologist can usually orient the eye with the help of the tendon of the lateral rectus. Since it is used by the surgeon to gain purchase during enucleation, it is in general left longer than any other muscle; it can also be marked by a suture. The fact that the distance between the corneal limbus and the optic

Les difficultés de préparation des coupes du globe oculaire tiennent surtout à la consistance différente de ses divers éléments anatomiques: la sclère et la cornée sont dures et résistantes, de même que le cristallin après fixation, alors que la rétine et la choroïde sont minces et extrêmement fragiles. Afin d'éviter plissements et déchirures, il faut choisir un matériel d'inclusion adéquat. La celloïdine utilisée pendant longtemps donnait de belles coupes, mais trop épaisses (12μ) pour une bonne étude cytologique, nécessitait une inclusion prolongée de plusieurs semaines, enfin ne permettait pas toutes les colorations du fait de la persistance du support de collodion. Elle a été remplacée par des paraffines spéciales, de consistance plus élastique que les paraffines habituelles, avec un point de fusion de 56–58°.

La section du globe se fait après déshydratation, qui le rend plus ferme, donc plus facile à couper.

L'axe de section, sagittal, est choisi selon la localisation géographique de la lésion à étudier. S'il s'agit d'un examen intéressant l'ensemble du globe la meilleure section sera horizontale, car elle inclura dans la même coupe papille et macula. En cas de tumeur intra-oculaire, si sa localisation n'est pas précisée sur la fiche de demande d'examen, son repérage est possible grâce à la transillumination du globe. Cette dernière se pratique en chambre noire avec une lumière focalisée très puissante qui traverse les tissus oculaires, et est arrêtée par toute masse opaque, tumeur ou hémorragie.

L'orientation du globe se fait le plus souvent grâce au muscle droit externe dont le tendon sert de prise au moment de l'énucléation et

Die Schwierigkeiten bei der Herstellung von Bulbusschnitten rühren vor allem von der unterschiedlichen Konsistenz seiner verschiedenen anatomischen Bestandteile her: Sklera und Cornea sind ebenso wie der Glaskörper nach der Fixierung hart und widerstandsfähig, während Retina und Choroidea dünn und außerordentlich zerreißlich sind. Um ein Knittern oder Zerreißen zu verhindern, muß ein geeignetes Einschlußmaterial gewählt werden. Das lange Zeit benutzte Zelloidin ergab schöne, aber für eine zufriedenstellende zytologische Untersuchung zu dicke Schnitte (12μ), verlangte eine mehrere Wochen dauernde Einbettungszeit und eignete sich nicht für alle Färbungen. Es wurde durch Spezialparaffine, die elastischer als die normalen Paraffine sind und ihren Schmelzpunkt bei 56–58° haben, ersetzt.

Der Bulbusschnitt erfolgt nach Dehydratierung, die diesen festigt und so den Schnitt erleichtert.

Die Wahl der sagittalen Schnittachse hängt von der Lokalisation der zu untersuchenden Läsion ab. Bei einer dem gesamten Augapfel geltenden Untersuchung werden Papille und Macula in denselben horizontalen Schnitt mit einbezogen. Ist im Fall eines intra-okularen Tumors dessen Lokalisation nicht auf dem Untersuchungsauftrag angegeben, so ist diese mit Transillumination des Augapfels auszumachen. Diese letztere erfolgt in der Dunkelkammer mit einem sehr starken gebündelten Lichtstrahl, der die Augengewebe durchdringt und von jeder lichtundurchlässigen Masse (Tumor oder Hämorrhagie) aufgehalten wird.

Am Augapfel orientiert man sich nach dem

nerve is shorter nasally than laterally may also be used for the orientation of the globe.

Two parallel calottes are taken off with the razor blade on both sides of the intra-ocular lesion. In cases of retinoblastoma, the optic nerve is cut where it emerges sclerally, included separately and examined in cross sections. The same technique is applied to a malignant melanoma of the choroid if it is close to the optic disc.

In cases of melanoma of the choroid or ciliary body, it will be useful, before the inclusion, to measure its dimensions as accurately as possible. The volume of these tumours is decisive in prognosis.

The paraffin-wax block containing the eye is fixed on the microtome so that the equatorial sclera is touched first by the razor (and not the cornea or the area of the optic disc); the risk of artefacts is thus reduced. Given a relatively slow rotation of the microtome wheel, a well-sharpened razor, frequent cooling of the block and of the razor with ice, it is possible to obtain sections of not more than 7μ. For correct mounting of the sections, the ribbons must be floating on water at 56°C containing a small amount of albumin: the sections thus stretch out and can be mounted without folds.

Intra-ocular tumours require serial sections. Occult trans-scleral growths along the track of ciliary vessels and nerves are well known, and only detectable in this way. The presence of a trans-scleral extension will require additional therapy.

reste ainsi plus long que celui des autres muscles, sectionnés au ras du globe. Sinon, on peut repérer le côté nasal grâce au fait que le nerf optique quitte le globe du côté nasal; ainsi la distance entre le bord de la cornée et le nerf optique est plus courte nasalement que temporalement.

Deux calottes parallèles sont enlevées au rasoir de part et d'autre de la lésion à étudier. En cas de rétinoblastome, le nerf optique est sectionné au ras du globe et traité séparément, en coupes frontales. Cette même technique sera appliquée devant un mélanome malin de la choroïde juxta-papillaire; lui aussi peut quitter le globe en suivant les vaisseaux ou les gaines méningées du nerf optique.

En cas de mélanome choroïdien ou ciliaire, il sera bon avant d'inclure le globe en paraffine de pratiquer des mensurations aussi précises que possible; le volume de la tumeur a en effet une valeur pronostique.

Le bloc contenant le globe oculaire est fixé dans le porte-objet du microtome de façon que le rasoir attaque la sclère équatoriale (et non la cornée ou la papille); on a ainsi un minimum de risque d'artéfacts. Avec un mouvement relativement lent du volant, un rasoir bien affûté et un refroidissement fréquent du bloc et du rasoir à la glace, on arrive à réaliser des coupes ne dépassant pas 7μ. Autre détail technique: pour le montage, il est indispensable de faire flotter les rubans sur un bain d'eau maintenue à 56°, contenant un peu d'albumine; les coupes s'étalent ainsi et sont plus faciles à monter sans plis.

Les coupes en série de toutes les tumeurs intra-oculaires sont indispensables car rien ne permet de prévoir une atteinte sclérale profonde ou une fusée intra-sclérale le long d'un pédicule vasculaire ciliaire. Une extériorisation transsclérale impose une thérapeutique complémentaire.

äußeren Muskel, dessen Sehne man bei der Enukleation hält und die deshalb länger ist als die anderen direkt am Augapfel abgetrennten Muskeln. Ansonsten ist der nasale Teil an dem auf dieser Seite aus dem Bulbus austretenden Sehnerv zu erkennen; der Abstand zwischen dem Kornea-Rand und dem Sehnerv ist auf der nasalen Seite kürzer als auf der Schläfenseite.

Zwei parallele Kalotten werden mit dem Rasiermesser beiderseits der zu untersuchenden Läsion entfernt. Im Fall eines Retinoblastoms wird der Sehnerv direkt am Augapfel abgetrennt und separat in Frontalschnitten behandelt. Dieselbe Technik wird bei einem malignen Melanom der Chorioidea in unmittelbarer Nähe der Papille angewandt; auch dieses kann entlang den Opticusgefäßen oder den Optikusscheiden aus dem Bulbus auswachsen.

Im Fall eines Choroidea- oder Ziliarkörpermelanoms sollten vor dem Einbetten des Bulbus möglichst genaue Messungen vorgenommen werden; in der Tat hängt vom Tumorvolumen die Prognose ab.

Der Block mit dem Augapfel wird so auf dem Objektträger des Mikrotoms befestigt, daß das Messer die äquatoriale Sklera (und nicht die Cornea oder die Papille) anschneidet; das Artefaktrisiko wird damit so klein wie möglich gehalten. Bei einer verhältnismäßig langsamen Radbewegung des Mikrotoms, einer gut geschliffenen Klinge und häufiger Abkühlung des Blocks und des Messers mit Hilfe von Eis gelingen Schnitte von nicht mehr als 7μ. Ein weiteres technisches Detail: zum Aufziehen der Schnitte ist es unerläßlich, die Streifen auf einem bei 56° gehaltenen Wasserbad, das ein wenig Albumin enthält, schwimmen zu lassen; die Schnitte breiten sich so flach aus und sind leichter knitterfrei aufzuziehen.

Nur mit Serienschnitten kann eine tiefe Schädigung der Sklera oder ein extra-sklerales Ausbreiten eines intra-okulären Tumors erkannt werden. Letzteres macht eine zusätzliche Behandlung unumgänglich.

List of the histopathological staining techniques quoted in this atlas

These techniques may stain certain tissues or certain well defined components of the tissues specifically. They are often of great help in the histopathological diagnosis.

Alcian Blue – Acid mucopolysaccharides are stained pale blue.

Fontana – In this technique a silver-ammoniacal complex is used to demonstrate melanogenesis (black staining).

Giemsa – A complex stain, (azur, eosin, methylene blue) it is used either on blood smears or on paraffin sections, mostly in haematology.

Grimelius – Technique of argyrophilic impregnation demonstrating the cytoplasmic granules of the majority of cells of the APUD type (Amine Precursor Uptake and Decarboxylation). The presence of these granules, brown or black in appearance, suggests neurosecretory activity.

Liste des colorations d'histopathologie citées dans cet atlas

En colorant spécifiquement certains tissus ou composants tissulaires, elles s'ajoutent à la coloration classique à l'hématéine – éosine et constituent souvent une aide précieuse au diagnostic.

Bleu Alcian – Colore en bleu les mucopolysaccharides acides.

Fontana – Utilisation d'un complexe argent ammoniacal pour la mise en évidence melanogénèse (coloration noire).

Giemsa – Colorant composite (Azur – éosine – bleu de méthylène), utilisé sur frottis ou sur coupes, particulièrement dans le diagnostic hématologique.

Grimelius – Méthode d'imprégnation argyrophile mettant en évidence les granulations cytoplasmiques de la plupart des cellules de la série APUD (Amin Precursor Uptake and Decarboxylation). Ces granulations, témoins de la neurosécrétion, apparaissent en brun ou en noir.

Liste der in diesem Atlas erwähnten histopathologischen Färbemethoden

Spezifische Färbungen bestimmter Gewebe oder Gewebebestandteile zusätzlich zu der klassischen Hämatein-Eosin-Färbung sind oft eine wertvolle diagnostische Hilfe.

Alcian-Blau – Färbt saure Mukopolysaccharide blau.

Fontana – Verwendung eines Ammoniak-Silber-Komplexes für den Nachweis einer Melanogenese (schwarze Färbung).

Giemsa – Farbgemisch (Azur – Eosin – Methylenblau), das bei Ausstrichen oder Gewebsschnitten, insbesondere zur hämatologischen Diagnose verwendet wird.

Grimelius – Anfärbmethode mit Silberpräparaten zum Nachweis von Zytoplasmagranula der meisten Zellen der APUD-Reihe (Amin Precursor Uptake and Decarboxylation). Die bei Neurosekretion vorhandenen Granula erscheinen braun oder schwarz.

Laidlaw – A stain for reticulin, using ammoniacal silver nitrate. Reticulin fibres appear black.

Leder – Histo-enzymological technique for demonstration of non-specific esterases. The cytoplasmic granules are stained dark red.

Mucicarmin – Natural stain used for certain types of mucous secretions. (In ophthalmology, especially the mucus-secreting cells of the conjunctiva.)

PAS – (Method using periodic acid Schiff.) Among other glucidic substances, glycoproteins are stained red to violet. This technique is used commonly to stain epithelial basement membranes, and the content of certain mucus-secreting cells.

Perls – This technique uses Prussian Blue (Potassium ferrocyanide). Ferric iron contained in haemosiderin appears dark blue.

Reticulin – The reticulin fibres are argyrophilic and thus stain black (after oxidation) by silver impregnation. Several techniques use this affinity.

Congo Red – Stains the amyloid substance from pink to red. The nuclei are stained with haematein.

Sudan III – This technique is rarely used nowadays. It is based upon the dissolution in the lipids of a stained substance (a 'lysochrom'), in this case an azo compound. With Sudan III the lipids appear red orange.

Thioflavin T – This method is based on the affinity of the amyloid substance for fluorochromes (Thioflavine T is one of them). The technique is sensitive and reliable. The amyloid substance appears bright green.

Masson's trichrome – It uses acid fuchsin, phosphomolybdic acid (or phosphotungstic acid), and anilin blue (or light green). Nuclei, chromatin and nucleoli appear black, the cytoplasm red, collagen fibers blue (or green), erythrocytes red.

Crystal violet – It is generally mixed with methyl violet and produces when applied to amyloid substance a red to purple metachromasia. This is not a specific reaction.

Laidlaw – Technique de coloration de la réticuline à base de nitrate d'argent et d'ammoniaque. La réticuline apparaît en noir.

Leder – Méthode histo-enzymologique pour la mise en évidence des estérases non spécifiques. Les granulations cytoplasmiques sont colorées en rouge foncé.

Mucicarmin – Colorant naturel utilisé pour mettre en évidence certains types de mucus (en ophtalmologie, en particulier celui des cellules caliciformes de la conjonctive).

PAS – (Méthode à l'acide périodique – Schiff). Parmi d'autres substances glucidiques, les glycoprotéines sont colorées en rouge – violet. Technique utilisée couramment pour les basales épithéliales et le contenu de certaines cellules à mucus.

Perls – Méthode au Bleu de Prusse (ferrocyanure de potassium) colorant en bleu le fer ferrique de l'hémosidérine.

Reticuline – Les fibres de réticuline sont argyrophiles et se colorent de ce fait en noir (après oxydation) par imprégnation argentique. Diverses techniques se fondent sur cette affinité.

Rouge Congo – Colore la substance amyloïde en rose – rouge. Les noyaux sont colorés à l'hématéine.

Soudan III – Peu utilisée actuellement, cette méthode utilise la dissolution dans les lipides d'un corps coloré (un "lysochrome"), ici du groupe des azoïques. Avec le Soudan III les lipides prennent une teinte rouge orangée.

Thioflavine T – Méthode fondée sur l'affinité de la substance amyloïde pour le fluorochrome qu'est la Thioflavine T. C'est un procédé sensible et spécifique. Elle donne lieu à une très belle teinte verte.

Trichrome de Masson – Utilise la Fuchsine acide, l'acide phosphomolybdique (ou phosphotungstique) et le bleu d'aniline (ou le vert lumière). Noyaux, chromatine et nucléole apparaissent en noir; le cytoplasme en rouge; le collagène en bleu (ou en vert); les érythrocytes en rouge.

Violet cristal (violet de Paris) – Généralement mélangé au violet de méthyle, donne lieu avec l'amyloïde à une métachromasie rouge – pourpre. Ce n'est pas une méthode spécifique.

Laidlaw – Retikulin-Färbetechnik auf der Basis von Silbernitrat und Ammoniak. Das Retikulin erscheint schwarz.

Leder – Histo-enzymologische Methode für den Nachweis nicht spezifischer Esterasen. Die Zytoplasmagranula färben sich dunkelrot.

Mucicarmin – Natürlicher Farbstoff, der für den Nachweis bestimmter Schleimzelltypen (in der Ophthalmologie vor allem für die Becherzellen der Conjunctiva) verwendet wird.

PAS – (Perjodsäuremethode – Schiff). Neben anderen Glucosesubstanzen werden Glykoproteide damit rot-violett gefärbt. Die Technik wird üblicherweise für die Epithelbasalschichten und den Inhalt bestimmter Schleimzellen angewandt.

Perls – Berliner Blau (Ferrozyaneisen), mit dem das Ferrieisen des Hämosiderins blau gefärbt wird.

Retikulin – Die Retikulinfasern sind argyrophil und färben sich daher (nach Oxydierung) durch Silbereinwirkung schwarz. Verschiedene Techniken beruhen auf dieser Affinität.

Kongorot – Färbt Amyloidsubstanz rosa-rot. Die Kerne werden mit Hämatein angefärbt.

Soudan III – Bei dieser heute selten verwendeten Methode wird ein farbiger Körper (ein "Lysochrom"), hier von der Gruppe der Azokörper, in den Lipiden aufgelöst. Mit Soudan III nehmen die Lipide eine rot-orangene Färbung an.

Thioflavin T – Die Methode beruht auf der Affinität zwischen der Amyloidsubstanz und dem Fluorochrom Thioflavin T. Es handelt sich um ein empfindliches, spezifisches Verfahren. Es ergibt eine sehr schöne Grünfärbung.

Masson-Trichrom – Verwendet saures Fuchsin, Phosphormolybdänsäure (oder Phosphorwolframsäure) und Anilinblau (oder Lichtgrün). Kern, Chromatin und Nukleolus erscheinen schwarz, das Zytoplasma rot, das Kollagen blau (oder grün), die Erythrozyten rot.

Kristallviolett – Meist mit Methylviolett vermischt, ergibt mit Amyloid eine Purpur-Rot-Metachromasie. Es ist keine spezifische Methode.

Literature

Littérature

Literatur

Considering that the purpose of this atlas is essentially practical, the authors deemed it unnecessary to provide a detailed bibliography: only works of a general purport have been listed hereafter.

Compte-tenu du caractère essentiellement pratique de cet atlas, une bibliographie détaillée a semblé superflue: seuls des ouvrages de référence d'intérêt général figurent ci-dessous.

Da dieser Atlas im Wesentlichen für den praktischen Gebrauch bestimmt ist, schien eine ausführliche Bibliographie überflüssig: nur Referenzwerke die von allgemeinem Interesse sind wurden nachstehend aufgeführt.

Lever W.H., Schaumberg-Lever G.: *Histopathology of the skin*. Lippincott 1983.

Naumann G.O.H.: *Pathologie des Auges*. Springer Verlag 1980.

Naumann G.O.H., Apple D.J.: *Pathology of the eye*. Springer Verlag 1986.

Nicholson D.H., Green W.R.: *Pediatric ocular tumours*. Masson 1981.

Offret G., Dhermy P., Brini A., Bec P.: *Anatomie pathologique de l' oeil et de ses annexes*. Rapport de la Société Française d'Ophtalmologie. Masson 1974.

Spencer W.H.: *Ophthalmic pathology* (3 volumes). W.B. Saunders 1985 (3e edition).

Types histologiques des tissus mous. Classification histologique internationale des tumeurs – No. 3. Organisation Mondiale de la Santé, Genève 1970.

Types histologiques des tumeurs cutanées. Classification histologique internationale des tumeurs – No. 12. Organisation Mondiale de la Santé, Genève 1975.

Types histologiques des tumeurs de l' oeil et de ses annexes. Classification histologique internationale des tumeurs – No. 24. Organisation Mondiale de la Santé, Genève 1980.

Yanoff M., Fine Ben S.: *Ocular pathology*. Lippincott 1989 (3e edition).

Alphabetical index of subjects

Adéno-acanthoma *see* Squamous cell carcinoma adenoid type
Adenocarcinoma
    anaplastic of the lacrimal gland *84*
    of the ciliary epithelium *98*
    meibomian *see* meibomian carcinoma
    mucus secreting of the lacrimal gland *84*
    of the retinal pigment epithelium *132*
    of the sweat glands *see* Carcinoma of the sweat glands
Adenoma
    of the ciliary epithelium *98*
    of the iris pigment epithelium *92*
    meibomian *14*
    oxyphilic
        of the caruncle *18*
        of the lacrimal sac *86*
    pleomorphic
        of the lacrimal gland *see* benign mixed tumour
    of the retinal pigment epithelium *132*
    sebaceous of Pringle *124*
Albright-Fuller Syndrome *70*
Amyloidosis *56*
Angiography 106, 107, 112
Angioma
    "strawberry" *see* Benign haemangio-endothelioma
    tuberous *see* Benign haemangio-endothelioma
Angiomatosis
    encephalo-trigeminal *see* Sturge-Weber-Krabbe's syndrome
Angiosarcoma *see* Malignant haemangio-endothelioma
Antoni A and B patterns *72*
Astrocytoma of the retina *124*

Birbeck granules 88
Botryomycoma *see* Pyogenic granuloma
Bourneville's disease *see* Tuberous sclerosis
Bowen's disease 22, 28
Breslow's criteria 42
Brill-Symmers lymphoma 79
Brown tumour of Recklinghausen *68*
Burkitt's lymphoma 78

Callender's classification *110*
Calcospherites 74
Carcinoma
    adenoid cystic of the lacrimal gland *84*
    basal cell *24*
        adenoid *24*
        cystic *24*
        morphealike 24, *26*
        nodular *24*
        pigmented 24, *26*
        pilar type *24, 25, 26*
        ulcerated 24, *26*
    epidermoid *see* Carcinoma, squamous cell
    of the glands of Zeis *32*
    within a pleomorphic adenoma *84*
    in situ *22, 30, 56*
    of the lacrimal sac *86*
    meibomian *32*
    muco-epidermoid of the conjunctiva *30*
    sebaceous *32*
    squamous cell *28*
        adenoid type *28*
        of the conjunctiva 22, *30*
        of the eyelid *7, 28*
        spindle cell type *28*
    sweat glands *32*
    trabecular *see* Merkel cell tumour
Chalazion *32, 46, 48, 52, 54*
Chloroma *see* Granulocytic sarcoma
Choristoma *50*, 112
    complex *52*
    osseous epibulbar *see* Epibulbar osteoma
Clark's classification *42*
Clear cell hidradenoma *see* Eccrine acrospiroma
Clumped cells 22
Coats's disease *126*

Cutaneous horn *21*
Cylindroma
    skin *see* Basal cell carcinoma, adenoid type
    of the lacrimal gland *see* Adenoid cystic carcinoma of the lacrimal gland
Cyst(s)
    aneurysmal of bone *70*
    conjunctival *8*
    dermoid 12, *50*
    epidermal *8*
    infundibular *see* Epidermal cyst
    of the iris *92*
    "lymphatic" *8*
    pilar *8*
    tricholemmal *8*

Dermis like choristoma *50*
Dermoid of the limbus *50*
Dermolipoma *52*
Destombes disease *see* Sinus hystiocytosis
Diktyoma *see* Medullo-epithelioma
Disciform retinal degeneration 106
Drusen
    of the optic disc *136*
    of the retina 102

Eccrine acrospiroma *18*
Emperopolesis 89
Epithelioma
    calcifying (Malherbe) *see* Pilomatricoma
    cystic adenoid (Brooke) *10*

Fasciitis
    nodular *60*
Fibrohistiocytoma
    atypical *60*
    benign *60*
    malignant *60*
Fibrous dysplasia of bone *70*
Fibroxanthoma *see* Fibrohistiocytoma
Fleurettes (T'so) *123*
Flexner-Wintersteiner
    rosettes *122*
Francois's triad *48*
Fuchs's adenoma *98*

Gamel and Mac Lean's method *110*
Ganglioneuroma *102*
Gardner and Richard's syndrome *68*
Ghost cell 13
Giant cell tumour of bone *68*
Glial tumours of the retina *124*
Glioma
    of the optic nerve *74*
    periphal *72*
    of the retina *124*
Goldenhar's syndrome *50*
Granular cell
    tumour *72*
    myoblastoma *see* Granular cell tumour
Granuloma
    eosinophilic of bone *88*
    pyogenic 53, 54
    telangiectatic *see* Pyogenic

Haemangio-endothelioma
    benign *64*
    intravascular vegetating *66*
    malignant *64*
Haemangioma
    of the bone *68*
    cavernous *64*
    cerebellar *128*
    choroïdal 10(), *112*
    flat *66*
    of the retina *128*

Haemangio-pericytoma 60, *66*
    of bone *68*
Hand-Schüller-Christian disease *88*
Hematoma of the choroid 106
Hidrocystoma *16*
Histiocytosis X *88*
Homer-Wright rosettes 72
Hutchinson's syndrome 72
Hyaline verrucosities *136*
Hyperplasia
    adenomatoid sebaceous *14*
    of the retinal pigment epithelium *132*
Hyperplastic primary vitreous *122*
Hypertrophy of retinal pigment epithelium 106

Immunocytoma *see* Lymphoplasmacytic lymphoma
Islets of Fuchs *55*

Kahler's disease *80*
Kaposi's sarcoma *46*
Kerato-acanthoma 4, *6*
Keratosis
    actinic *20*, 28, 30
    senile *see* Keratosis, actinic
Kissing naevus *34*
Knapp-Rönne type of melanoma *109*
Koïlocytes *5*

Langerhans's histiocytosis *see* Histiocytosis X
Langerhans rods *88*
Leiomyoma *96*
Leucocoria *118*, 122
Leukaemia
    and choroid *114*
    and retina *130*
Lindau's disease *128*
Linear naevus verrucosus 2
Lipofuscin *see* Orange pigment
Lipoma
    of the conjunctiva *46*
    of the orbit *66*
Liposarcoma *66*
Lisch nodules *94*
Lymphangioma of the eyelid and conjunctiva *46*
Lymphoma 56, *76*
    B immunoblastic *80*
    B lymphoblastic *78*
    lympho-plasmacytic *78*, 114
    centroblastic *78*
    centrocytic *78*
    centrocyto-centroblastic *78*
    giant follicular *79*
    lymphocytic *78*
    malignant cerebro-retinal *114*

Malherbe's calcifying epithelioma *see* Pilomatricoma
Medullo-epithelioma
    of the ciliary body *98*
    teratoid *98*
Melanocytic tumours of the iris stroma *92*
Melanocytoma
    of the choroid *102*
    of the ciliary body *100*
    of the iris *94*
    of the optic disc 104, *134*
Melanocytosis
    of the iris *94*
    oculo-dermal *see* Naevus of Ota
Melanoma
    choroïdal *106*, 132, 134
    of the ciliary body *100*
    of the iris *94*
    juvenile of Spitz 34, *38*
    lentigo maligna *40*
    malignant of the eyelid and conjunctiva *40*
    nodular *42*
    superficial spreading *42*
Melanomalytic glaucoma *100*
Melanosis
    acquired *40*
    oculi *104*
    precancerous (Hutchinson Dubreuilh) *see* Melanosis, acquired
    Reese *see* Melanosis, acquired

Meningioma *74*
Merkel cell tumour 32, *48*
Mesenchymatous chondro-sarcoma *68*
Metastases
    in the choroid 106, *114*
    in the ciliary body *100*
    in the iris *96*
Mixed tumour of the lacrimal gland
    benign *82*
    malignant *see* Carcinoma within a pleomorphic adenoma
Molluscum contagiosum *4*
Morning glory syndrom *122*
Muco-epidermoid tumour of the lacrimal gland *84*
Myeloma *see* Plasmacytoma

Naevoxantho-endothelioma *see* Xanthogranuloma, juvenile
Naevus
    ballooncell 34, *36*
    benign cystic *36*
    blue cellular *38*
        of Tièche *see* Mesenchymal naevus
    choroidal *102*, 106
    ciliary body *100*
    combined *38*
    compound *34*
    dysplastic *40*, 102, 106
    fusco-caeruleus ophtalmo maxillaris *see* Naevus of Ota
    giant pigmented, 34, *38*
    halo *102*
    intradermal 34, *36*
    of the iris *94*
    junctional *34*
    magno-cellular *100*, 134
    mesenchymal 34, *38*
    naevo-cellularis partim lipomatodes *37*
    of Ota *104*
    pilosus *36*
    "senile" sebaceous *14*
    unpigmented *35*
    with epithelioid and/or spindle-shaped cells *see* Juvenile melanoma of Spitz
Neuroblastoma *see* Sympathoblastoma
Neurofibroma
    of the eyelid and conjunctiva *48*
    of the choroid *102*
    of the orbit *72*
Neurofibromatosis 48, 72, 74, 94, 102, 106, 124
Neurilemmoma *see* Schwannoma, orbital
Neurinoma *see* Schwannoma, orbital
Neuromatous elephantiasis *see* Pachydermatocele
Nodular fasciitis *60*
Norrie's disease *123*

Oncocytoma
    of caruncle *18*
    of lacrimal sac *86*
Orange pigment 102, 106, 107, 108
Ossifying fibroma of bone *70*
Osteoclastoma *see* Giant cell tumour of bone
Osteoma
    choroidal *112*
    epibulbar *52*
    episcleral *see* Epibulbar
    orbital *68*
Osteosarcoma *68*

Pachydermatocele *48*
Paget's disease *68*
    extra-mammary *32*
Papilloma
    basaloid cell *see* Seborrheic keratosis
    of conjunctiva *4*
    of eyelid *2*
    of lacrimal sac *86*
Parinaud's dermo-epithelioma *see* Benign cystic naevus
Phakoma *124*
Phakomatoses *124*, 128
Phleboliths *65*
Pilomatricoma *12*
Pinguecula *54*
Plasmacytoma *80*
Plexiform neuroma *48*
Psammoma *74*, 75
Pterygium *54*

Reticulosarcoma *see* B immunoblastic lymphoma
Retinal dysplasia *122*
Retinoblastoma *118*, 124
    trilateral *118*
Retrolental fibroplasia *122*
Rhabdomyosarcoma
    alveolar *62*
    botryoid *62*
    embryonal *62*
Richter's syndrome *131*
Ring melanoma *100*
Rosai and Dorfman disease *see* Sinus histiocytosis
Rosenthal's fibres *75*
Roth's spots *130*

Sarcoma
    alveolar soft part *72*
    granulocytic *80*, 114
    myeloid *see* Sarcoma granulocytic
Schwannoma
    choroidal *102*
    orbital *72*
    palpebral *48*
Seborrheic
    keratosis *2*
    wart *see* Seborrheic keratosis
Sinus histiocytosis 88
Shadow cells 13
Sjögren's syndrome 78
Snowballs *120*
Solomon's syndrome *52*
Spiderweb cells 63
Sturge-Weber-Krabbe's syndrome *66*, 112

Sympathoblastoma *72*
Syringadenoma, papillary *16*
Syringocystadenoma papilliferum *16*
Syringoma *18*

Touton cell *45*, 96
Trichilemmoma *10*
Trichoepithelioma *10*
Tuberous sclerosis *124*
Tumours
    of the non pigmented ciliary epithelium *48*
    of the pigment epithelium of the retina *132*

Ulcus rodens *see* Ulcerated basal cell carcinoma

Verocay's bodies *73*
Von Hippel's disease *128*
Von Hippel-Lindau's disease *128*

Waldenström's disease 78
Working formulation *76*

Xanthelasma *44*
Xanthogranuloma
    juvenile of the eyelid and conjunctiva *44*
    of the iris *44*
Xanthoma tuberous *44*
Xanthomatosis *44*
    hypercholesterolemic *44*
    normocholesterolemic *44*
    normolipidemic of Montgomery-Polano *44*
Xeroderma pigmentosum *22*

Index alphabétique des sujets

Acrospirome eccrine *18*
Adéno-carcinome
    anaplasique de la glande lacrymale *84*
    de l'épithélium ciliaire *98*
    de l'épithélium pigmentaire de la rétine *132*
    meibomien *cf* Carcinome meibomien
    mucosécrétant de la glande lacrymale *84*
    sudoral *cf* Carcinome sudoral
Adéno-acanthome *cf* Carcinome épidermoïde adénoïde
Adénome
    de l'épithélium ciliaire *98*
    de l'épithélium pigmentaire irien *92*
    de l'épithélium pigmentaire de la rétine *132*
    meibomien *14*
    oxyphile de la caroncule *18*
    oxyphile du sac lacrymal *86*
    pléomorphe de la glande lacrymale *cf* Tumeur mixte de la glande lacrymale
    sébacé de Pringle *124*
    sébacé de la caroncule *14*
    sébacé de la paupière *14*
Albright-Fuller, syndrome de *70*
Amylose palpébro-conjonctivale *56*
Angiographie *106, 107, 112*
Angiomatose encéphalo-trigéminée *cf* Syndrome de Sturge-Weber-Krabbe
Angiome
    caverneux *64*
        de l'os *68*
    "fraise" *cf* Hémangio-endothéliome bénin
    plan *66*
    tubéreux *cf* Hémangio-endothéliome bénin
Angiosarcome *64, 66*
Antoni types A et B *72*
Astrocytome *124*

Birbeck, granules de *88*
Botryomycome *cf* Granulome pyogénique
Bourneville, maladie de *cf* Sclérose tubéreuse
Bourgeon charnu télangiectasique *cf* Granulome pyogénique
Bowen, maladie de *22, 28*
Breslow, critères de *42*

Calcosphérite *74*
Callender, classification de *110*
Carcinome
    adénoïde kystique de la glande lacrymale *84*
    basocellulaire *24*
        adénoïde *24*
        kératinisant *24*
        kystique *24*
        nodulaire *24*
        pigmenté *24, 26*
        pilaire *24, 25, 26*
        sclérodermiforme *24, 26*
        tatoué *cf* Carcinome basocellulaire pigmenté
        ulcéreux *24, 26*
    dans un adénome pléomorphe *84*
    des glandes de Zeis *32*
    épidermoïde *cf* Carcinome spinocellulaire
        adénoïde *28*
    in situ *22, 30, 56*
    meibomien *32*
    muco-épidermoïde de la conjonctive *30*
    du sac lacrymal *86*
    sébacé *32*
    spinocellulaire
        de la conjonctive *30*
        de la conjonctive à cellules fusiformes *28*
        palpébral *7, 28*
    sudoral *32*
    trabéculaire *cf* Tumeur à cellules de Merkel
Cellules
    "en toile d'araignée" *63*
    momifiées *13*
    de Touton *45, 96*
Chalazion *32, 46, 48, 52, 54*
Chlorome *cf* Sarcome granulocytaire

Choristome *50*, 112
    complexe *52*
    épibulbaire osseux *cf* Ostéome épibulbaire
Chrondrosarcome mésenchymateux *68*
Chromhidrose *16*
Clark, classification de *42*
Clumped cells 22
Coats, maladie de *126*
Corne cutanée *21*
Corps meissneriens *36*, 37
Cylindrome cutané *cf* Carcinome basocellulaire adénoïde
    de la glande lacrymale *cf* Carcinome adénoïde kystique de la glande lacrymale

Dermoïde du limbe *50*
Dégénérescence disciforme de la rétine 106
Dermis like choristoma *50*
Dermo-épithéliome de Parinaud 34, *36*
Dermolipome *52*
Destombes, maladie de *cf* Histiocytose sinusale
Diktyome *cf* Médullo-épithéliome du corps ciliaire
Druses de la papille *cf* Verrucosités hyalines
    de la rétine *102*
Dysplasie
    fibreuse de l'os *70*
    rétinienne *122*

Echographie 106
Elephantiasis névromateux *cf* Pachydermatocèle
Emperopolesis 89
Epithelioma adénoïde kystique *cf* Tricho-épithéliome
    basocellulaire *cf* Carcinome basocellulaire
        kératinisant *10*
    calcifié *cf* Pilomatrixome

Fasciite nodulaire *60*
Fibres de Rosenthal 75
Fibrohistiocytome
    atypique *60*
    bénin *60*
    malin *60*
Fibrome ossifiant *70*
Fibroplasie rétrolentale *122*
Fibroxanthome *cf* Fibro-histiocytome
Fleurettes de T'so 123
François, triade de *48*
Fuchs, adénome de 98

Gamel et Mac Lean, méthode de 110
Ganglioneurome de la choroïde *102*
Gardner et Richards, syndrome de *68*
Glaucome mélanolytique 100
Glioblastome malin *74*
Gliome
    du nerf optique *74*
    périphérique *cf* Schwannome
    vrai de la rétine *124*
Goldenhar, syndrome de *50*
Granulome éosinophile de l'os *88*
Granulome pyogénique 53, *54*
    télangiectasique, *voir* pyogénique

Hand-Schuller-Christian, maladie de *88*
Hémangio-endothéliome
    bénin *64*
    malin *64*
    végétant intravasculaire *66*
Hémangiome
    cérébelleux *128*
    de la choroïde 106, *112*
    de l'os *68*
    de la rétine *128*
Hémangio-péricytome 60, *66*
    de l'os *68*
Hématome de la choroïde 106
Hématosarcomes *76*
Hidradénome à cellules claires *cf* Acrospirome eccrine

Hidrocystome *16*
Histiocytose(s)
    X *88*
    Langerhansiennes *cf* Histiocytoses X
    macrophagique lymphocytaire *cf* Histiocytose sinusale
    sinusale *88*
Hutchinson, syndrome de *72*
Hyperplasie de l'épithélium pigmenté de la rétine *132*
Hypertrophie de l'épithélium pigmenté de la rétine 106

Ilots de Fuchs *55*
Immunocytomes *cf* Lymphomes lymphoplasmocytaires

Kahler, maladie de *80*
Kérato-acanthome 4, *6*
Kératose
    actinique *20*, 28, 30
    sénile *cf* Kératose actinique
Kiel, classification de *76*
Kissing naevus *34*
Knapp-Rönne, mélanome de 109
Koïlocytes *5*
Kyste
    anévrysmal de l'os *70*
    conjonctival *8*
    dermoïde 12, *50*
    épidermique *8*
    infundibulaire *8*
    irien *92*
    "lymphatique" *8*
    pilaire *8*
    tricholemmique *8*

Lames foliacées *cf* Corps meissnériens
Langerhans, bâtonnets de *88*
Leiomyome de l'iris *96*
Lentigo malin *40*
Leucémie(s)
    et choroïde *114*
    et rétine *130*
Leucocorie 118, 122
Lindau, maladie de *128*
Lipofuscine *cf* Pigment orange
Lipome
    de la conjonctive *46*
    de l'orbite *66*
Liposarcome *66*
Lisch, nodules de *94*
Lymphangiomes palpébro-conjonctivaux *46*
Lymphoedème *46*
Lymphome(s) 56, *76*
    de Burkitt 76, *78*
    centroblastique *78*
    centrocytique *78*
    centrocyto-centroblastique *78*
    gigantofolliculaire de Brill-Symmers *79*
    immunoblastiques B *80*
    lymphoblastique B *cf* Lymphome de Burkitt
    lymphocytique *78*
Lymphoplasmocytaire *78*, 114
    malin cérébro-rétinien *114*

Malherbe, tumeur momifiée de *cf* Pilomatrixome
Médullo-épithéliome
    du corps ciliaire *98*
    tératoïde du corps ciliaire *98*
Mélanocytome
    de la choroïde *102*
    du corps ciliaire *100*
    de l'iris *94*
    de la papille 104, *134*
Mélanocytose
    de l'iris *94*
    oculo-dermique *cf* Naevus de Ota
Mélanome
    annulaire (Iris et corps ciliaire) *100*
    de la choroïde *106*, 132, 134
    du corps ciliaire *100*
    de l'iris *94*
    juvénile de Spitz 34, *38*
    et mélanose précancéreuse de Hutchinson-Dubreuilh *40*
    nodulaire *42*
    palpébro-conjonctival bénin *34*
    palpébro-conjonctival malin *40*

    superficiel extensif *42*
Mélanose acquise *cf* Mélanose précancéreuse de Hutchinson-Dubreuilh
    précancéreuse de Hutchinson-Dubreuilh *40*
    de Reese *cf* Mélanose précancéreuse de Hutchinson-Dubreuilh
Melanosis oculi *104*
Méningiome *74*
Métastases
    choroïdiennes 106, *114*
    ciliaires *100*
    iriennes *96*
Milium *cf* Kyste épidermique
Molluscum contagiosum *4*
Morning glory syndrome 122
Myélome *80*
Myoblastome à cellules granuleuses *cf* Tumeur à cellules granuleuses

Naevo-xantho-endothéliome *cf* Xanthogranulome juvénile
Naevus
    achrome *35*
    bleu cellulaire *38*
    bleu de Tièche *cf* Naevus mésenchymateux profond
    à cellules ballonisantes 34, *36*
    à cellules épithélioïdes et/ou fusiformes *cf* mélanome juvénile de Spitz
    choroïdien *102*, 106
    du corps ciliaire *100*
    combiné *38*
    composé *34*
    dysplasique *40*, 102
    fusco-caeruleus ophtalmo-maxillaris *cf* Naevus de Ota
    en halo *102*
    intradermique 34, *36*
    irien *94*
    jonctionnel *34*
    kystique bénin *36*
    magno-cellulaire *100*, 134
    mésenchymateux profond 34, *38*
    naevo-cellularis partim lipomatodes *37*
    de Ota *104*
    pigmentaire géant 34, *38*
    pileux *36*
    verruqueux linéaire *2*
Neurilemmome *cf* Schwannome
Neurinome *cf* Schwannome
Neuroblastome *cf* Sympathoblastome
Neurofibromatose de Recklinghausen *48*, 72, 74, 94, 102, 106, 124
Neurofibrome
    de la choroïde *102*
    de l'orbite *72*
    palpébro-conjonctival *48*
Neuro-naevus de Masson *36*
Névrome plexiforme *48*
Nodule de Verocay *73*
Norrie, maladie de *123*

Oncocytome *cf* Adénome oxyphile
Ostéo-chondro-sarcome de l'orbite *69*
Ostéoclastome *cf* Tumeur à cellules géantes de l'os
Ostéome
    choroïdien *112*
    épibulbaire *52*
    épiscléral *cf* Ostéome épibulbaire
    de l'orbite *68*
Ostéosarcome de l'orbite *68*

Pachydermatocèle *48*
Paget extra-mammaire *cf* Carcinome sudoral
    maladie de *68*
Papillome
    baso-cellulaire *2*
    conjonctival *4*
    palpébral *2*
    du sac lacrymal *86*
Persistance et hyperplasie du vitré primitif 122
Phacomatose(s) *124*, 128
Phacomes *124*
Phlébolithes *65*
Pigment orange 102, 106, *107*, 108
Pilomatrixome *12*
Pinguécula *54*
Plasmocytomes *80*
Premier arc, syndrome du *50*, 52
Psammome 74, *75*
Ptérygion *54*

Réticulosarcome *cf* Lymphome immunoblastique B
    cérébro-rétinien *cf* Lymphome malin cérébro-rétinien
Rétinoblastome *118*, 124
    trilatéral *118*
Rhabdomyosarcome
    alvéolaire *62*
    botryoïde *62*
    embryonnaire *62*
Richter, syndrome de 131
Rosai et Dorfman, histiocytose de *cf* Histiocytose sinusale
Rosettes
    de Flexner-Wintersteiner *122*
    de Homer-Wright *72*
Roth, taches de *130*

Sarcome
    alvéolaire des parties molles *72*
    granulocytaire *80*, 114
    de Kaposi *46*
    myéloïde *cf* Sarcome granulocytaire
Schwannome
    de la choroïde *102*
    de l'orbite *72*
    palpébral *48*
Sclérose tubéreuse *124*
Sjögren, syndrome de 78
Solomon syndrome de *52*
Sturge-Weber-Krabbe, syndrome de *66*, 112
Sympathoblastome *72*
Syringadénome papillaire *16*
Syringocystadénome papillifère *cf* Syringome papillaire
Syringome *18*

Thèques *34*
Trichilemmome *10*
Tricho-épithéliome *10*

Tumeur(s)
    brune de Recklinghausen *68*
    à cellules géantes de l'os *68*
    à cellules granuleuses *72*
    de l'épithélium non pigmenté du corps ciliaire *98*
    de l'épithélium pigmenté de la rétine *132*
    gliales papillo-rétiniennes *124*
    mélaniques choroïdiennes *102*
        du stroma ciliaire *100*
        du stroma irien *92*
    de Merkel 32. *48*
    mixte de la glande lacrymale *82*
    maligne de la glande lacrymale *cf* Carcinome dans un adénome pléomorphe
    muco-épidermoïde de la glande lacrymale *84*
    à myéloplaxes *cf* Tumeur à cellules géantes de l'os

Ulcus rodens *cf* Carcinome basocellulaire ulcéreux

Verrucosités hyalines de la papille *136*
Verrue séborrhéique *2*
Von Hippel, maladie de *128*
Von Hippel-Lindau, maladie de *128*

Waldenström, maladie de 78
Working formulation 76

Xanthelasma *44*
Xanthogranulome
    juvénile de l'iris 96
    palpébro-conjonctival *44*
Xanthome
    plan *cf* Xanthelasma
    tubéreux *44*
Xanthomatose
    hypercholestérolémique *44*
    normocholestérolémique *44*
    normolipidémique de Montgomery-Polano *44*
Xeroderma pigmentosum 22

Alphabetisches Sachwörterverzeichnis

Adeno-Akanthom (Lever) *siehe* Adenoides Plattenepithelkarzinom
Adenokarzinom
    des Pigmentepithels der Netzhaut *132*
    der Talgdrüsen *siehe* Meibomsches Karzinom
    anaplastisch oder undifferenziert der Tränendrüse *84*
    schleimbildendes der Tränendrüse *84*
    der Schweissdrüsen *siehe* Schweissdrüsenkarzinom
    des Ziliarepithels *98*
Adenom
    der meibomschen Drüsen *14*
    oxyphiles
        der Karunkel *18*
        des Tränensacks *86*
    des Pigmentepithels der Regenbogenhaut *92*
    des Pigmentepithels der Netzhaut *132*
    der Talgdrüsen nach Pringle *124*
    der Talgdrüsen der Lider *14*
    der Talgdrüsen der Karunkel *14*
    pleomorphes der Tränendrüse *siehe* Gutartiger Tumor der Tränendrüse
Akrospirom, ekkrines *18*
Albright-Fuller Syndrom *70*
Amylose der Lider und der Bindehaut *56*
Angiographie 106, 107, 112
Angiomatose, enzephalotrigeminale *siehe* Sturge-Weber-Krabbe Syndrom
Angiosarkom *64, 66*
Antoni, Typ A und B *72*
Astrozytom *124*

Birbecksche Granula 88
Botryomycom *siehe* Granuloma pyogenicum
Bourneville *siehe* Tuberöse Sklerose
Bowen der Konjunctiva *22, 28*
Breslow, Kriterien nach *42*

Callender, Klassifizierung nach *110*
Carzinoma in situ der Konjunctiva *22, 30, 56*
Chalazion *32, 46, 48, 52, 54*
Chlorom *siehe* granulozytäres Sarkom
Chondrosarkom, mesenchymatöses *68*
Choristom 50
    komplexes *52*
    epibulbäres ossöses *52*
Chromhidrose *16*
Clark, Prognose Kriterien *42*
Clumped cells 22
Coats, Morbus *126*

Dermis like choristoma *50*
Dermo-Epitheliom nach Parinaud 34, *36*
Dermoid des Limbus *50*
Dermolipom *52*
Destombes, Krankheit *siehe* Histiocytose macrophagique lymphocytaire *und* Sinus Histiozytose
Diktyom *siehe* Medullo-epitheliom des Ziliarkörpers
Drusen
    der Papille *136*
    der Netzhaut 102
Dysplasie
    der Netzhaut 122
    fibröse des Knochens *70*

Echographie 106
Elefantiasis, neuromatöse *48*
Emperopolesis 89
Epithelioma
    verkalkendes nach Malherbe *siehe* Pilomatrixom
    zystisch, adenoides nach Brooke *siehe* Trichoepitheliom

Fasciitis nodularis 60
Fibrohistiozytom
    atypisches *60*
    bösartiges *60*
    gutartiges *60*
Fibrom, verknöcherndes *70*
Fibroplasie, retrolentale 122
Fibroxanthom *siehe* Fibrohistiozytom

Fleurettes nach T'so 123
François, Trias von *48*
Fuchs, Ziliarkörperadenom 98
Fuchssche Inseln *55*

Gamel und Mac Lean, Methode von *110*
Ganglioneurom, der Aderhaut 102
Gardner-Richards, Syndrom *68*
Glaukom, melanolytisches *100*
Gliobastom, bösartiges 74
Gliom
    echtes der Netzhaut *124*
    peripheres *siehe* Schwannom
    des Sehnervs und des Chiasmas 74
Goldenhar, Syndrom *50*
Granulom, eosinophiles des Knochens *88*
Granuloma pyogenicum 53, *54*
    telangiectaticum *siehe* pyogenicum

Hand-Schüller-Christian, Krankheit *88*
Haemangio-Endotheliom
    bösartiges *64*
    gutartiges *64*
    wucherndes intravasales *66*
Haemangiom
    der Aderhaut 106, *112*
    flaches *66*
    kavernöses des Knochens *64, 68*
    des Knochens *68*
    der Netzhaut *128*
    tuberöses *siehe* Gutartiges Haemangio-endotheliom
    zerebellares *128*
Haemangio-Perizytom 60, *66*
    des Knochens *68*
Haematosarkome *76*
Hämatom der Aderhaut 106
Hauthorn *21*
Hidradenom, klarzelliges *siehe* Ekkrines Akrospirom
Hidrozystom *16*
Histiozytosen
    X *88*
    Langerhanssche *siehe* X Histiozytose
    macrophagique lymphocytaire *siehe* Sinus Histiozytose
Hutchinson Syndrom *72*
Hyaline Drusen *siehe* Drusen der Papille

Immunozytome *siehe* Lymphoplasmozytäre Lymphome

Kahler Krankheit *80*
Kalkospherite *74*
Karzinom
    adenoid *siehe* Plattenepithelkarzinom des Lides
    zystisch der Tränendrüse *84*
    basalzell *24*
        adenoid *24*
        knötchenförmig *24*
        pigmentiertes *26*
        ulzeröses 24, *26*
        sklerodermie-artiges *26*
        tätowiertes *siehe* pigmentiertes
        zu Verhornung neigende Form *24, 25, 26*
        zystisch *24*
    der meibomschen Drüsen 32
    muko-epidermoid der Bindehaut 30
    Plattenepithelkarzinom der Bindehaut 30
    des Lides 28
        adenoides *28*
        mid Spindelförmigen Zellen *28*
    in einem pleomorphen Adenom *84*
    der Schweissdrüsen 32
    Stachelzellkarzinom *siehe* Plattenepithelkarzinom des Lides
    der Talgdrüsen *32*
    Trabekelkarzinom *siehe* Merkel Zell Tumor
    des Tränensacks *86*
    der Zeisschendrüsen *32*
Keratoakanthom 4, *6*

Keratose
aktinische
der Konjunctiva 20
des Lides 28, 30, *20*
senile, *siehe* aktinische
Kiemenbogensyndrom, erster *50*, 52
Kissing Naevus *34*
Knapp-Rönne Typ, Aderhautmelanom *109*

Langerhans Stäbchen *88*
Leiomyom der Regenbogenhaut *87*
Lentigo maligna 40
Leukokorie *118*, 122
Leukämien
und Netzhaut *130*
und Uvea *114*
Lindau Krankheit *128*
Lipofuscin *siehe* Orange farbenes Pigment
Lipom
der Bindehaut *46*
der Orbita *66*
Liposarkom *66*
Lisch, Knötchen *94*
Lymphangiome, palpebro-konjunktivale *46*
Lymphödem *46*
Lymphome 56, *76*
Burkitt 76, *78*
Grossfollikel Lymphome nach Brill-Simmers *79*
B immunoblastär *80*
B lymphoblastär *siehe* Burkitt
lymphozytär *78*
plasmozytär *78*
malignes zerebroretinales *114*
zentroblastisch *78*
zentrozytisch *78*
zentrozyto-zentroblastisch *78*

Malherbe, verkalkendes Epithelioma *siehe* Pilomatrixom
Medullo-Epitheliom
des Ziliarkörpers *98*
teratoide Form *98*
Meissnersche Körperchen (Masson) *36*
Melanom
der Aderhaut *106*, 132, 134
der Iris *94*
des Ziliarkörpers *100*
Iris und Ziliarkörper (Ringmelanom) *100*
der Lider und Bindehaut
gutartig *34*
bösartig *40*
juveniles Spitz Melanom 34, *38*
noduläres *42*
sich oberflächlich ausbreitendes *42*
auf prekanzeröser erworbener Melanose *40*
Melanose
erwobene *siehe* prekanzeröse Melanose
nach Hutchinson-Dubreuilh *40*
nach Reese *siehe* Hutchinson-Dubreuilh
Melanosis oculi *104*
Melanozytom
der Aderhaut *102*
der Papille 104, *134*
der Regenbogenhaut *94*
des Ziliarkörpers *100*
Melanozytose
oculodermale *siehe* Naevus von Ota
der Regenbogenhaut *94*
Meningiom des Sehnervs *74*
Merkel-Zell Tumore, *siehe* Tumor
Metastasen
in die Aderhaut 106, *114*
in die Regenbogenhaut *96*
in den Ziliarkörper *100*
Milium *siehe* Epidermiszysten
Molluscum contagiosum *4*
Morning glory Syndrom 122
Myelom *80*

Naevoxantho-endotheliom *siehe* juveniles xanthogranulom
Naevus
achromer *35*
der Aderhaut *102*, 106
Ballonzell 34, *36*

bleu nach Tieche *siehe* tiefer mesenchymaler Naevus
compound *34*
dysplastisch 40, 102, 106
mit epitheloid oder spindelförmigen Zellen *siehe* juveniles Spitz Melanom
fusco-caeruleus ophtalmo-maxillaris *siehe* Naevus von Ota
gutartig zystisch *36*
halonaevus *102*
intradermaler 34, *36*
junktionaler *34*
lineares Warzennaevus *2*
magnozellular *100*, 134
naevo-cellularis partim lipomatodes *37*
von Ota *104*
pili *36*
der Regenbogenhaut *94*
Riesenpigmentmal 34, *38*
tiefer mesenchymaler 34, *38*
zellulär blauer *38*
des Ziliarkörpers *100*
zusammengesetzter *38*
Nester, Zellnester in Naevus *34*
Netzhaut
disziforme Degeneration *106*
Hyperplasie des Pigmentepithels *132*
Hypertrophie des Pigmentepithels 106
Neurilemmom *siehe* Schwannom
Neurinom *siehe* Schwannom
Neuroblastom *siehe* Sympathoblastom
Neurofibrom
der Aderhaut *102*
der Lider und Bindehaut *48*
der Orbita *72*
Neurofibromatose Von Recklinghausen 48, 72, 74, 94, 102, 106, 124
Neurom, plexiformes *48*
Neuronaevus nach Masson 36, 37
Norrie Krankheit *123*

Onkozytom *siehe* oxyphiles Adenom
Osteo-chondro-sarkom der Orbita *69*
Osteoklastom *siehe* Riesenzelltumor des Knochens
Osteom
der Aderhaut *112*
epibulbäres *52*
episclerales *siehe* epibulbäres Osteom
der Orbita *68*
Osteosarkom der Orbita *68*

Paget
extramammäres *siehe* Karzinom der Schweissdrüsen
Krankheit *68*
Papillom
basalzellen *2*
der Bindehaut *4*
des Lides *2*
des Tränensacks *86*
Persistenz mit Hyperplasie des primären Glaskörpers 122
Phakomatose *124*, *128*
Phakome *124*
Phlebolith *65*
Pigment, orangefarbenes 102, 106, 107, 108
Pilomatrixoma *12*
Pinguecula *54*
Plasmozytome *80*
Psammom *74*, 75
Pterygium *54*

Retikulosarkom *siehe* B immunoblastäre Lymphome
zerebroretinales *siehe* malignes zerebroretinales Lymphom
Retinoblastom *118*
trilateral *118*
Rhabdomyosarkom
alveoläres *62*
botryoides *62*
embryonales *62*
Richter Syndrom *131*
Ringmelanom der Iris und des Ziliarkörpers *siehe* Melanom
Rosai und Dorfman, Histiozytose von *siehe* Sinushistiozytose
Rosenthal-Fasern *75*
Rosetten
nach Flexner-Wintersteiner *122*
nach Homer-Wright *72*
Roth-Flecken *130*

Sarkom
  alveoläres Weichteilsarkom 72
  granulozytäres 80, 114
  Kaposi 46
  myeloides siehe Granulozytäres
Schwannom
  der Aderhaut 102
  des Lides 48
  der Orbita 72
Sjögren Syndrom 78
Sklerose, tuberöse 124
Sturge-Weber-Krabbe Syndrom 66, 112
Sympathoblastom, orbitale Lokalisation 72
Syringom 18
Syringozystadenom, papillares 16

Trichilemmom 10
Trichoepitheliom 10
Tumor
  bösartiger Mischtumor der Tränendrüse siehe Tränendrüse Karzinom in
    einem pleomorphen Adenom
  brauner Recklinghausen 68
  glial der Netzhaut und Papille 124
  granulosazell 72
  melanotische
    der Aderhaut 102
    des Stromas der Iris 92
    des Stromas des Ziliarkörpers 100
  Merkel-Zell 32, 48
  Mischtumor der Tränendrüse 82
  mukoepidermoid der Tränendrüse 84
  myeloplaxtumor siehe Riesenzellentumor des Knochens
  des nicht pigmentierten Ziliarepithels 98
  des Pigmentepithels der Netzhaut 132
  Riesenzellentumor des Knochens 68

Ulcus rodens siehe ulceröses Basalzellkarzinom

Verocay-Knötchen 73
Von Hippel Krankheit 128
Von Hippel-Lindau Krankheit 128

Waldenström Krankheit 78
Warze, seborrhoische 2
Working formulation 76

Xanthelasma 44
Xanthogranulom
  juveniles
    der Lider und Bindehaut 44
    der Regenbogenhaut 96
Xanthom
  flaches siehe Xanthelasma
  tuberöses 44
Xanthomatose
  hypercholesterolämisch 44
  normocholesterolämisch 44
  normolipidämisch nach Montgomery-Polano 44
Xeroderma pigmentosum 22

Zellen
  Touton 45, 96
  mumifizierte Zellen 13
  Spinngewebzellen 63
Zylindrom
  des Lides siehe adenoide Variante Basalzellkarzinom
  der Tränendrüse siehe adenoidzystisches Karzinom der Tränendrüse
Zysten
  aneurysmatische des Knochens 70
  konjunktivale 8
  dermoid 12, 50
  der Epidermis 8
  des Infundibulums 8
  "lymphatische" 8
  der Regenbogenhaut 92
  der Haarhülle oder Tricholemzysten 8

Monographs in Ophthalmology

1. P.C. Maudgal and L. Missotten (eds.): *Superficial Keratitis.* 1981
   ISBN 90-6193-801-5
2. P.F.J. Hoyng: *Pharmacological Denervation and Glaucoma.* A Clinical Trial Report with Guanethidine and Adrenaline in One Eyedrop. 1981
   ISBN 90-6193-802-3
3. N.W.H.M. Dekkers: *The Cornea in Measles.* 1981
   ISBN 90-6193-803-1
4. P. Leonard and J. Rommel: *Lens Implantation.* 30 Years of Progress. 1982
   ISBN 90-6193-804-X
5. C.E. van Nouhuys: *Dominant Exudative Vitreoretinopathy and Other Vascular Developmental Disorders of the Peripheral Retina.* 1982
   ISBN 90-6193-805-8
6. L. Evens (ed.): *Convergent Strabismus.* 1982
   ISBN 90-6193-806-6
7. A. Neetens, A. Lowenthal and J.J. Martin (eds.): *The Visual System in Myelin Disorders.* 1984
   ISBN 90-6193-807-4
8. H.J.M. Völker-Dieben: *The Effect of Immunological and Non-Immunological Factors on Corneal Graft Survival.* A Single Centre Study. 1984
   ISBN 90-6193-808-2
9. J.A. Oosterhuis (ed.): *Ophthalmic Tumours.* 1985
   ISBN 90-6193-528-8
10. O. van Nieuwenhuizen: *Cerebral Visual Disturbance in Infantile Encephalopathy.* 1987
    ISBN 0-89838-860-0
11. E.A.C.M. Sanders, R.J.W. de Keizer and D.S. Zee (eds.): *Eye Movement Disorders.* 1987
    ISBN 0-89838-874-0
12. R. Živojnović: *Silicone Oil in Vitreoretinal Surgery.* 1987
    ISBN 0-89838-879-1
13. A. Brini, P. Dhermy and J. Sahel: *Oncology of the Eye and Adnexa.* Atlas of Clinical Pathology / *Oncologie de l'Œil et des Annexes.* Atlas Anatomo-Clinique / *Onkologische Diagnostik in der Ophthalmologie.* Vergleichender Klinisch-Pathologischer Atlas. 1990
    ISBN 0-7923-0409-8

KLUWER ACADEMIC PUBLISHERS – DORDRECHT / BOSTON / LONDON